Family Violence in

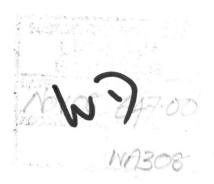

Whilst every effort has been made to ensure that the contents of this book are as complete, accurate and up-to-date as possible at the date of writing, Oxford University Press is not able to give any guarantee or assurance that this is the case. Readers are urged to take appropriately qualified medical advice in all cases. The information in this book is intended to be useful to the general reader, but should not be used as a means of self-diagnosis or for the prescription of medication.

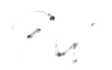

Family Violence in Primary Care ·

Edited by

Stephen Amiel
Caversham Group Practice
4 Peckwater Street
London

and

Iona Heath
Caversham Group Practice
4 Peckwater Street
London

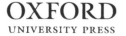

OXFORD
UNIVERSITY PRESS

OXFORD
UNIVERSITY PRESS

Great Clarendon Street, Oxford OX2 6DP

Oxford University Press is a department of the University of Oxford.
It furthers the University's objective of excellence in research, scholarship,
and education by publishing worldwide in

Oxford New York

Auckland Cape Town Dar es Salaam Hong Kong Karachi
Kuala Lumpur Madrid Melbourne Mexico City Nairobi
New Delhi Shanghai Taipei Toronto
With offices in
Argentina Austria Brazil Chile Czech Republic France Greece
Guatemala Hungary Italy Japan South Korea Poland Portugal
Singapore Switzerland Thailand Turkey Ukraine Vietnam

Oxford is a registered trade mark of Oxford University Press
in the UK and in certain other countries

Published in the United States
by Oxford University Press Inc., New York

ISBN 0-19-262828-3

Antony Rowe Ltd., Eastbourne

Preface

Family violence presents very particular difficulties to general practitioners because of their role as doctors to whole families. Each individual consultation is confidential and, to be effective, is predicated on the principle of the doctor having unconditional positive regard for the patient. The patient must have confidence that the doctor will act, to the limit of his or her ability, entirely in the patient's best interest. Violence and abuse within families necessarily bring conflicts of interest and if the doctor is to act in the best interest of the victim he or she may need to take steps which will undermine the confidence of the abuser and may even betray his confidence. The ethical dilemmas proliferate and the doctor is fearful of doing more harm than good.

In the past, the acceptance of an imbalance of the physical, social and economic power within a family relationship has been thought to legitimate violence against children, women and older people. But today the overt imbalance of power and status, let alone the violence, is less and less acceptable. Attitudes have altered considerably and society is gradually making clear its determination to treat all forms of family violence as seriously as any other form of violence.

There are many factors which make it difficult for general practitioners to respond adequately and appropriately to a presentation of family violence. The time constraints of busy practice exacerbate the fear of revealing a problem which is going to be difficult and time-consuming to tackle. The presentation is often hidden behind a range of 'calling card' symptoms and this offers the general practitioner the chance to collude. The difficulty of first voicing the suspicion of violence or abuse within the family is often daunting and information about other services or agencies which can offer help, expertise and support is often not immediately available at the moment of the consultation.

On the other hand, there are factors which make it easier for a general practitioner to deliver an effective response. The long-term relationship between the general practitioner and the family can provide a basis of trust and the general practitioner consultation is accessible, acceptable and free of stigma. There is increasing knowledge and expertise about the different areas of family violence among a wide range of agencies, both statutory and voluntary. Support should be readily available with the potential to enable the general practitioner to work effectively within a network of agencies.

This book is aimed primarily at the general practitioner, but family violence can present to any member of the primary care team. Sharing knowledge and concerns within the team and planning coordinated ways of working can make each individual's response more effective and it is hoped that most of this book will have usefulness and relevance to all the members of the team.

The aim of this book is to empower the general practitioner to respond effectively by providing information about the presentation of the various forms of family violence, by encouraging the high index of suspicion, which is probably the most important single aid to diagnosis, and by mapping a way through the onward referral process once the diagnosis has been made. The damage inflicted by family violence in terms of physical, psychological and social morbidity is enormous. The endeavour of striving to respond effectively is more than worthwhile; it has the potential to save and salvage lives.

Many people have helped to make this book happen, and we should like to thank them all. First, of course, we thank our contributors, whose expertise in the field of family violence we have found as in valuable as it is humbling. The example and wise counsel of local medical, nursing and social work colleagues have also, we hope, found expression in this book: particular thanks to Judy Barker and Kyra Haydon and stories that have taught us so much of what we ourselves have learned about family violence: we owe them a debt of gratitude too.

Finally, we should like to thank Olivia Amiel and David Heath for their insights, for their forbearance and for reminding us that it was past our bedtime. This book is dedicated to them.

December 2002

Iona Heath
Stephen Amiel

Contents

List of Contributors

Amiel, Stephen
Caversham Group Practice,
4 Peckwater Street,
London NW5 2UP, UK

Bennett, Gerry
Barts and The London Queen Mary's
School of Medicine and Dentistry,
1st floor Alderny Building,
Mile End Hospital,
London E1 ADG, UK

Cloke, Christopher
Child Protection Awareness Unit,
National Society for the Prevention of
Cruelty to Children,
Weston House,
42 Curtain Road,
London EC2A 3NH, UK

de Zulueta, Felicity
Department of Forensic Psychiatry,
King's College London,
De Crespigny Park,
Denmark Hill,
London SE5 8AF, UK

Edwards, Sarah
Chartered Institute of Housing, UK

Glaser, Danya
Department of Psychological Medicine,
Great Ormond Street Hospital for
Children,
Great Ormond Street,
London WC1N 3JH, UK

Goodman, Wendy
Eastbourne Downs NHS Primary
Care Trust,
Avenue House,
The Avenue,
Eastbourne, BN 21 3XY

Hanmer, Jalna
International Centre for the Study of
Violence and Abuse,
University of Sunderland,
Sunderland, UK

Harwin, Nicola
Women's Aid Federation of England,
PO Box 391,
Bristol BS99 7WS, UK

Heath, Iona
Caversham Group Practice,
4 Peckwater Street,
London NW5 2UP, UK

Hendry, Enid
Child Protection Training Centre,
National Society for the Prevention of
Cruelty to Children,
3 Gilmour Close,
Beaumont Leys,
Leicester LE4 1EZ, UK

Hodes, Deborah T
Child and Adolescent Services,
City and Hackney Primary Care Trust,
Nuttall Street,
London N1 5LZ, UK

Ismach, Madeline
Formerly National Society for the
Prevention of Cruelty to Children,
NSPCC National Centre,
42 Curtain Road,
London EC2A 3NH

Jenkins, Ginny
Formerly Action on Elder Abuse,
Astral House,
1268 London Road,
London SW16 4ER, UK

Kingston, Paul
School of Health,
University of Wolverhampton,
Gorway Road,
Walsall WS1 3BD, UK

Lindley, Bridget
Centre for Family Research,
University of Cambridge,
Free School Lane,
Cambridge, CB2 3RF, UK

Lowton, Alison
Camden Council,
Camden Town Hall,
Judd Street,
London WC1H 9LP, UK

Mayer, Vera
4 Brick Court,
Temple,
London EC4 9AD, UK

McCreadie, Claudine
Age Concern Institute of Gerontology,
King's College London,
Waterloo Road,
London SE1 9NN, UK

McDonald, Ann
School of Social Work and Psychosocial
Studies,
University of East Anglia,
Norwich NR4 7TJ, UK

McFarlane, Gloria
Formerly London Borough of Southwark
Legal Services Division,
South House,
30/32 Peckham Road,
London SE5 8UB, UK

Morris, Tamson
31 Private Road,
Sherwood,
Nottingham NG5 4DD, UK

Penhale, Bridget
Department of Social Work,
University of Hull,
Cottingham Road,
Hull HU6 7RX, UK

Phair, Lynne
AgeCare,
47 Great Russell Street,
London WC1B 3PB

Phillipson, Chris
School of Social Relations,
Keele University,
Keele ST5 5BG, UK

Pritchard, Jacki
Beyond Existing,
PO Box 1779,
Sheffield S6 37B, UK

Reed, Susan
Metropolitan Police,
London, UK

Siddiqui, Hannana
Southall Black Sisters,
52 Norwood Road,
Southall,
Middlesex UB2 4DU, UK

Smith, Lorna J. F.
Research Development and Statistics,
Home Office,
Queen Anne's Gate,
London SW1H 9AT, UK

Stainton Rogers, Wendy
The Research School,
The Open University,
Walton Hall,
Milton Keynes MK7 6AA, UK

Trowell, Judith
Tavistock Clinic,
120 Belsize Lane,
London NW3 5BA, UK

Ussher, Jane
School of Psychology,
University of Western Sydney,
Penrith South DC, NSW 1797,
Australia

Vizard, Eileen
The Young Abusers' Project,
6 Peckwater Street,
London NW5 2TX, UK

Wakley, Gill
School of Psychology,
Staffordshire University,
Brindley Building,
Leek Road,
Stoke-on-Trent ST4 2DF, UK

Weir, Amy B.
Children and Families Service,
London Borough of Harrow,
Civic Centre,
Harrow, Middlesex HA1 2UL, UK

Wynne, Jane
Department of Child Health,
Belmont House,
Leeds General Infirmary,
Leeds LS2 9NJ

Part 1

Introduction to family violence

Chapter 1

Violence in society and in the family

Lorna J. F. Smith

Introduction

Violence harms not only those upon whom it is inflicted but the communities and societies in which it takes place. Its effects are far-reaching, going beyond the physical harm sustained to psychological and emotional suffering, which is often long-lasting. It diminishes the quality of our lives as social beings.

What is meant by violence is problematic, as is defining the point at which violence is deemed to be crime. Most people would agree that 'killing people is wrong'; but this statement is open to changing definitions. Although the act involved—taking someone's life—is the same, it opens up questions of legitimate and illegitimate violence. In war, taking lives is expected. Is a punch a violent act or does its definition as such depend on the circumstances? If the same person punches in the boxing ring and in the pub will the act be defined differently? If a man punches his wife or children in his home will it again be defined differently? Would everyone in any one particular society define or classify the same act in the same way?

What is regarded as criminal is place—and time—specific. Moreover, there may be no universal consensus on the definitions embodied within the criminal law at any particular point. What is seen to constitute violence is subject to disagreement and to change over time. Some forms of behaviour will be more generally agreed to be intrinsically criminal than others—murder, for instance, is likely to be universally condemned. But other types of behaviour are subject to more disagreement and to shades of opinion dependent upon perceptions of situations, circumstances, participants and the values of those who make the perceptions and definitions. The physical chastisement of children is a case in point. Many would regard this as a parental right, provided it is not over-excessive and does not become abusive—although there would be differences in opinion on what is excessive and what is abusive. Indeed, an increasing number of countries are now criminalizing all forms of this behaviour. Perceptions, thus definitions and remedial action, can change over time. Legal and social definitions do not necessarily correspond exactly.

'Family violence' is a nebulous concept lacking a clear and standardized definition, either of 'family' or 'violence'. The term can encompass a range of activities and behaviour that may be included or excluded by different researchers. In this chapter, family has been interpreted widely to include cohabitants and relatives as well as relationships made by remarriage. It is concerned with violence against family members by family members. In practice, family violence has tended to be studied in three discrete strands: child abuse, domestic violence and elder abuse. This may change as knowledge develops and there is greater recognition of the links between these strands. The terms themselves suggest the lack of agreed definition and conceptualization. Why child and elder *abuse* but domestic *violence*? The term violence emphasizes a link with the criminal law; abuse does not necessarily do so. All terms have been subject to criticism for masking as much as they reveal. Child abuse tends to cover a range of behaviour dependent on the purposes for which the definition is sought. Since 'reasonable physical chastisement' of children is not prohibited in this country, legitimate punishment has to be distinguished from physical assaults involving intention and from assaults caused by neglect or by accident. Research into child abuse can embrace physical and sexual assault, emotional abuse and neglect. Similarly, domestic violence research has examined a range of behaviours. This moves through physical and sexual assaults to psychological, emotional or verbal abuse involving threats, harassment and denigration. Some research includes deliberate social isolation from friends and family and economic abuse where control of all financial resources is by one partner (almost invariably the male partner). In elder abuse, too, similar aspects are found. In this type, neglect is more central than in domestic violence and economic abuse tends to refer to the unauthorized and improper use of the financial resources of the older person.

Although not wishing to detract from the very real harm caused by all forms and types of family violence, concentration in this chapter will be on the sexual and physical abuse of children, spouses and parents, which are the categories most closely approximating what would be classified as violence in criminal law. The literature referred to is in the main English or from English-speaking countries. It must be recognized at the start that the necessary information for all categories is not always readily available and that the three strands of family violence have received uneven attention.

A fundamental point to keep in mind is that many of these acts coexist in one family. Women who report physical abuse by their partners often also report sexual abuse. Similarly, children and parents who are subject to one form of abuse often experience other forms too. In many families, where the woman is abused, the children are also abused. Research, too, points to the fact that many abusers were themselves abused as children or witnessed such abuse. Furthermore, elder abuse can be the continuation into old age of domestic violence between partners. Finally, it has to be stressed that although there are differences between and within the three strands of family violence, in the main women and girls are the victims, men the perpetrators.

Historical perspective

In the last three decades or so, there has been a burgeoning of interest in family violence as evidenced by increasing media attention, research activity, public inquiries, activities of lobbying groups, and so forth. It might be thought—erroneously—that this form of violence was a comparatively new phenomenon. Just as violence has always existed in our history and culture so, too, has family violence. What has happened is that family violence has attracted greater or lesser attention as attitudes, values and definitions have changed. The subject has moved on and off the political and social agenda in competition with other social problems. Nor has its recognition as a social problem shared an equal and even history over its three strands. Interest was first generated in child abuse, followed by domestic violence. Elder abuse has only come to be recognized comparatively recently.

Child abuse

It has been argued that religious, legal, political, social and cultural structures have long condoned and sanctioned the exploitation, abuse and acceptance of violence against children.[1] In Roman law, a father had the right to sell, abandon, offer as sacrifice, devour, kill or otherwise dispose of his offspring. Closer to home, until the last century, English law held that women and children were the property of husbands and fathers.[2,3] The Industrial Revolution brought the issue of child abuse into focus when the conditions in which they were forced to work were revealed. Writers such as Dickens and Roberts[4] drew further attention to the plight of children, their working conditions and routine beatings. The Society for the Prevention of Cruelty to Children was established in Britain in 1889 and its work over the years did much to gain recognition of the problem.

Radiologists in the 1940s, however, are generally credited as the major discoverers of child physical abuse.[5,6] With improved technology, many unexplained fractures in young children were detected. Perhaps ironically, the medical profession in general is viewed as one of the bodies that impeded discovery.[5] There was desire to retain the confidential doctor–patient relationship; a reluctance to believe that parents could inflict such injuries; and a reluctance to become involved in possible criminal proceedings. This ceased, in 1962, with the publication of an influential article in the *Journal of The American Medical Association*.[7] It brought the issue once more into public discussion and the harm inflicted on children was gradually recognized. Well-publicized horrific cases—Maria Caldwell and Jasmine Beckford—caused public outcry and brought calls for greater recognition and improved responses.

Child sexual abuse, by contrast, has a rather shorter history as a recognized social problem. Although rape, sodomy and bestiality have long been recognized by common law, cases involving incest were traditionally dealt with by the ecclesiastical courts until the passage, in 1908, of the Punishment of Incest Act.[8] As the concept of what constitutes child maltreatment broadened, especially among professionals charged with the protection of children, child sexual abuse gradually came on to the political and social agenda. This was in part fuelled by the increasing numbers of physically abused and neglected children who revealed that they were also victims of sexual abuse. Further impetus came from the increasing influence of the women's movement in the 1970s. Through their efforts, it came to be understood that many adult women had been sexually abused in childhood and much of that abuse had been perpetrated by family members. Gradually, the sexual abuse of young boys by people they knew and trusted came to light also. Child sexual abuse was firmly on the political agenda in the United States by the mid-1970s and, a decade later, in the United Kingdom. Again, public outcries which fuelled the Cleveland Inquiry and later the Orkney Inquiry helped keep the subject in the public eye.

Following the publication of the highly influential report by Lord Justice Butler-Sloss on the Cleveland Inquiry,[9] there followed a period of intense official action on child abuse, including sexual abuse. Circulars by the then Department of Health and Social Security and by the Home Office, providing guidance to all appropriate agencies and professions, were published simultaneously with that report. The emphasis of the response lay heavily on interagency cooperation as epitomized by the title of the DHSS publication *Working Together*.[10] The next milestone was the passage of the Children Act 1989. At the same time, a wide-ranging programme of research into all aspects of child protection was set in train and is ongoing (for details, see [11]).

Domestic violence

The sociohistorical roots of domestic violence are equally deep. The subjugation of women to their husbands was sanctioned by the church and wives were counselled that increased devotion and submissiveness were the means of avoiding 'disciplinary' chastisement.[12] The Dobashes maintain that for centuries husbands have used violence, systematically and severely, to dominate, punish and control their wives simply as a husband's prerogative.[13] A husband's rights over his wife were clearly articulated in English common law and extended to control over her property and daily affairs, and to correct and chastise her. Blackstone[14] believed that the right to beat one's wife had become obsolete but Freeman[5] contends that some 75 years after Blackstone's pronouncements, the legality of the privilege was being upheld and was not finally abolished until 1891.

Pressure to reform the law started in the latter half of the nineteenth century. Influential proponents of change included John Stuart Mill, Caroline Norton and Frances Power Cobbe. The latter's systematic collection of evidence of abuse, published in the pamphlet 'Wife torture in England',[15] did much to raise awareness. Pressure for change continued with the suffrage movement but declined between 1920 and 1970, when a strong women's movement was absent. By the 1970s, the movement had revived, child abuse had been 'discovered' and a network of refuges had grown to which women who were victims of domestic violence fled. Demonstrable evidence existed of a real and potentially considerable problem. This combination of influences led to the establishment in 1974 of the House of Commons Select Committee on Violence in Marriage which was followed fairly shortly afterwards by three important pieces of legislation dealing with the problem.[16]

Again, there followed a period of relative inactivity until the Women's National Commission[17] considered domestic violence in the context of violence against women more generally, and called for action on a number of fronts.

The Home Office set in train a wide-ranging critical review of the research literature to inform policy-making across government departments.[16] At the national level, the next main impetus was the House of Commons Home Affairs Select Committee, *Inquiry into Domestic Violence*[18] which led to the establishment of the interdepartmental Ministerial and Official Group on Domestic Violence.

Elder abuse

In contrast, abuse of the elderly has been little researched, so much so that McCreadie[19] had to rely largely on North American material. Ironically, as Bennett and Kingston[20] note, the first article in English language literature of recent origin was British.[21] In common with child abuse and domestic violence, there is no reason to believe that elder abuse has not always been endemic. Anthropological literature contains many references to the ill treatment of elders, including matricide and patricide.[22]

The attention drawn to 'granny battering' by Baker[21] was scarcely followed up in this country, whereas in the United States the topic was established on the political agenda by 1984.[20] Indeed the term 'elder abuse' rather than 'granny bashing' was first coined in 1979 in the United States in recognition that the latter term refocused enquiry and thus action.[23] A conference organized by Age Concern England in 1982 stirred research interest once more and led to Eastman's publication.[24] Policy-making, however, remained unaffected.[20,25] Another conference, organized in 1988 by the British Geriatrics Society, was the next major step in the history of elder abuse as a social problem. This event brought together professionals from various fields—medicine and nursing, social work and policing—and led to a publication on the prevention of this type of family violence.[26]

Biggs places formal recognition of elder abuse in the United Kingdom in the context of the National Health Service and Community Care Act 1990.[25] Certainly, this was swiftly followed by action from the Social Services Inspectorate.[27,28] Almost simultaneously, Age Concern England launched a new pressure group—Action on Elder Abuse—in an endeavour to keep the subject on the political agenda.

Violence in society

Society attempts to set limits to violence through the legal definition of violent crime. The barometer of the level of violent crime in England and Wales is generally taken to be that contained in *Criminal Statistics*. Traditionally, offences classified as 'violence against the person' and 'robbery' were regarded as the measurement of violence. However, it has become increasingly recognized that rape and some other sexual offences are associated more with the exercise of power than with uncontrollable sexual urges, and these offences are now viewed as crimes of violence. It has to be borne in mind, however, that some sexual offences are consensual. For example, petting between an adolescent boy and girl where the girl is under 16 and thus, in law, deemed incapable of giving informed consent may, if reported and recorded, be classified as an indecent assault. Similarly, an offence of indecency between males may be recorded as an offence if both or one of the consenting males is under 21 and also if the behaviour is not conducted in private. The range of behaviour embraced in the categories of 'violence against the person', 'sexual offences' and 'robbery' is wide. They include the most serious on the statute book—murder, rape and armed robbery—but they also include attempts to commit these crimes and abetting and inciting others to commit them.*

The proportion of all recorded crime which is defined as violence has remained relatively stable over many years (at around 6 per cent). However, as the trend in crime levels has generally risen over the years, inevitably so, too, has the level of violent crime. For example, the average annual percentage change between 1984 and 1994 for all offences of violence against the person showed an increase of 6 per cent; that for sexual offences, an increase of 5 per cent; and that for robbery, an increase of 9 per cent (*Criminal Statistics* 1994). But these average annual percentages can conceal significant year-on-year comparisons, and, indeed, can obscure significant increases or decreases within subcategories of these very broad classifications. For example, quite dramatic increases for the subcategory of rape were shown in 1984–85 and 1985–86: 29 and 24 per cent, respectively. Was this a real increase? Newspaper headlines certainly treated these rises as real, but it is doubtful if that was the case. Changes in police recording practices are likely to account for most of the increase (for a discussion see [29]). Similarly, there were quite large increases in both more and less serious categories of violence against the person between 1986–87 and 1987–89. More serious offences increased by 22 and 16 per cent, respectively, and less serious offences by 12 per cent in each of these years. This was a period in which police-recording practices on domestic violence were reviewed and victims were encouraged to report such offences. It is arguable that at least some of the increases stemmed from these changes.

What appears in *Criminal Statistics* is not necessarily an accurate measure of the true incidence of crime since they are subject to, among other things, changes in public reporting to the police and police crime-recording practices. There are many reasons

---

* *Criminal Statistics* do not include all offence categories, only those known as notifiable offences. Broadly these are the more serious offences—those that are indictable or triable either way. Summary offences, which are tried only in the Magistrates' Courts, are not included. *Criminal Statistics* are published annually by the Home Office.

why people do not report crimes to the police.[30,31] Included among these are that they may regard the matter as too trivial; or something the police would not do anything about; or that they would not be believed; or that they do not define what has happened to them as a crime. In recording offences, police officers have to be satisfied that the incidents reported to them meet the legal criteria of what constitutes an offence. Their judgement is bound to a large extent by the criminal law, police procedures and evidential requirements, but the exercise of any judgement is also influenced by subjective interpretation of what has happened. Crime figures can also be affected when chief constables decide to target or have a 'blitz' on certain types of offence. Home Office advice may also suggest changes in the criteria by which decisions are made as to whether or not reported incidents have to be recorded—and thus appear in *Criminal Statistics*—as crimes.

Levels of violence as measured by *Criminal Statistics* do not take us very far, however, in thinking about the problem and how to tackle it. These statistics reflect legal categories that, in themselves, are not particularly informative or meaningful. Such categories as 'wounding or other acts endangering life' or 'malicious wounding' or even 'grievous bodily harm' and 'actual bodily harm' do not reveal anything about what is happening, to whom, by whom, where, and in what circumstances. Neither family violence nor its various strands—child abuse, domestic violence and elder abuse—are distinct nominate crimes and do not appear in *Criminal Statistics*. Some crimes specifically concerning children are identifiable—infanticide, child destruction, abandoning a child, gross indecency with a child, unlawful sexual intercourse—but some of these can be committed by people other than family members. In general, as neither the sex nor age of the victim, nor the relationship between victim and offender, is routinely recorded by the police nor presented in *Criminal Statistics*, they are not a good source of information about the extent and direction of family violence.

The statistics on homicide (i.e. murder, manslaughter and infanticide), however, are classified by age, sex and relationship to the principal suspect and shed some light on the familial nature of violent crime. But these offences are comparatively rare. In 1994, there were only 677 offences of homicide (*Criminal Statistics* 1994). Risk ratios per million population for different age groups showed that in common with most previous years, children under 1 year of age were the most likely to be victims of homicide—usually cases of infanticide. But children aged 5 and under 16 were the least likely victims, and the elderly (aged 70 and over) also had comparatively small risks. The majority of victims of homicide were male (60 per cent) and those aged over 16 and under 50 years were most at risk. In two-thirds of all homicides, victims were killed by people known to them but the pattern differs between the sexes: 31 per cent for male victims and 77 per cent for female victims. Almost two-fifths of female homicide victims were killed by present or former partners (spouses, cohabitants and lovers) compared with less than one-tenth of male victims. Women, too, were killed more frequently by other family members than were men (22 per cent compared with 12 per cent). In contrast, about three-tenths of male victims but only one-tenth of females were killed by strangers. If partners and lovers (former or current) are added to family members, one-fifth of male victims but three-fifths of female victims were killed by those in a relationship. The homicide figures thus attest to the domestic or family nature of this most serious form of violence. This is especially so for women.

To overcome some of the inherent limitations in *Criminal Statistics* and to flesh out the picture of violence, the Home Office Research and Statistics Directorate has, in the last few years, carried out a series of special exercises with police forces. They were asked to provide information on violence offence characteristics such as age of victim, relationship of victim to suspect and the location of the offence. Watson[32] combined and analysed information from 1990–92 and 1992–94, which covered data provided by up to 28 of the 43 police forces in England and Wales.* She found that for violence against the person offences, almost two-thirds of victims were male and the majority of all victims were aged between 16 and 39. The elderly (aged over 60) were rarely victims (2 per cent of both men and women) and children (aged under 16) comprised 14 and 12 per cent, respectively, for males and females. The location of these offences had quite a different pattern for male and female victims: almost one-half of offences against women were carried out in either their own home or that of the suspect. The comparable figure for men was just under one-fifth. This, Watson suggests, reflects the greater 'domestic' nature of violence against women.

Almost two-thirds of rape victims were aged between 16 and 39, and only 1 per cent were over 60. Just over one-quarter were children under 16, of whom 4 per cent were under 10 years of age. Again there are indications of the domestic or familial nature of some rape offences. Only just over a quarter were committed by strangers and almost a further third by acquaintances (friends, colleagues, neighbours, etc.). Spouses and lovers accounted for 15 per cent, as did parents or other family members (in 13 per cent of cases no relationship was recorded). Although the figure is not quoted, it is noted that additional information provided on child victims showed the risk of attack by strangers was very low.

The majority (70 per cent) of male victims of indecent assault (including buggery) were children under the age of 16, of whom about a quarter were under 10; none were recorded in adults over 60. Although female victims tended to be older, one-half were children under 16 and in 17 per cent of cases, the girl was under 10. Elderly victims aged over 60 were rare (1 per cent). Relationship patterns for indecent assault were somewhat different from rape. Given the high number of child victims, spouses and lovers did not feature prominently (4 per cent and 2 per cent for male and female victims, respectively). Female victims were more likely to be indecently assaulted by a stranger (37 per cent) than were male victims (27 per cent). Parents or other family members

---

* Since the level of information provided by police forces varied considerably across different offence categories and characteristics, caution has to be exercised in interpreting Watson's findings.

were implicated in 15 per cent of cases involving female victims and 13 per cent of male cases. Not surprisingly, given the higher percentage of females who were assaulted by strangers, offences committed out of doors were higher for females (35 per cent) than for males (22 per cent). But about half the offences were committed at the home of the victim or suspect (56 per cent for male victims and 48 per cent for female victims), and a further 15 per cent in the home of a friend or relative, again suggestive of a domestic familial link.

Violence in the family

Although Watson's analysis furthers some understanding of family violence, it does not take us very far.[32] Moreover, when it is recalled that many offences are never reported to the police or recorded by them, it will be recognized that the true extent of any type of crime is unknown. The gap between the 'real' or 'true' level of crime and that indicated by recorded crime statistics has been termed the 'dark figure of crime' by criminologists. The *British Crime Survey*[33] has shown that, overall, crime is three to four times greater than that recorded by the police and that there is some four to five times more violence. There is every reason to believe that the dark figure of family violence is particularly high. By its intrinsic nature, violence in the family remains an elusive research topic: it takes place behind closed doors; is concealed from the public eye; and is often unknown to anyone outside the immediate family.[34] Research cannot be undertaken unless victims are willing to disclose their experiences to someone. But much family violence is secret and victims may be subject to a variety of pressures not to tell outsiders about it—fear, loyalty, embarrassment, even self-blame and guilt. Just as importantly, where victims do tell, they may be offered little help (as in the case of women who are abused) or may be disbelieved (as in the case of children who say they have been sexually abused). There may be no obvious person to tell if extreme social isolation exists—the case for many elderly people. All sources of information, therefore, are underestimates. Only a very small minority of cases are disclosed to any agency and these may not be representative of all cases. We have little insight into how pervasive violence is within 'functioning' or 'normal' families.

A variety of techniques and sources have been used to estimate the extent of family violence. Specific surveys have been carried out with special groups within the general population such as students or residents of refuges. Newspapers and magazines have run surveys of their readership. Methods used have included face-to-face interviews, telephone and postal surveys and other types of self-completion questionnaires. Analyses have been carried out of records of different agencies, for example, the police, social work departments, hospital emergency rooms and general practitioners' surgeries.

All methods and sources, however, pose problems both individually and collectively. There are the problems of definition already referred to: What is used as the basis for measurement? What type of behaviour is taken to comprise violence? Unfortunately, the definition employed is not always made explicit yet it is self-evident that different measures will yield different rates. In addition, victims' perceptions and definitions of what happened to them may not fit with the definitions offered by the researchers.[35] Questions, for example, asking 'have you ever been forced to have sex' produce higher incidence rates than asking women 'have you ever been raped?' Then there are questions of which relationships 'count' as family and at what age does childhood end or people come to be classified as elderly. There are also problems of measurement. Measurements of incidence have to be distinguished from those of prevalence. Estimates of the number of families affected by family violence tell us little about how often they are so affected. Individual research studies are bedeviled by the difficulties of generalizing from their findings to the general population. Studies drawn from special populations may represent quite different types of cases and may be biased towards those who are more likely to come to the attention of formal agencies. Problems of definition, measurement, reliability, representativeness, concealment and subjectivity plague attempts to build up a picture of the extent of family violence from the various sources of information.

It is also impossible, because of these problems, to be precise about whether or not particular phenomena are increasing or decreasing. Family structure has changed significantly over the last century, becoming much smaller and more isolated. This may mean that violence is more likely to remain invisible. On the other hand, increased awareness, particularly through media attention, may mean that it has become more visible, although not necessarily more common. There is no reliable way of knowing the 'true' situation. Despite these reservations, information from diverse sources can provide some clues about the extent and, importantly, the direction of family violence.

Child abuse

Estimates of the physical and sexual abuse of children are high. Although each local authority in England has registered children suffering from or at risk of abuse for some time, national statistics were produced first in 1990 covering the year ending 31 March 1989. These provide an indication of extent but they are not exact. Some children on the register will not have been victims of actual abuse whereas some who have will not be on the registers. There were 34 954 children and young people on the registers at 31 March 1995: a rate of 32 children per 10 000 in the population aged under 18 years.[36] Rates for girls on the register were slightly higher than for boys (32 and 31 per 10 000, respectively) and considerably higher for sexual abuse (10 and 6 per 10 000, respectively), though rates for boys were slightly higher for physical abuse (12 and 11 per 10 000, respectively). There was no difference between the sexes for neglect or emotional abuse.

Studies of sexual abuse in childhood suggest that it is not a rare occurrence, although there is no agreement on estimates. A low estimate by Mrazek et al.[37] suggested that three children per 1000 were sexually abused at some point during childhood (i.e. about one in 6000 children a year). Baker and Duncan[38] estimated that over

4.5 million adults were sexually abused as children—12 per cent of girls and 8 per cent of boys. La Fontaine[39] concluded that a 10 per cent prevalence rate for sexual abuse involving physical contact was likely. Some studies have put the figure much higher. Nash and West[40] suggest that almost one in two will be sexually abused but they used a very inclusive definition. Kelly et al.[41], using a similarly broad definition, suggested that one woman in two and one man in four had been subjected to an unwanted sexual event or interaction before they were 18. When the most common reported experiences—flashing and touching—were excluded, the figure dropped to one woman in five and one man in 14. But even when calculations were based on only the most serious forms of abuse—rape, forced sex and coerced masturbation—experiences were frequent: one in 25 women and one in 50 men.

Many studies point to the familial nature of much sexual abuse of children. La Fontaine[39] found that twice as many children were abused by known people within their own homes as by outsiders although again there are varying estimates. Mrazek et al.[42] found that over two-fifths of victims were abused by members of their immediate family. Macleod and Saraga[43] put the number of girls who have been incestuously abused at between one in ten and one in three.

Domestic violence

Numerous studies have attempted to put a figure on the extent of domestic violence. These vary considerably (see [44]). Some put the figure of women experiencing at least one act of violence by a partner in their life time at one in four, others at one in ten. Marriages suffering serious violence are thought to range from one in 20 to one in 100. It has been suggested that one in three marriages experience physical violence and one in three divorces result from violence by husbands against wives. The range of estimates stems from different definitions, measurements and research methods used.

Crime surveys ask people directly about their experiences as victims but there are still problems in estimating domestic violence.[16,45,46] The only national crime survey in this country is the *British Crime Survey* (BCS) conducted by the Home Office. It employs a wider definition of domestic violence than some other surveys in that the incident need not have taken place at home and includes other relatives and household members within domestic relationships. On the other hand, it is more restricted in that sexual violence is not included. In the 1991 survey, three-quarters of the domestic violence uncovered did in fact occur at home and nine-tenths of incidents involved partners.

Domestic violence was found to be more frequent than street, work or pub/club violence. Eight out of ten domestic violence incidents were against women. A third of the domestic assaults against women involved a current husband or partner, one-fifth a current boyfriend and one-third a former husband or partner. In contrast, six out of ten domestic assaults on men were actually by non-partner relatives or non-partner household members.[47] The 1994 BCS found that just over half of all violence against women was domestic.[48]

The 1992 BCS also looked at lifetime prevalence of domestic violence among women. It focused on partners and physical violence. Overall, 11 per cent of women who had lived with a partner at some time said there had been some degree of physical violence. This figure is lower than that obtained from other surveys. Mooney's survey[45] in north London found a 30 per cent prevalence rate of lifetime experience, whereas Painter's study[49] of married women from 12 town centres produced figures of 24 per cent for currently married women and 59 per cent for divorced/separated women. Again, differences in definition, measurement, methods and populations studied are at work.

Elder abuse

There are no precise figures on the extent of abuse of the elderly. In comparison with 'spouse' and child abuse, it remains a relatively unexplored area (for a review, see [50]). On the whole, studies have been conducted with very small samples and drawn from special populations based, for example, on cases reported to agencies or from clinical populations. A study of 51 carers of partners receiving respite care, found that almost half admitted to some form of abuse.[51]

Some information is also available, from two large-scale surveys of the general population: the BCS and research by Ogg and Bennet[52] using the vehicle of the Omnibus Survey conducted by the Office of Population, Censuses and Surveys. In 1991, the BCS found that the elderly were significantly less at risk of physical violence from other household members than younger age groups.[47] They comprised only 2 per cent of domestic violence victims. In contrast to findings for younger age groups, men were almost as likely as women to be victims. On the basis of the Omnibus Survey's 593 respondents of pensionable age, prevalence rates were calculated of 15 in 1000 elderly for physical abuse, 54 in 1000 for verbal abuse, and 15 in 1000 for financial abuse.[20]

The nature of family violence

Scale, severity and effects

Despite disagreement over many aspects of family violence by various researchers, one of the few things about which there is almost universal agreement is that there is an escalation both in frequency and intensity over time. Research conducted in the 1960s and 1970s suggested that three-fifths of physically abused children were re-abused. More recent research, however, puts the figure lower at between a quarter and a third.[11] Sexually abused children are similarly at risk of re-abuse. La Fontaine[39] concludes that in many cases there is a progression from exhibitionism or touching and fondling to masturbation and then intercourse: anal, oral and vaginal. Cooper[53] also argues that abuse in incestuous relationships is regular and lasts over several years.

Spousal violence usually enters the relationship early: often within the first year of marriage or cohabitation. It may even predate cohabitation. A growing body of American research points to the frequency of violence in dating relationships. Few cases are cited in the research literature where the violence only emerged after the first 3 years of cohabitation. Moreover, the violence is frequent, but again estimates vary. Mooney's north London research[45] found that four times was the average for a woman who had been physically abused in the previous 12 months. On the other hand, Pahl[54] and the Dobashes[55,56] found that, in their samples of women who had fled to refuges, attacks occurred approximately twice a week. McCreadie[50] also concludes that elder abuse occurs in relationships that are very longstanding and that it may have existed for many years.

The injuries sustained by family members are severe—the homicide figures point to this. The specific details of the type of violence described in numerous studies include slaps, punches, kicking, choking, burning, stabbing and so on. In violence against wives, rape is commonly cited as coexisting with assaults. The inquiry into child abuse in Cleveland[9] cited examples of a girl of 7 having tea squirted up her vagina from a syringe and a boy of 4 having an iron bar pushed up his anus. Farmer and Owen's study[57] of child abuse demonstrates clearly that victims are often subjected to many different types of abuse. In one-third of cases primarily of neglect, there were also concerns about physical abuse; in one-fifth of cases where the main concern was with physical abuse, there were concerns about neglect; one-quarter of those principally concerned with sexual abuse also had concerns about neglect; and one-sixth of sexual abuse cases also raised questions about physical abuse.

Many individual studies chronicle the degree of severe physical injury suffered by victims of family violence. Indeed, in domestic violence between spouses, Morley and Mullender[58] claim that victims typically suffer a higher degree of violence relative to victims of other violent crimes. In addition to the physical injuries sustained, it is common for victims to also suffer psychological damage such as depression, stress, lack of sleep, weight loss or gain, ulcers, nervousness, loss of self-esteem and thoughts of suicide. Feelings of embarrassment, shame, humiliation and even self-blame are common.[16,50] Children who are the subject of abuse often display forms of psychological disorder, emotional and conduct disorder, and school and relationship difficulties (see, for example, [59]). These effects can be long lasting and can lead to attempted suicide, sexual promiscuity, running away, chemical dependency, self-destructive behaviour and withdrawal from sexual relationships.[40] Not all victims experience these, however, and it is not clear how to account for this.

Physical or sexual assault by someone known to the victim is sometimes perceived as in some way 'less serious' than assault by a stranger. The evidence contradicts this. Russell,[60] for example, found that 59 per cent of the women raped by husbands or ex-husbands were extremely distressed by this and that the long-term effects of rape by a husband were considerably greater than the effects of rape by a stranger; 52 per cent of women raped by a husband or relative reported that the rape had a profound effect on their lives, as compared with 39 per cent of the women raped by a stranger. A women raped (or, indeed, physically abused) by her husband cannot seek comfort or safety in her home. The impact of the sexual abuse of children, especially where no direct violence was involved, is also sometimes minimized. But this contrasts sharply with the feelings of incest survivors who describe feelings of fear and guilt.

The social and economic costs entailed in family violence are sometimes overlooked. Costs include strain on agency resources, such as medical services, social workers, police, solicitor and court costs, emergency housing provision, childcare facilities and state benefits. Although there has been no attempt to measure such costs in the United Kingdom, some countries have tried to put a figure on these costs in relation to domestic violence. In Canada, for example, Macleod[61] estimated that, in 1980, Canadian tax payers spent the equivalent of £17 billion on police intervention and related support and administration for wife battering. In Queensland, Australia, an attempt was made to produce a comprehensive economic audit of the costs of domestic violence for 20 women.[62] Including all services used by these 20 women, state benefits, compensation and super-annuation pay-offs, in addition to indirect costs in lost productivity in having to take time off work or indeed cease to work, produced an average lifetime cost for each of the 20 women of approximately £27 500. Economic costs would be even greater if child and elder abuse were also included.

Who are the perpetrators?

It is inescapable that it is primarily, although not exclusively, men—whether as husbands, fathers or stepfathers, sons or brothers—who are perpetrators of family violence. Apart from this one factor there is no single profile of abusers. They come from all cultural, racial, socio-economic, religious and age groups.

Department of Health statistics on children on at-risk registers provide no information on suspected perpetrators, unlike those previously published by the National Society for the Prevention of Cruelty to Children (NSPCC). An analysis of the years 1988–90 at first suggested that natural mothers were implicated in physical abuse more frequently than any other category of suspected perpetrator. However, a different picture emerged when the figures were adjusted to take account of who the child was living with at the time. Natural fathers and father substitutes then dominated. Where the child was living with his or her natural mother, she was implicated in one-third of physical injury cases; where the home was with the natural father, he was implicated in just over three-fifths of cases.[63]

Although there are a few mothers who sexually abuse their children, NSPCC statistics show this is very rare. Almost half of all reported sexual abuse cases involved natural fathers, stepfathers and male cohabitants; natural mothers comprised only 2 per cent of sexual abusers. The research literature[39,59,64] also confirms that most child sexual abusers are male and most studies (with the exception of the Northern Ireland study) confirm that they are family members. Men are also the majority of perpetrators of domestic violence according to most research. Two studies suggest the opposite. Straus *et al.*[65] and Straus and Gelles[66] claim that in the United States women are about as violent as men. In 1991 a United Kingdom Market and Opinion Research International survey—using the Conflict Tactics Scale developed by Straus—suggested that women were more violent than men. However, this scale has attracted considerable criticism for ignoring the differences in strength and fighting skills between men and women and for failing to distinguish between offensive and defensive behaviour (see, for example, [67]). Even Straus[68] argues that women, on the whole, fight back in self-defence and do not resort to severe violence until they have been the victim of a virtually continual stream of violence by their husbands.

A possible exception to this male monopoly was thought to be abuse of the elderly. Early studies indicated that the majority of abusers were female—primarily daughters and daughters-in-law. Eastman[24] suggested that they made up 60 per cent of perpetrators. As research into elder abuse has developed, it has become clear that, again, men are more likely to be abusers.[50] However, differences have been observed in the types of abuse perpetrated: men are more likely to physically and sexually abuse, women to use psychological abuse.

Who are the victims?

Family violence is primarily perpetrated against women and children. Female children are particularly vulnerable to sexual abuse, but as research in this field develops more male children are beginning to disclose their abuse. However, particularly when the assault occurs within the family, it is questionable whether boys are sexually abused because they are *boys*. Smith and Morris[69] argue that they are assaulted by heterosexual men because they are *children*. Amongst elderly victims, too, the majority are female, although as McCreadie[50] has pointed out, there are substantially more women than men in the older age groups so that even if the rates of abuse to men and women were the same, women would comprise the majority of victims.

Victims of family violence, like their abusers, come from all walks of life. Social class, family income, level of education, occupation and ethnic or racial background make little difference. These factors may, however, affect the likelihood of disclosure. The common assumption, for example, that family violence is largely a working class phenomenon may stem from the fact that researchers have often made use of police and social welfare records and working class families are more likely to come to the attention of these agencies. Middle class families, on the other hand, may be less willing to admit the occurrence of family violence, and to draw outsiders' attention to their problems, and may make more use of private, medical or other resources.

Explanations of family violence

Many attempts have been made to delineate the causes of family violence but no single explanation seems all powerful. Why men are primarily the abusers and women and children the victims requires explanation. There are, as has been demonstrated, some women who abuse their partners and their parents (usually mothers) and who sexually abuse their children, but they are comparatively rare. Women also physically abuse their children although not as commonly as previously thought. Explanations of family violence thus need to be responsive to the gendered nature of that violence but, in fact, few are.

Most of the theories reviewed here are drawn from research on child abuse and domestic violence. Given the relative infancy of research into elder abuse, especially in England and Wales, theoretical explanations are, by comparison, underdeveloped and tend to extrapolate from those on other forms of family violence.

Individualistic explanations

For a long time, explanations of family violence focused on individualistic explanations. That is, the behaviour was viewed as exceptional, unusual or deviant, and abusers were seen as mentally ill, pathological, neurotic or psychotic. In the case of domestic violence, they were often described as suffering from low self-esteem, insecurity and high marital dissatisfaction.[70,71] Child physical abusers were thought to be immature, self-centred and lacking in impulse control. In all likelihood they suffered from role reversal, expecting their children to be the providers of love, approval and a sense of importance.[72] Similarly, child sexual abusers were described as suffering from diminished intellectual and communication skills, paedophiliac sexual orientation, and psychosis.[73] Drug addiction, alcohol and gambling problems have also been identified as major contributors to violence. Those attempting to explain elder abuse have pointed to similar factors among the abusers (see, for example, [20,50] for reviews and discussion).

In this approach, there has been as much, if not more, concern with the individual pathology of the victim as with the abuser. Victims of domestic violence have been variously described as passive, aggressive, domineering, masochistic, frigid or emotionally deprived and are characterized as being neurotic or mentally ill.[70] So too with child sexual abuse, but here the descriptions are of a child behaving in a 'seductive' manner, acting out fantasies and welcoming fathers' and uncles' attention as expressions of love.[74] In short, women and children precipitate their own victimization. Blaming the victim is very evident. In relation to wife abuse the question is posed 'Why doesn't she leave?'; with child abuse it is 'Why doesn't she tell him to stop?' Without the victim's actions, the violence would not have occurred. Another line of blame attaching to child abuse is that of maternal collusion. Psychological literature has tended to place the responsibility for a child's care and upbringing on mothers; therefore, if a child is abused it must be due to something the mother did or did not do.

These characterizations are too simplistic. 'Why doesn't she leave?' ignores the emotional, social and economic conditions in which a female victim of domestic violence lives. It ignores the fact that she may have sought help where it was often not forthcoming, thus further increasing her sense of isolation and powerlessness. The basic assumption underlying the question 'Why does the child not tell him to stop?' also ignores the reality of the situation, which includes fear and helplessness. The Butler Sloss report[9] cites the various types of threats that are made to ensure silence—threats of violence to the child, or that the child will be taken away from home and put into care, or that the abuser will commit suicide. Silence may simply be due to a feeling that no-one will believe them or that the consequences would be too great. Maternal collusion, as Wilson[75] remarks, explains nothing; the behaviour is the man's responsibility. How does a poor sexual relationship between a man and a woman explain his decision to have sex with their child?

As recognition of the extent of family violence—and, indeed, of its dark figure—has increased, so too has the recognition that such individualistic and exceptionalistic explanations do not fit well with the universal nature of the problem. This type of explanation may be useful in understanding a few specific cases but it cannot provide a broad theory to explain the general phenomenon of the gender differential. Most of the research has been based on small unrepresentative samples using few or no control groups. It is simply not known whether the characteristics identified are not also commonly observed among those who do not commit or experience violence within the family, or whether the 'explanations' proffered are merely rationalizations. Importantly, such theories do not address the question of why these men abuse their wives and children rather than, say, their bosses or neighbours.

Sociostructural explanations

As knowledge about family violence increased, in particular about the extent of the problem, explanations that were individually based were seen as inadequate. Instead, the phenomenon came to be viewed as a response to sociostructural factors: for example, a response to frustration, stress or blocked goals. Circumstances such as poverty, unemployment, low occupational status, poor housing and low educational attainment, were seen as sources of stress which, combined with pressures in the family, led to violent outbursts. These external stresses, although not contributing directly to family violence, were seen as contributing to internal stresses within individuals and families and thus to violence. The work of the Family Violence Research Program at the University of New Hampshire was particularly influential in directing attention to the importance of sociostructural factors seen to be essentially male-dominated (see, for example, [65]). Role expectations are such that men are expected to be successful outside the home and to be the 'breadwinners', the 'head of the household', the 'master' within it. By contrast, women are expected to look to men for economic support and to be 'good wives and mothers'.

Faced with stressful situations, individuals seek mastery over the situation and this is often expressed in violence in the home, even where the sources of stress are outwith the home. Violence is 'a response to perceived powerlessness' and the greater the power differential within the home, the greater the likelihood of abuse.[76,77]

The socialization patterns within such families not only affirm traditional sex roles but teach children that violence is normal under certain circumstances. Linked to this, is an explanation based on the existence of a 'cycle of violence' established by intergenerational transmission. The contention is that people who observed violence between their parents or who were themselves victims of family violence are more likely to become abusers and victims in their own adulthood. This is thought to be true of domestic violence, child physical and sexual abuse, and there is also some suggestion that those who abuse their parents were themselves victimized by them as children—thus the cycle becomes complete.

The evidence for these hypotheses is equivocal. It propounds an essentially deterministic view of family violence. Later studies have questioned this stance, especially its relevance to victims. Even with regard to abusers, however, it is questionable. Widom's longitudinal study[78] of adults who were abused as children found that adult men had a higher frequency of arrest for violent offences than non-abused adult men. Nevertheless, it was a minority who were violent. Moreover, such a difference was not observed for adult women who had been abused or neglected as children. Its explanatory power is thus only partial. The family may act as a training ground for violence or form part of that training ground but, clearly, violence is committed by those who neither witnessed nor experienced such violence as children and not all those who had such violent childhood experiences commit acts of violence in adulthood.

As individual explanations blamed first the victim and then the abuser, the sociostructural approach indicts society—the structure and norms of society are to blame. What is not adequately explained by these approaches is why violence is seen as an appropriate response to various stresses or as acceptable behaviour in a particular culture. But the notion of pathology still prevails. As Bograd[79] has commented 'sociologists replicate the same error at the social level that psychologists make at the individual level'. The social structural approach also tends to be gender neutral; that is, it sees violence as a problem of both sexes equally and it places insufficient emphasis on the fact that it is females—whether as wives, mothers or children—who are disproportionately the victims of abuse.

Sociocultural–political explanations

Whilst the sociological explanations discussed above draw attention to both larger social factors and individual reactions to these, they fail to examine the societal power structure. With regard to explaining family violence, this necessitates explaining the acceptance and condoning of male power over women and children as the norm. This has been explored most fully by feminist researchers working in the area. For them, gender is a critical variable and family violence too prevalent to be explained as the result of individual problems experienced by a group of pathological men. Their views are not necessarily antithetical to those of sociostructural theorists, but they are often critical of one another. Feminists share some of the emphases of sociostructural theorists—for example the importance of socialization and cultural values, the relevance of social stresses, use of alcohol, sexual problems and so on—but they argue that their explanatory power is not sufficient. Explicitly, they take the view that all violence is a reflection of unequal power relationships and that violence in the family is a reflection of the unequal power of men and women in society and, therefore, also in their personal relationships.

Their argument is that the ideology of the family and the privacy accorded the family in our society mean that women are, and are seen to be, subordinate to the men they live with. They serve and service men's emotional, domestic and sexual needs. Many feminist writers, perhaps most notably the Dobashes,[55,67] make use of the notion of patriarchy to explain women's subordinate status. Put simply, patriarchy is the power of men over women and, consequently, of husbands over wives, fathers over children, sons over mothers. Using both historical analysis as well as sociological study, the Dobashes demonstrate how ingrained are the notions of husbands' authority and wives' subservience to it. Because women, children and the elderly are relatively powerless and dependent, they are vulnerable to abuse within the family. This is particularly so when the husband/father holds traditional views about the role of wives and daughters. The predominant sources of conflict in families in which wives are abused are possessiveness and jealousy, the provision of services and money. Research has also found that men are most likely to become violent when women question their authority or challenge their behaviour. It is also true that paternal sexual abuse tends to occur in families where the father is dominant.[40] In feminist writings, the pathology is moved from that of the individual or even of the individual family to the family structure itself and its unequal power structure. Moreover, the family is seen as a microcosm of an unequal society.

In this school of thought, violence typifies the cultural style of society, as socially learned behaviour, traditionally condoned in large measure by such institutions as religion and the law and as about *taking*, not losing, control. As Smith and Morris[69] argue, men are responding to the dictates of culturally constructed concepts of masculinity—what it is to be a 'real man'. They abuse within the family because they are allowed to and, until recently, social institutions condoned it. They are not abnormal men; rather feminists suggest that they are acting within the mainstream of normal male behaviour.

The fact that not all men are violent within the family is irrelevant to the feminist thesis. Some men choose not to abuse their power by violence, which is seen as being at the extreme end of a continuum of control—or to abuse it in non-violent ways (for example, restricting freedom of movement or access to resources)—but the fact remains: they have the power to choose. The widespread acceptance of the rationalizations of men who abuse their partners, not least in the clinical literature and amongst criminal justice and social welfare professionals, points to male privilege being endemic in our culture. Whilst many feminists agree on the importance of such factors as unemployment, lack of advancement at work, poor living conditions or whatever, they argue that family members are the victims of violence rather than anyone else because the family structure gives men the power to act violently and, equally importantly, to get away with it in large measure. If it did not, then, regardless of the state of their finances, levels of stress or whatever, their violence would not be concentrated in the family.

Feminists also argue that the small amount of family violence that is perpetrated by women can be explained by power. Cole,[80] for example, contends that women express their powerlessness by abusing the only ones within the family more vulnerable and dependent than they are—their children and elderly parents.

Although feminist explanations may be uncomfortable reading for some, their contribution has been to question taken-for-granted assumptions and to begin to explore the ways in which social institutions and traditional relationships between the sexes interact to produce and condone family violence. There is some empirical research which points to their significance. Straus, in a paper presented to the American Society of Criminology in 1987, examined the rate of husband to wife assaults in 45 states in the United States. He found the greater the degree of equality between men and women, the lower the degree of wife beating.

Conclusion

Family violence is common; it can be severe and long lasting; it can have profound long-term effects; and is primarily perpetrated by men. A variety of explanations ranging from a focus on individual aspects of offenders and victims to broad socio-structural/cultural/political factors has been advanced. Yet, there is still no precise understanding and an integration of all three explanatory approaches is probably needed.

References

1 **Korbin JE**, ed. *Child Abuse and Neglect—Cross Cultural Perspectives.* Berkeley and Los Angeles: University of California Press, 1983.

2 **Gil DG.** *Violence Against Children.* Cambridge, MA: Harvard University Press, 1970.

3 **Steele BF.** Violence in the family. In: Herfer RE, Kempe CH, eds. *The Abused Child.* Cambridge, MA: Ballinger Publishing Co., 1976.

4 **Roberts R.** *The Classic Slum: Salford Life in the First Quarter of the Century.* Manchester: Manchester University Press, 1971.

5 **Freeman M.** *Violence in the Home.* Farnborough, UK: Saxon Hall, 1979.

6 **Dwyer K.** *Violence Against Children.* Australian National Committee on Violence, Violence Today Series, Paper 3. Canberra: Australian Institute of Criminology, 1989.

7 Kempe CH, Silverman FN, Steele BF, Silver HK. The battered child syndrome. *Journal of the American Medical Association* 1962; **181**: 17–24.

8 Turner JWC, ed. *Kenny's Outlines of Criminal Law.* Cambridge, UK: Cambridge University Press, 1952.

9 Butler Sloss E. *Report of the Inquiry into Child Abuse in Cleveland, 1987.* London: HMSO, 1988.

10 Department of Health & Social Security. Home Office, Department of Education & Science. Working Together under the Children Act 1989. London: HMSO, 1991.

11 Department of Health. *Child Protection Messages from Research.* London: HMSO, 1995.

12 Martin D. Battered women: society's problem. In: Chapman JR, Gates M, eds. *The Victimisation of Women.* Beverley Hills: Sage, 1978.

13 Dobash RE, Dobash RP. Community response to violence against wives: charivari, abstract justice and patriarchy. *Social Problems* 1981; **28** (5): 563–81.

14 Blackstone W. *Commentaries on the Laws of England* (first published 1765). London: Dawsons, 1966.

15 Cobbe FP. Wife torture in England. *Contemporary Review* 1878; **April**: 55–87.

16 Smith LJF. *Domestic Violence: an Overview of the Literature.* Home Office Research Study No. 107. London: HMSO, 1989.

17 Women's National Commission. *Violence Against Women.* London: Cabinet Office, 1985.

18 Home Affairs Select Committee. *Inquiry into Domestic Violence.* London: HMSO, 1993.

19 McCreadie C. *Elder Abuse: an Exploratory Study.* London: Age Concern Institute of Gerontology, Kings College, 1991.

20 Bennet G, Kingston P. *Elder Abuse.* London: Chapman & Hall, 1993.

21 Baker AA. Granny battering. *Modern Geriatrics* 1975; **8**: 20–4.

22 Sumner WG. *Folkways: a Study of the Sociological Importance of Usage, Manners, Customs, Mores and Morals.* New York: New American Library, 1960.

23 O'Malley T, Segal H, Perez R. *Elder Abuse in Massachusetts.* Boston, MA: Legal Research and Services to the Elderly, 1979.

24 Eastman M. *Old Age Abuse.* London: Age Concern England, 1984.

25 Biggs S. A family concern. Elder abuse in British social policy. *Critical Social Policy* 1996; **47** (16): 63–88.

26 Tomlin S. *Abuse of Elderly People: An Unnecessary and Preventable Problem.* London: British Genetics Society, 1989.

27 Social Services Inspectorate. *Confronting Elder Abuse.* London: HMSO, 1992.

28 Social Services Inspectorate *No Longer Afraid.* London: HMSO, 1993.

29 Smith LJF. *Concerns about Rape.* Home Office Research Study No. 106. London: HMSO, 1989.

30 Hough JM, Mayhew P. *Taking Account of Crime: Key Findings from the 1984 British Crime Survey.* Home Office Research Study 85. London: HMSO, 1985.

31 Hough JM, Mayhew P. *The British Crime Survey: First Report. Home Office Research Study 76.* London: HMSO, 1983.

32 Watson L. *Victims of Violent Crime Recorded by the Police, England and Wales 1990–94.* Home Office Statistical Findings 1/96. London: Home Office, 1996.

33 Mayhew P, Mirlees-Black C, Aye Maung N. *Trends in Crime: Findings for the 1994 British Crime Survey.* Home Office Research Findings No. 14. London: Home Office, 1994.

34 Smith LJF. *Family Violence: its Extent, Nature and How it is being Tackled.* World Health Organisation Consultation on Preventive Interventions in Social Violence Copenhagen: 1989.

35 Kelly L. *Surviving Sexual Violence.* London: Sage, 1988.

36 **Department of Health.** *Children and Young People on Child Protection Registers, England.* London: HMSO, 1996.

37 **Mrazek PB, Lynch MA, Bentovim A.** Sexual abuse of children in the United Kingdom. *Journal of Child Abuse and Neglect* 1983; 7 (2): 147–53.

38 **Baker A, Duncan S.** Child sexual abuse: a study of prevalence in Great Britain. *Child Abuse and Neglect* 1986; **9**: 4.

39 **La Fontaine J.** *Child Sexual Abuse.* ESRC Research Briefing. London: ESRC, 1988.

40 **Nash C, West D.** Sexual molestation of young girls. In: West D, ed. *Sexual Victimisation.* Aldershot, UK: Gower, 1985.

41 **Kelly L, Regen L, Burton S.** An explanatory study of the prevalence of sexual abuse in a sample of 1244 16–21 year olds. Find Report to ESRC. London: ESRC, 1991.

42 **Mrazek PB, Lynch MA, Bentovim A.** Recognition of child sexual abuse in the United Kingdom. In: Mzarek PB, Kempe GH, eds. *Sexually Abused Children and Their Families.* Oxford: Pergamon, 1981.

43 **MacLeod M, Saraga E.** Challenging the orthodoxy. *Feminist Review* 1988; **28**: 16.

44 **Smith LJF.** Domestic Violence: the Wider Context. Paper presented at St Catherines Conference on responding to Domestic Violence: where are the gaps?, 1994.

45 **Mooney J.** *The Hidden Figure: Domestic Violence in North London.* London: Islington Council, 1993.

46 **Mirlees-Black C.** *Estimating the Extent of Domestic Violence: Findings from the 1992 BCS.* Home Office Research Bulletin No. 37. London: Home Office, 1995.

47 **Mayhew P, Maung N, Mirlees-Black C.** *The 1992 British Crime Survey.* Home Office Research and Planning Unit Study 132. London: HMSO, 1992.

48 **Home Office RSD.** *Domestic Violence Fact Sheet Issue 3.* London: Home Office, 1996.

49 **Painter K.** *Wife Rape, Marriage and the Law. Survey Report: Key Findings and Recommendations.* Manchester: University of Manchester, Faculty of Economics and Social Sciences, 1991.

50 **McCreadie C.** *Elder Abuse: Update on Research.* London: Age Concern Institute of Gerontology, Kings College, 1996.

51 **Homer A, Gilleard C.** Abuse of elderly people by their carers. *British Medical Journal* 1990; **301**: 1359–62.

52 **Ogg J, Bennet G.** Elder abuse in Britain. *British Medical Journal* 1992; **305**: 998–9.

53 **Cooper L.** Decriminalisation of incest—new legal-clinical responses. In: Eckelaar J, Sandford K, eds. *Family Violence.* Toronto: Butterworths, 1978.

54 **Pahl J.** *Private Violence and Public Policy.* London: Routledge & Kegan Paul, 1985.

55 **Dobash RE, Dobash RP.** *Violence Against Wives.* New York: The Free Press, 1979.

56 **Dobash RE, Dobash RP.** The nature and antecedents of violent events. *British Journal of Criminology,* 1984; **24**(3): 269–88.

57 **Farmer E, Owen M.** *Child Protection Practice: Private Risks and Public Remedies—Decision Making, Intervention and Outcome in Child Protection Work.* London: HMSO, 1995.

58 **Morley R, Mullender A.** *Preventing Domestic Violence to Women.* Police Research Group Crime Prevention Unit Series, Paper 48. London: Home Office, 1994.

59 **The Research Team (N).** *Child Sexual Abuse in Northern Ireland.* Antrim: Greystone Books, 1990.

60 **Russell D.** *Rape in Marriage.* New York: Collier Books, 1982.

61 **MacLeod L.** *Battered but not Beaten . . . Preventing Wife Battering in Canada.* Ottawa: Canadian Advisory Council on the Status of Women, 1987.

62 **Roberts G.** Domestic violence: costing of service provision for female victims—20 case histories. In: *Beyond These Walls. Report of the Queensland Domestic Violence Task Force.* Brisbane: Queensland Domestic Violence Task Force, 1988.

63 **NSPCC.** *Child Abuse Trends in England and Wales 1988–1990.* London: NSPCC, 1992.

64 **Waterhouse L, Dobash R, Carnie J.** *Child Sexual Abusers.* Edinburgh: Scottish Office Central Research Unit, 1994.

65 **Straus MA, Gelles R, Steinmetz SK.** *Behind Closed Doors.* New York: Anchor, 1980.

66 **Straus MA, Gelles R.** Societal change and change in family violence, 1975 to 1985, as revealed in two national surveys. *Journal of Marriage and the family* 1986; **48**: 465–79.

67 **Dobash RE, Dobash RP, Wilson M, Daly M.** The myth of sexual symmetry in marital violence. *Social Problems* 1992; **39** (1): 71–91.

68 **Straus MA.** Victims and aggressors in marital violence. *American Behavioural Scientist* 1980; **23** (5): 681–704.

69 **Smith LJF, Morris A.** Physical and sexual assaults in the family. Paper presented at International Colloqiumin on Violence in our Cities, Munster, Germany, 1988.

70 **Gayford JJ.** Wife battery: a preliminary summary of 100 cases. *British Medical Journal* 1975; 1(5951): 194–7.

71 **Roy M.** Four thousand partners in violence: a trend analysis. In: Roy M. ed. *The Abusive Partner.* New York: Van Nostrand Reinhold, 1982.

72 **Gelles RJ.** An exchange/social control theory of intrafamily violence. In: Finkelher D, Gelles RJ, Hotaling GT, Straus MA, eds. *The Dark Side of Families.* Beverley Hills: Sage, 1993.

73 **Berlin FS, Krout E.** Paedophilia: diagnostic concepts, treatment and ethical considerations. American Journal of Forensic Psychiatry, 1986; 7: 13–30.

74 **Erikson EL, McEvoy AW, Colucci ND.** Jr. *Child Abuse and Neglect: a Guide Book for Educators and Community Leaders,* 2nd edn. Holmes Beach: Learning Publications, 1984.

75 **Wilson E.** *What is to be Done About Violence Against Women.* Harmondsworth: Penguin, 1983.

76 **Finkelhor D.** Common features of family violence. In: Finkelhor D, Gelles RJ, Hotaling GT, Straus MA, eds. *The Dark Side of Families.* Beverly Hills: Sage, 1983.

77 **Finkelhor D.** *Child Sexual Abuse.* London: The Free Press, 1984.

78 **Widom C.** Child abuse, neglect, and violent criminal behaviour. *Criminology* 1998; **27**: 251–71.

79 **Bograd M.** Feminist perspectives on wife abuse: an introduction. In: Yllo K, Bograd M, eds. *Feminist Perspectives on Wife Abuse.* Beverly Hills: Sage, 1988: 11–26.

80 **Cole SG.** Child battery. In: Guberman C, Wolfe M, eds. *No Safe Place: Violence Against Women and Children.* Toronto: Womens Press, 1985.

EDITORS NOTE: This historical review of the literature was prepared in 1997. The more recent evidence is summarised in Chapters 4, 10, and 15.

Chapter 2

Psychological causes of family violence

Felicity de Zulueta

Introduction

It is useful to see family violence as a continuum—ranging from neglect and disregard of emotional and material needs, through lesser forms of physical aggression, such as slapping, hitting, kicking and beating, up to maiming or even murder. Gelles,[1] a noted researcher in the field of domestic violence, defines it as an 'act carried out with the intention, or perceived intention, of physically injuring another person'. I find it more useful to expand this definition to include the intention of physically or psychologically injuring another person, since the sexual abuse of children often results in severe long-term emotional consequences for the victims but does not necessarily involve physical injury.

The essential ingredient in family violence is fear, fear for the victim's safety or fear for the safety of other family members. It is partly because of this fear that family violence is still so much of a secret. However, this is not the only reason why domestic violence impinges still so little upon most of our personal or professional lives: becoming aware of the extent of this problem is painful because of the emotions it arouses in us. As a consultant psychotherapist in the National Health Service, I have had a lot of contact with the victims of family violence. At least half our patients were known to have been physically and/or sexually abused, but it is only through focusing on the terrible fear that these people experience that I have come to know what the term 'family violence' really means. Both victims, and often abusers, live for years in the shadow of an all pervading terror. They have learnt to cope with it, as we all do, through denial and dissociation and all the other defence mechanisms most people use to keep going in the face of helplessness and fear. One adult patient speaking of her father's repeated rejections stated: 'I am taking it all as normal but it's so wrong!' She could only see what was going on once her experience of abuse had been validated and defined for what it was. Another young patient explained how her violent drunken father had so abused her she used to go to bed wearing a crash helmet, just in case.

Once we begin to listen to these individuals' terrifying and often humiliating experiences, once we begin to recognize the magnitude of the pain and fear which goes on in the privacy of people's homes, we balk. Professionals and public alike do not really want to know how terrible it can be for some families, particularly if we feel helpless and unable to do anything about it. We are exposed to more than enough violence in the media. We were repelled and horrified by what we saw on the video of the Bulger case, by the horrifying descriptions of child torture and murder during Rosemary West's trial, by the cold-blooded cruelty which produced the Dunblane massacre. We cry out for more security, an end to the use of handguns, longer prison sentences, and it is natural that we do so.

However, it is important for us to realize that the violence of these horrible crimes is but the tip of the iceberg. At the base is the secret violence of family life: the abuse and attacks that take place in the homes of those we meet as we go about our daily business. Many of the victims of family violence visit their general practitioners. They complain of tension, insomnia, fatigue, alcoholism, anxiety, depression, panic attacks, irritability and physical symptoms . . . the list is endless. The doctor may not recognize the source of these symptoms and may feel confused and frustrated when these patients do not get better.

If the reality of family violence has been, and still is, one of our society's best kept secrets, it is simply that we cannot often see what we cannot bear to see. For the victims of such violence, shame, guilt, denial or, more often than not, real fear prevents them from telling professionals what they are going through. And as for the professionals, how many really want to know what lies behind some of their patients' symptoms? Hidden behind a woman's 'depression' may lurk a reality that is so disgusting, frightening or out of control that her doctor cannot allow him or herself to think beyond the need for an antidepressant pill. Whatever our medical specialty, we feel the need to wrap our patients' tragedies into symptoms and syndromes we can understand and manage. We want to feel in control and to know what we are dealing with, particularly when we work in the context of a very busy surgery. In addition, we are also human beings like everyone else. Most of us cherish the idea that home can be a refuge from the pains and traumas of everyday life. The family is still seen by society as a nurturing microcosm where children are brought up by caring parents to become good responsible citizens. And yet how true is this belief?

My aim in this chapter is to outline a new way of understanding of human destructiveness supported by recent research findings (summarized in [2]). This theory of violence assumes that, like other mammals, we are driven by a fundamental instinct to form attachments. Investigation of the effects of separation, loss, abuse and psychological trauma on both children and adults shows that the individual can only exist in relation to the 'other', and that it is the nature of this relationship that is at the heart of our understanding of human behaviour, be it loving or destructive. From birth, the human infant needs to establish and maintain proximity to some other preferred and differentiated individual, usually, but not necessarily, the mother. The need to form attachments is a form of human motivation as fundamental as the drive for food or sex.

Once we have recognized the importance of the affiliative bonds which link us to one another, it will come as no surprise to discover that it is the disruption of these powerful attachments and the accompanying shattering of the self which is the source of human destructiveness.

The relationship between attachment behaviour and violence

John Bowlby[3–5] and his colleagues in the United States have made us aware of this hitherto unrecognized and yet fundamental motivational system in the life and development of human beings. Although there is clearly insufficient space here to present the vast literature in this field, which has been reviewed elsewhere, I will attempt to provide a brief review of the most important ideas and findings with reference to family violence, and how if affects individuals.

In the infant, attachment behaviour is activated by either an internal cue, such as an illness, or by external threats, both of which drive the child to seek protection from his or her caregiver, usually, but not always, the mother. If the latter is not available the infant will protest before showing despair, finally becoming detached. What happens then is that the infant will no longer respond to the return of his or her mother and might even appear to ignore her. As we shall see later, this *avoidant* response is crucial to our understanding of some types of violent behaviour.

The development of these attachment bonds is achieved by a complex process of physical and emotional attunement which, if disrupted in childhood through deprivation, loss or any other form of trauma, has long-term effects on the way the individual feels about him or herself and how he or she behaves towards others. Although very evident in childhood, when attachment behaviour provides for the infant both protection and an interactional pathway for the development of the self, attachment behaviour characterizes humans throughout their lifespan.

Studies on separation (with the sequential response of protest, despair and detachment) carried out on primate infants and their mothers reveal that: (i) attachment behaviour has a psychobiological substrate; and (ii) it is a form of behaviour mediated by opiates, so much so that one researcher describes social bonding as an 'opiate addiction'. Indeed the symptoms of distress produced by separation are similar to those seen in narcotic withdrawal states and involve aggressive behaviour. This implies that emotions are at the root of social bonding. Pleasure is the outcome of attachment mediated by endogenous opiates. Separation produces distress and aggression. These findings lead us to postulate that the mechanisms underlying love and hate may be related reciprocally.

Studies on human development show that infants are born with this innate predisposition to form strong attachments to their primary caregiver and subsequently to their secondary caregivers such as father, siblings, childminders, the extended family, etc. This process allows young infants early physiological and hormonal systems to be regulated by their primary caregiver, functions that the infants gradually acquire themselves as they develop. This is achieved through the formation of what Hofer[6] describes as internal 'biologic regulators'. He maintains that it is the presence of these biological regulators within the interaction that determines an infant's behaviour following separation.

> If bonnet macaque monkeys are obliged to forage for food rather than receiving it *ad libitum*, the mother–infant relationship becomes more tense with increased maternal rejection and increased infant independence. When separated from their mothers these infants show the normal protest response of the acute phase but become markedly depressed in the second week of separation. This does not occur in their usual environment.[7]

This study, amongst others, shows how the nature of the mother–infant relationship can be disrupted through deprivation or trauma and can produce an altered response to separation and loss. Hofer maintains that these 'biologic regulators' have an important function throughout life.

These important physiological changes are accompanied by parallel emotional and behavioural developments arising from the interaction between mother and infant that lead to the development of the self and the creation of an inner psychic world of internal object relations or working models. The latter are probably the equivalent of what Hofer describes as 'psychologic regulators'. He goes on to demonstrate how these may be so intimately linked with their physiological counterparts as to ensure normal behavioural patterns during periods of planned seperation: we do not grieve every time we part from our loved ones for a day's work. Having acquired the capacity to hold the 'other' within our mind, we can thus survive temporary losses. Hofer suggests that our 'psychologic' regulators achieve this through their control of our 'biologic' regulators.[6]

This complex process of psychobiological 'attunement' between the infant and caregiver is replayed throughout the individual's subsequent relationships and is at the heart of his or her attachment to others. This implies that any disruption of this essential developmental process leads to serious long-term effects, both at a physiological and psychological level. Thus, the traumas of loss, deprivation and abuse, whether physical, sexual or emotional, can all have longstanding effects on our capacity to form relationships, our sense of self and, in particular, the potential for violent or destructive behaviour.[2]

Recent research on the effects of chronic stress on children shows that the dysregulation of the normal stress response through chronic abuse, for example, can result in a set of highly dysfunctional and maladaptive brain activities.[8] Perry also believes that there may be a link between childhood trauma and many medical and psychiatric conditions relating to the cardiovascular, neuroendocrine and immune systems. The damage to the brain resulting from child abuse also interferes with normal parenting in the next generation.[9]

Harlow's research on maternally deprived rhesus monkeys produced, among other abnormalities, inappropriate aggressive behaviour, which has been attributed by some researchers to the reciprocal manifestation of a damaged attachment system.[10]

Studies on loss, deprivation and abuse in children and adults, in terms of their psychobiology and attachment behaviour, clearly show that the individual can only exist in relation to the 'other'. Satisfactory attachments that are essential for our emotional well-being are dependent on the capacity to become attuned to the 'other'.

Different types of attachment behaviour

During development, infants learn to be alert to the physical and emotional availability of their caregivers. Mothers may be experienced as either rejecting or unpredictable, in which case different strategies for gaining access will be developed. These different responses to the caregiver (mother and/or father) have become the focus of much research in the field of attachment behaviour.

Mary Ainsworth and her colleagues[11] in the United States were the first to demonstrate that the way 1-year-old infants behaved when reunited with their parent (in this case, the mother) after an enforced separation depended on how sensitively she had responded to their needs during infancy. This was assessed by first observing infants in their home surroundings and then by devising a laboratory experiment called the 'strange situation'. The procedure is as follows:

> A mother and child are put together in a room full of toys, under observation (Episode 1 and 2). A stranger is introduced to see how the infant responds (Episode 3). Then the mother leaves the room unobtrusively so that her infant is alone with the stranger (Episode 4). How does the infant respond to mother's first departure? Mother returns, greeting and comforting the infant, encouraging her to play again. Mother then leaves the room saying 'bye, bye' (Episode 5). The infant is alone for the second separation episode (Episode 6). The stranger returns (Episode 7) and then the mother and the infant are reunited (Episode 8).

What Ainsworth and her team found using the 'strange situation' was that 63 per cent of their middle class infants showed a secure attachment; they usually cried on separation from their mother but responded rapidly to her warm hug on her return. In the nursery or in the home these children were able to form good relations and to tune into the needs of others, that is to empathize. The 'other' for such an individual is perceived and treated as another human being whose needs can be attended to.

However, 12 per cent of the infants tested were described as showing an anxious/ambivalent form of attachment behaviour. These babies were very distressed when separated from their mothers and took a long time to settle down when they returned. These insecurely attached infants had been exposed to inconsistent parenting.

Of particular interest to us are the 20–25 per cent of insecurely attached infants who were found to show an avoidant response to their mother on her return. In other words, they showed no distress when the mothers left and ignored them on their return.

However, these infants' rapid heartbeats betrayed how anxious they felt. They had either been deprived or rejected and their avoidant behaviour appears to have arisen because they had been placed in an intolerable conflict situation by their caregivers. Usually, if threatened in any way infants will run to their mothers for security. But what if the mother becomes threatening or forbids physical contact? These infants learn to displace their attention elsewhere and thereby 'cut themselves off' from feelings of anger and fear so as to be able to remain as close as possible to the parent they totally depend on. These avoidant children show poor self-esteem and frequent hostility, which means that their peer interactions are generally negative. These findings were confirmed in a study on 19 pairs of children aged 4–5 years.[12] The investigators found that victimization occurred in all the pairs where one or both children were found to show an avoidant attachment response and the other was also insecurely attached, either avoidant or anxious/ambivalent. Children with secure attachment patterns were not observed to be either abusers or victims.

This study is of particular interest to our study of human violence because it shows two things: (i) secure children do not show needless aggression, whereas (ii) avoidant children can become either abusers or victims. This means that they internalize a behavioural template (working model or internal object relation) based on the actual relationship they have been subjected to, and can enact either the role of victim or victimizer depending on the circumstances.

In subsequent studies carried out by Mary Main in the United States, another group of infants were identified using Ainsworth's 'strange situation'. These infants displayed a disorganized response to their returning parent, a mixture of avoidant and anxious/ambivalent behaviour. On their mothers' return, they behaved in a bizarre and unpredictable manner. Some infants suddenly 'froze', others withdrew to another side of the room, others fell to the ground or crawled under their mother's chair, etc. This new category of infants appear to have mothers who are either abusive to their children or who have themselves been traumatized and therefore tended to dissociate.[13] Research in this area suggests that when these infants become adults some of them may be diagnosed as suffering from borderline personality disorders,[14,15] Further evidence is needed to establish whether these same individuals can resort to the more extreme forms of violent criminal behaviour seen in the forensic population.

These studies on attachment behaviour patterns have been replicated in many different countries producing very similar results. Where there are differences, these have been ascribed to cultural differences in upbringing. It is important to note that the same child can develop different attachments with each parent.[16]

Attachment behaviour and family violence

What is becoming clear is that patterns of attachment are self-perpetuating, allowing an individual to preserve a sense of identity and continuity. For this to be maintained, cognitive distortions need to take place so that the individual deals with the world and others very much in the way he or she was dealt with. For example, avoidant children when faced with a crying peer, will respond negatively and may even hit the other child. This response may be determined by the fact that these children find the crying unbearable because it elicits their own unresolved pain or because that it is how adults dealt with their tears. They show little or no capacity to empathize. A battered woman I knew reported that when she was a child and cried her father would beat her and then say 'Now you have something to cry about'. An example of such perceptual distortion is provided by Frodi's study[17] on the effect of infant crying on different caregivers. The human baby's cry is always aversive, the equivalent of being repeatedly insulted or receiving an electric shock. A smiling baby elicits a positive reaction from most of us, but for an abusive mother suffering from a so-called borderline personality disorder (the adult form of disorganized attachment) both smiling and crying can be aversive. Her insensitivity to her infant's signals may correspond to her own need as a parent to preserve a particular organization of information or state of mind that, in some cases, can actually lead to an active need to alter infant signals or to inhibit them.[18]

What studies on attachment behaviour demonstrate is that the avoidant and disorganized infants grow up with a sense of worthlessness. These individuals are so insecure that they have a desperate need to have some sense of control over others, who can thereby become objects of contempt, abuse and exploitation.

The *avoidant infant* learns to cut off his or her feelings of fear and anger in order to obey and thereby please his or her parent. The price this child pays is that he or she cannot integrate the feelings of fear and rage that can be triggered by the pain of another. For these individuals, to do unto others what was done unto them is a way of being in charge and getting satisfaction or even excitement. When they grow up they can find their needs for control and revenge fulfilled within the confines and secrecy of the family home or under the orders of an able group leader who knows how to command and channel their rage to his ends. For these individuals, the more 'legitimate' or socially approved the context of their activity, the more manifest their use of power and control.

The *disorganized infant* grows up in a state of recurring terror and with a desperate need to feel that he or she is in control. If these individuals do not feel in control, they fear they will be reduced to the state of helpless terror and pain of their past or even become insane. To understand them better we need to consider research on psychological trauma and what it has to teach us regarding the origins of violence. However, before moving to this subject let us look at another important aspect of the research in attachment.

Transgenerational transmission of attachment behaviour

What we know so far is that the experience of loss, deprivation and child abuse, whether physical, sexual or emotional, can all have long-term effects on the capacity to form relationships and a sense of identity and, in particular, on the potential for destructive or violent behaviour. Recent research based on interviews with adults using the Adult Attachment Interview is beginning to show that we can determine what attachment patterns these individuals have (i.e. secure, anxious/ambivalent, avoidant or disorganized). Of even greater interest is the finding that these adults will tend to have infants with the same attachment pattern.[13] This means that mothers assessed prior to the delivery of their child can be helped, through psychotherapy, to avoid repeating their destructive attachment behaviour. These findings are very important since they provide us with another way of understanding the transgenerational transmission of violence, hitherto attributed mainly to genetic transmission.

Psychological trauma and violence

If psychological trauma is defined as the 'sudden uncontrollable disruption of affiliative bonds'[19] it is not surprising to find that there is considerable overlap between attachment disorder and psychological trauma—both result from a disruption of the attachment system. Post-traumatic stress disorder (PTSD) involves the wounding of the human psyche during states of terrifying helplessness. An understanding of its manifestations is important in the treatment of its victims, whether they were affected through prolonged traumatic experiences during childhood (complex PTSD) or through more recent trau-matization. The psychobiological manifestations of PTSD are similar to those seen with disrupted attachments only even more severe.

It is important to emphasize here that whether someone develops PTSD depends not only on the severity of the trauma and the meaning it has for the individual but also on the sociocultural context in which it is experienced. The strength of community attachments is an important factor in determining whether an individual develops PTSD.

PTSD presents as a biphasic response involving, on the one hand, the reliving of traumatic events and, on the other, a sense of numbness and a reduced responsiveness to the outside world as the individual attempts to 'cut himself off' or to dissociate from his or her source of terror and pain.

Dissociation and re-enactment

Traumatized individuals find themselves reliving their traumatic experience mainly through intrusive thoughts, such as flashbacks, nightmares, recurrent memories or, of particular relevance here, through the actual re-enactment of the event. In the latter, the subject may play the role of the victim or the victimizer, as in avoidant infants discussed above.[20] It is this particular consequence of psychological trauma that is an important cause of violence. It can be at the root of what appears to be unprovoked violence occurring many years after the original trauma. In these individuals, damage to the attachment system results in such intense terror and accompanying rage that it is often 'split off' or dissociated from consciousness: this means that the individual has no idea why he is doing what he is doing.

Painful memories can be lost to consciousness because of a failure to integrate traumatic experiences into declarative memory. They can then be triggered back into action (although not necessarily consciousness) by some external or internal stimulus to recreate the pain the individual was once subjected to, either in himself or in the other, as we see in many parents who abuse their children. These traumatized individuals are thereby exposed to states of high arousal which cannot be handled because of an associated inability to modulate such experiences, both psychologically and physiologically. Indeed, victims of chronic trauma often cannot use symbols to cope with their feelings, a condition referred to as 'alexathymia'. In addition, if subject to early emotional deprivation, they develop less opiate receptors and therefore need higher levels of opiates than they can produce to feel soothed. This may well result in all kinds of addictive behaviour including compulsive re-exposure to trauma, which in itself releases endogenous opiates. This is the reason why many so-called 'borderline patients' with a background of sexual abuse take to cutting themselves: it gives them relief when exposed to inner states of inexpressible pain or emptiness.

It is becoming clearer that psychological trauma is a psychobiological reaction involving various aspects of the brain, for example the amygdala, hippocampus and prefrontal cortex. The hippocampus of people who have been chronically traumatized is smaller than normal.[21]

In a recent study, Van der Kolk and his team[22] showed how, when exposed to a traumatogenic stimulus such as a tape recording of a traumatic experience, the brains of patients suffering from PTSD display considerable changes under positron emission tomography. The speech area in the left dominant hemisphere closes down and the right hemisphere becomes more active, particularly in the limbic and paralimbic areas as well as in the visual cortex. These findings correspond with clinical observations: patients with PTSD often report a failure to speak when they relive traumatic experiences and many 'see things' relating to these experiences, i.e. flashbacks. The research on PTSD is only at its infancy but is extremely important in the study of traumatogenic violence. It is beginning to confirm already existing evidence that psychological trauma does alter the neurophysiology of the brain and even its anatomical appearance. In a sense, one could say that psychological trauma is a disease with both psychological and physiological manifestations, one of which is violence.

Case

A 27-year-old woman presented to her psychiatrist suffering from severe anxiety, breathing difficulties, tingling and even paralysis of the hands and insomnia. She said she lived in permanent fear and was unable to cope with work and to relate to people from whom she felt alienated, or even at times 'in another world'. She was worried she was going mad and, at times, her anguish was so unbearable she wanted to cut herself. On being interviewed, she quickly declared that she was quite sure her problems had nothing to do with her past. However, on being questioned, she revealed a childhood of extraordinary emotional neglect. Neither parent had had any time for her nor had they shown any affection. Our patient and her brother were never given proper meals or help with their school work, and were even not allowed to play, as this meant making a mess. If they did, their mother would suddenly lose all control and start screaming abuse at them and destroy their furniture and toys. The children were terrified of their mother's outbursts. But, thanks to a good aunt and grandmother, she found the strength to cope by switching off all these disturbing memories and getting on with her life.

It was only when she became involved with a boy friend who started to be emotionally abusive towards her, reminding her unconsciously of her mother, that she had her first breakdown at the age of 23. She was on a train going home when she suddenly collapsed in a state of terror and paralysis. She found herself too terrified to go out and, when she finally did get herself to her general practitioner, he gave her beta-blockers for her panic attacks. She did not take them but, gradually over a year or so, she got herself back to work by using Valium to which she became addicted.

In this case, the patient's childhood trauma remained a well-guarded secret. As a little girl, she had difficulties at school and, from the age of 5 onwards she would often run away from home to be brought back by the police. Her mother had a severe breakdown when the patient was little and was treated at home by a doctor. No one ever wondered what effect the mother's strange, violent behaviour might have had on her two children, one of whom later committed suicide.

What this case illustrates very clearly is how abused children will often protect their parents—denying both to themselves and to others the harm that has been done to them by those who are meant to love, care and protect them. This is the result of the child's desperate attempt to preserve their vital attachment to their caregiver. Knowing that their survival depends on remaining close to their parent, the abused child will dissociate him or herself from memories or experiences that threaten this fundamental precarious attachment. When severe, this dissociation can result in the development of a fragmented sense of self, now referred to as a dissociative identity disorder.[23]

Similar dynamics are at work with women who are physically abused by their partners. They can feel so terrified of their partner, frequently as a result of the PTSD they often suffer from, that they dissociate themselves from the memories of their partner's attacks. Their symptoms of PTSD will also make them feel utterly helpless and unable to think of a way out when under attack. The resulting mixture of terror and dissociation may make a battered woman quite unable to gage the extent of the danger she and her children are in. Often this is compounded by the belief that if she were to leave her abuser, he may well become more dangerous. Unfortunately, this is often the case as her male partner feels he is losing contol over the woman he considers as his.

Conclusion

The current levels of violence both outside and inside the home are now so high that many would describe it as an epidemic. Unfortunately, the measures that are being taken to address this problem have often little do with any scientific understanding of its cause and more to do with the political aspirations of those in power. However, if it can be established that violence is the psychobiological manifestation of a damaged attachment system with all that this implies, we are well on the way to arguing for the need for a medical campaign against violence. The facts speak for themselves: research in the field of attachment behaviour and psychological trauma is beginning to show important links with violence. Looking back at the attachment studies mentioned above, most humans are born with the capacity and the need to form loving attachments. In our society about two-thirds of 1 year olds are securely attached to their parents and are able to form loving relations with others. They will not be bullies or bullied. Another one-fifth or so of infants have experienced rejection and have the potential to bully and to hurt if and when they are given 'permission' or encouragement to do so. Finally, another one-tenth or so of individuals are already so damaged by abuse or terror that are destined for our mental hospitals or prisons. The misery they can cause is testimony of what they went through in their desperate struggle to love and be loved.

But what can a general practitioner do even if he or she is equipped with an understanding of the domestic origins of human violence? Some might say 'very little'. Though such a response is understandable, I think it denies the enormous importance of doctors in primary care. By being aware of what secret terrors can exist in their patients' homes, doctors can begin to make sense of their patients' coded messages, of what is not being said. They can make themselves available to those who dare to speak for the first time about their living nightmares. This very act of both listening to, and validating, the experiences of those whose suffering has meant a loss of all their self-esteem is perhaps the first and most important therapeutic measure in the treatment of family violence. It gives these patients a chance to feel that their lives are not normal, that their pain and terror need not be endured and that perhaps they can seek protection and help for themselves and those close to them. Their doctor in primary care can provide them with their first glimpse of hope and with the first assessment of the real danger faced by the various members of their family.

General practitioners need to be informed about the legal and support sources available for victims of family violence. They can undertake safety planning with the these victimized women and children and identify sources of support they can draw on. The task is daunting but necessary as family violence creates pathology and is life-threatening. Preventative or early work may be very effective as a group of general practitioners have shown in Dorset. They launched a successful 'Child and adolescent mental health service' from within their practice using a child and family counsellor.[43]

Once we have acknowledged and overcome the helplessness victims of family violence project onto their doctors, it can be most rewarding to break the terrifying cycle of family violence by enabling the victims, and sometimes the perpetrators, to find a more secure and fulfilling life, free from terror and pain.

References

1 **Gelles RJ.** Violence towards children in the United States. *American Journal of Orthopsychiatry* 1978; **48**: 580–92.

2 **Zulueta F de.** *From Pain to Violence. The Traumatic Roots of Destructiveness.* London: Whurr, 1993.

3 **Bowlby J.** *Attachment and Loss,* Vol. 1. *Attachment,* 2nd edn. London: Hogarth, 1969.

4 **Bowlby J.** *Attachment and Loss,* Vol. 2. *Separation, Anxiety and Anger.* London: Hogarth, 1973.

5 **Bowlby J.** *Attachment and Loss,* Vol. 3. *Loss, Sadness and Depression.* London: Hogarth, 1980.

6 **Hofer MA.** Relationships as regulators: a psychobiologic perspective on bereavement. *Psychosomatic Medicine* 1984; **46**: 183–97.

7 **Rosenblum L, Sunderland G.** Feeding ecology and mother infant relations. In: Hoffman LW, Gandelmann R, Schiffman HR, eds. *Biological Basis of Parental Behaviour.* London: Wiley, 1982.

8 **Perry BD.** Neurobiological sequelae of childhood trauma: post-traumatic stress disorders in children. In: Murberg M, ed. *Catecholamines in Post-traumatic Stress Disorder: Emerging Concepts.* Washington DC: American Psychiatric Press, 1994: 253–76.

9 **Teicher MH, Glod, CA, Surrey J, Swett C Jr.** Early childhood abuse and limbic system ratings in adult psychiatric outpatients. *Journal of Neuropsychiatry and Clinical Neurosciences* 1993; **5** (3): 301–6.

10 **Harlow HF, Mears C.** *Primate Perspectives.* London: John Wiley and Sons, 1979.

11 **Ainsworth MDS, Blehar MC, Waters E, Wall S.** *Patterns of Attachment: a Psychological Study of the Strange Situation.* Hillsdale, NJ: Erlbaum, 1978.

12 **Troy M, Sroufe LA.** Victimisation among pre-schoolers: role of attachment relation history. *Journal of American Academy of Child and Adolescent Psychiatry* 1987; **26**: 166–72.

13 **Main M, Hesse E.** Disorganised/disorientated infant behaviour in the Strange Situation, lapses in monitoring of reasoning and discourse during the parent's Adult Attachment Interview, and dissociative states. In: Ammanati M, Stern D, eds. *Attachment and Psychoanalysis.* Rome: Gius, Laterza & Figli, 1992.

14 **Patrick M, Hobson RP, Castle D, Howard R, Maughan B.** Personality disorder and the mental representation of early social experiece. *Developmental Psychopathology* 1994; **6**: 375–88.

15 **Fonagy P, Steele M, Steele H** *et al.* Attachment, the reflective self, and borderline states: the predictive specificity of the adult attachment interview and pathological emotional development. In: Goldberg S, Muir R, Kerr J, eds. *Attachment Theory: Social, Developmental, and Clinical Perspectives.* Hillsdale, NJ: The Analytic Press, 1995: 233–78.

16 **Steele M, Steele H, Fonagy P.** Associations amongst attachment classifications of mothers, fathers and their infants. *Child Development* 1996; **67**: 541–55.

17 **Frodi A.** Variations in parental and nonparental response to early infant communication. In: Reite M, Field T, eds. *The psychobiology of attachment and seperation.* London: Academic Press, 1985: 351–67.

18 **Main M, Kaplan N, Cassidy J.** Security in infancy, childhood, and adulthood: a move to the level of representation. In: Bretherton I, Waters E, eds. Growing Points of Attachment Theory and Research, *Monographs of the Society for Research in Child Development* 1985; **50**: 66–104.

19 **Lindemann E.** Symptomatology and management of acute grief. *American Journal of Psychiatry* 1944; **101**: 141–9.

20 **Van der Kolk BA.** The compulsion to repeat the trauma: re-enactment, re-victimisation and masochism. *Psychiatric Clinics of North America* 1989; **12**: 389–411.

21 **Bremner JD, Randall P, Scott TM** *et al.* MRI-based measurement of hippocampal volume in patients with combat-related posttraumatic stress disorder. *American Journal of Psychiatry* 1995; **152**(7): 973–81.

22 **Van der Kolk BA, McFarlane, Weisaeth L.** *Traumatic Stress, the Effects of Overwhelming Experience on Mind, Body, and Society.* New York: Guildford Press, 1996.

23 **Putnam FW.** Disturbances of 'self' in victims of childhood sexual abuse. In: Kluft RP, ed. *Incest-Related Syndromes of Adult Psychopathology.* Washington DC: American Psychiatric Press, 1990.

24 **Hayden A.** A GP based child and adolescent mental health service. *Young Minds Magazine* 1997; **30**: 12–13.

Chapter 3

Family violence: the general practice context

Iona Heath and Stephen Amiel

Introduction

The nature of general practice

The discipline of general practice is founded in the long-term relationship between doctor and patient,[1] which nurtures mutual respect and trust. Within this relationship, each has their own field of expertise. The patient has intimate knowledge of their own life situation and of the experience of illness or disease that brings them to the doctor; the doctor has expert knowledge of the science of disease.

> ... however pressed he may be for time, each patient should be made to feel that his illness is of real concern to the doctor. The general practitioner needs a deeply imaginative sympathy which enables him to understand his patient's fears, anxieties, pain and discomfort. ... He must be able to put himself in the patient's place.[2]

Illness is the patient's perception of something being wrong, a sense of unease in the functioning of the body or mind; disease is a theoretical construct which offers the benefits and risks of scientific medicine. Illness is what the patient has on their way to see the doctor and a disease is what they have on the way home. The former is subjective, the latter objective. Most disease involves illness, but by no means all illness involves disease. Both the disease and the illness can be more or less serious. The task of the general practitioner is to make these distinctions and to diagnose disease, to refer treatable disease requiring complex treatment to specialist colleagues, to treat less complex disease and to acknowledge and witness the suffering brought by illness. The interface between illness and disease is the point at which the vast undifferentiated mass of human distress and suffering meets the theoretical structures of scientific medicine, and the social sciences, which have been developed to enable humanity, to a still very limited extent, to understand and control the experience of illness.[3]

The overenthusiastic interpretation of illness as disease, borne of inexperience or fear of litigation, leaves patients open to the dangers but not the benefits of scientific medicine. Arthur Kleinman[4] writes: 'The physician's training also encourages the dangerous fallacy of over-literal interpretation of accounts best understood metaphorically.'

The demise of religious and philosophical explanations for the arbitrariness of human suffering has left the modern world with limited means of understanding and coping. Illness is one of the few valid outlets for human distress. But if that illness is wrongly interpreted as disease all kinds of damage can be done. Thus the general practitioner has two key roles. The first is to serve as interpreter and guardian at the interface between illness and disease.[5] The general practitioner as interpreter engages the patient in the necessary dialogue. The general practitioner as guardian safeguards the patient from the too ready interpretation of illness as disease. This guardian role is a parallel and prerequisite to the more widely acknowledged role as gatekeeper between primary and secondary care. The second key role is to serve as a witness to the patient's experience of illness and disease.[6]

The Swedish general practitioner Carl Edvard Rudebeck defines the core skill of general practice as bodily empathy.[7] This is the ability to identify imaginatively with the patient's subjective experience of illness to provide genuine recognition and validation of that experience. Only if the patient can believe that their experience is understood at a fundamental level by the doctor will that patient be able to trust in the doctor's interpretation of their illness. He distinguishes the subjective experience of 'body as self' from the objective experience of 'body as nature'. As doctors, we combine the subjective experience of our own bodies and minds, with the objective theoretical understanding of the science of their working. By straddling this divide within his or her own body, the generalist doctor is qualified to interpret the interface between illness and disease. The depth of understanding involved in this interpretation begins the process of witnessing, in which the doctor works with the patient to make sense of the patient's experience of both illness and disease in the context of the rest of their lives.[8]

The processes of imaginative and empathic understanding require the doctor to attempt to identify with the experience and attitudes of the patient: 'To be truly excellent clinicians we must love our patients'.[9]

However, if the doctor believes the patient to be the perpetrator of violence against a more vulnerable member of his or her own family, such identification can be very difficult and much of the basis and the power of the doctor–patient relationship will be seriously undermined.

The nature of the family

Human beings find sense and meaning in their experiences of life through the process of sharing these experiences with others. The foundation of this sharing is the family unit within which children are nurtured and protected by their parents. Family ties are often, and are meant to be, among the strongest that bind human beings together. Families share values, experience and history, and they are the setting for mutual love and reciprocal obligations to care for those who are least capable, either through youth or age or sickness. Yet families are also the setting of misery and violence.

> ... with the exception of the police and the military, the family is perhaps the most violent social group and the home, the most violent setting in our society.[10]

Hallett[11] argues that it is necessary to identify the family 'as a conflict-prone social institution with axes of conflict across gender and generation, that is between men and women and adults and children'.

Family violence

The reality of family violence cuts across, and profoundly disrupts, our notions of what both the family and the discipline of general practice should be. Not only is the family distorted by the experience of violence, but, struggling to make an effective response, the general practitioner is no longer able to summon unconditional positive regard, which is the optimal basis for the imaginative sympathy required for the full execution of his or her role. As a result, numerous difficulties and dilemmas arise: practical, interpersonal and ethical.[12]

In the remainder of this chapter we will explore some of these difficulties and dilemmas. Indeed, they surface time after time throughout this book, as contributors confront the complexities for general practitioners and other primary health care team members of dealing with the various manifestations of family violence.

We shall, however, attempt to show that the GP is also in some ways ideally placed to make a positive, sometimes pivotal contribution in dealing with family violence: to its prevention, to its early detection and to the mitigation of its consequences. This too is a theme throughout the book. We shall argue that, when confronting or being confronted by family violence, general practice possesses inherent strengths as well as weaknesses; and that the nature and structure of general practice confers on the GP and practice team unique opportunities when combating family violence. At the same time, we must acknowledge the threats that family violence poses for general practice, as well as other threats to general practice that may undermine its ability to respond to family violence.

Those familiar with change management techniques will be used to looking at things in these terms: strengths, weaknesses, opportunities and threats—the so-called SWOT analysis. We shall look at general practice with regard to family violence using these categories, but nothing in general practice is quite that simple, of course. Attributes can be strengths and/or weaknesses, opportunities and/or threats, depending on context, situation or point of view. General practice is also changing rapidly: at the time of writing, it is unclear whether the 'new NHS' will pose more opportunity or threat to the GP's response to family violence. We shall end this chapter by looking at recent and upcoming changes, attempting some sort of balance sheet in this regard.

Strengths

The 1974 Leeuwenhorst conference on the teaching of general practice[13] produced a now well-worn definition of the general practitioner:

> ... a licensed medical graduate who gives *personal, primary and continuing care* to *individuals, families and a practice population* irrespective of age, sex and illness. ... His aim is to make *early diagnoses*. He will include and *integrate physical, psychological and social factors* in his considerations about health and illness. This will be expressed in the care of his patients. ... *Prolonged contact* means he can use repeated opportunities to gain information at a pace appropriate to each patient and build up a *relationship of trust which he can use professionally*. ... He will practice in *co-operation with other colleagues*, medical and non-medical. ... He will know when and how to intervene through *treatment, prevention and education to promote the health of his patients and their families*. He will recognise that he also has a *professional responsibility to the community* [our emphasis].[13]

Whatever its limitations as a definition,[14] most UK general practitioners would recognize this as a fair description of what they aspire to do. A GP working to this job description should be well placed to understand the antecedents and dynamics of family violence at an individual and family level; and to respond proactively, responsibly and sensitively to family violence, working in cooperation with family members, other professionals and outside agencies.

To an extent, the training and education of general practitioners, and the structure (both professional and organizational) within which they traditionally work, already reflect and support their ability to meet these job requirements.

Training and education

- Medical sociology, ethics and communication skills comprise increasingly important parts of most medical schools' undergraduate curricula.

- Teaching at undergraduate level is increasingly community based, with medical students being attached to general practice teams for part of their paediatrics, care of the elderly and psychiatry modules.

- Vocational training schemes for UK general practitioners incorporate 18 months to 2 years minimum of experience in relevant post-registration hospital jobs. Often these will include general and/or developmental paediatrics, care of the elderly, psychiatry and/or accident and emergency.

- Post-registration training of general practitioners in the UK also comprises a 12–18-month period as a GP registrar in a training practice. This provides an opportunity for the registrar to develop clinical competencies, consultation skills and management strategies; to acquire an understanding of the health service and how to help patients to access it and other resources; to develop professional relationships with individual patients and their families, with colleagues and with other team members;

and to examine and learn from these relationships by a mixture of case analysis, study of videotaped consultations, and individual and group-based tutorials.

- Summative assessment of GP registrars, and the membership examination for the Royal College of General Practitioners, seek to test competencies and attitudes in all these areas of general practice. Satisfactory completion of summative assessment is now a prerequisite for independent practice.

- General practice has established itself over the past half century as an academic discipline in its own right, with departments of primary health care in all medical schools, a prolific research base and its own peer-reviewed journals. The day-to-day work of general practitioners is increasingly influenced by a quantitative and qualitative evidence base that helps them to integrate, and to mediate between, the breadth of biomedical science and patients' subjective and socially constructed experience of illness.[15]

- The vast majority of GPs participate in postgraduate education programmes, with financial incentives to do so.

Structure and organization

- UK general practice is a universal provider of primary health care: every resident member of the population is entitled and encouraged to be registered with a local general practitioner. The vast majority of people are registered with a GP, and in most cases, remain registered with the same GP until they move house.

- General practice is still used by most people as the first point of contact with the health services when they regard themselves as ill. General practice handles the vast bulk of illness episodes that are reported to the health services, managing in their entirety most diseases that are presented, or employing its gatekeeper role in both senses: as guardian both of the interface between illness and disease (see above), and of the interface between primary and secondary care.

- Of the independent contractor services to the NHS, general practice (in contrast to optometry and dentistry) is the only one currently free to all UK residents at the point of delivery. As a rule, social deprivation is associated with higher morbidity (including some family violence) and higher consultation rates. Ability to pay does not determine access to the GP and at least one inverse care law (at its simplest: 'people who need most get least)[16] is thereby attenuated.

- General practice operates traditionally on a list-based system: an individual patient is registered with an individual GP who is responsible for that person's care. That care may be delegated to another practitioner (e.g. a partner or deputy) or another team member, but even in many group practices, personal lists are encouraged to enable a patient to build up a relationship with a particular doctor, and vice versa.

- Home visits in the UK are still carried out by most GPs when necessary: health visitors will visit all new mothers at home at least once, and often carry out developmental checks in the home as a routine. These visits can be hugely revealing of home circumstances and can provide information important in the assessment of disabled and elderly housebound patients, or acutely ill children, such as evidence of neglect, substance abuse, postnatal depression, the return of an abusive partner and so on.

- The general practitioner is generally the custodian of the patient's health record, which in theory follows the patient when they change GP; it is not uncommon for a GP to be in possession of a patient's continuous health record going back five or six decades. Most GP practices have computerized age/sex and morbidity registers: many are moving towards a paperless system, with networked desktop systems allowing team members access and input to the entire medical record. Software systems based on standardized coding of data (Read codes[17]) allow accessible, legible, detailed, transferable and auditable recording of information, whether clinical, social or demographic. Some systems incorporate a genogram or family number system, allowing cross-referencing by team members: this may be of particular relevance to the mapping and risk evaluation of family violence.

- Either as a contractual obligation or in return for financial incentives, the GP, in addition to general medical services, often provides a wide range of preventative services targeted at specific age groups or risk groups. Some of these, for example developmental checks and immunization programmes for children, or regular checks offered to patients over 75, may have particular bearing on the recognition of family violence.

- The majority of UK general practitioners work as members of group practices comprising two or more GPs and a practice team. At a minimum, this team will include reception/secretarial staff and a practice nurse. Often, however, GPs work as part of a larger primary health care team (PHCT), generally comprising a practice manager, district nurses, health visitors and practice counsellor, but sometimes including other health professionals and social workers. These may be based in the same premises as the GP and their clientele may be coterminous with the GP's patient list; or they may work from separate centres aligned to a cluster of local practices. Regular team meetings, where patients and practice policies are discussed, are a normal part of many GPs' working week.

- GPs are traditionally independent contractors to the NHS and many work from premises which they own. These may vary from a downstairs room in the GP's own house, to an adapted flat on an estate, to a converted shop front, to purpose-built premises with advanced diagnostic and treatment facilities. The investment in premises and the ties of partnership are factors encouraging continuity of the carer as well as care: a GP with these roots in a community may well be less likely to move on after a few years.

- Such a GP is more likely to understand the family and community of which their patient is a part; is better able to achieve that 'imaginative sympathy' enabling them to understand their patient's experience; and is better able to achieve the long-term relationship based on mutual respect and trust that we have identified as a cornerstone of general practice.

- The proximity and domestic nature of many small GP premises is highly valued by many patients, particularly the elderly. Using a practice located within a community is convenient, and can also be reassuring and non-stigmatizing compared with a hospital or clinic setting where the purpose of a visit may be obvious to all.

- Domesticity, familiarity and continuity of practice personnel all help to foster confidence and trust, increasing the likelihood that patients will confide in the GP or other team member when in a crisis. Despite various high profile cases, not least the Shipman murders, GPs retain their position in the public mind as the most trusted of professionals, with 90 per cent ratings.[18]

- Underpinning that confidence and trust to an even greater extent is an expectation of clinical competence and an assumption of confidentiality. Patients widely and (largely) correctly assume a right to confidentiality when they visit their GP. The duty of any doctor 'to respect and protect' confidential information[19] extends to every member of the practice team: all clinical workers are governed by their professional bodies in this respect, and it is written in to employed staff's contracts. Many practices make this duty of confidentiality clear in their practice leaflets and posters, both in general terms and to cover specific groups, such as under 16s seeking contraception.

Weaknesses

Training and education

- The biomedical model of illness and disease dominates medical education, notwithstanding the broadening perspective that has been introduced over recent years. Medical students are still largely selected on their scientific and mathematical aptitude, and tend still to be recruited from relatively narrow class and cultural backgrounds.[20]

- Prevention (and palliation) figures far less in undergraduate medical education than the diagnosis and management of acute and—to a lesser extent—chronic disease.

- Many GPs report little or no undergraduate training in the recognition and management of child abuse (see Chapter 9d), let alone in the more recently acknowledged domestic violence and elder abuse.

- Undergraduate education for health professionals is still largely segregated: the understanding that many doctors at the beginning of their career have of what nurses or health visitors do is extremely limited. There is rarely if ever any joint training with social work students.

- Postgraduate education for GPs is a voluntary, haphazard affair: the huge range of competing educational priorities means that training on aspects of family violence, which after all represents only a small fraction of what GPs have to deal with in their daily work, is seen as a low priority. Many educational events are commercially sponsored by pharmaceutical companies who are naturally interested in hosting events that draw attention to their therapeutic field. Family violence figures low on their list too.

- The content of obligatory courses, such as those needed for accreditation in child health surveillance, is also variable—often the abuse dimension is omitted entirely.

- Postgraduate multidisciplinary training is on offer, usually promoted by social services, Area Child Protection Committees or organizations like CAIPE (Centre for the Advancement of Interprofessional Education). Attendance by GPs at these events is typically low, perhaps reflecting (and certainly not helping) the distrust that doctors and social workers traditionally have for each other. The take-up by GPs of multidisciplinary training with other health professionals is also poor: here, issues of assumed status and concerns about losing face might sometimes be relevant.

Structure and organization

- Whilst general practice is a universally available service, significant numbers of people are not registered with a GP where they currently reside. People who have recently moved address and who have not been ill enough to need to register may comprise the bulk of this group. More concerning, though, is the likelihood that amongst those not registered are a significant number of people whose health needs, sometimes including their risk of being involved in family violence, are greater than average: the street homeless, including children and young runaways; women and children escaping violent domestic situations, perhaps in hostel or hotel accommodation; mentally ill and substance-abusing adults; people with learning difficulties; sex workers; asylum seekers and refugees avoiding the authorities; recently arrived immigrants who are in the country legally but who cannot access health services because of language difficulties or lack of information; and a few perpetrators of abuse who wish to avoid detection.

- People in the above categories are more likely to access health services late and in a way more inappropriate to their needs (another example of an inverse care law), for example by using hospital casualty departments as their primary health care resource of choice or necessity. Even for those who are registered with a GP, many practices are not set up to provide equitable access, i.e. access proportionate to need. Appointment systems may be more difficult for them to understand or access, so that problems are dealt with more peremptorily in an emergency slot, and proactive care is not addressed at all. Language barriers may be insuperable in the absence of official interpreters or a health professional who speaks the same language: a woman may find it impossible to disclose violence in the home if her husband or child is the only interpreter at hand. The absence of a woman doctor may make it impossible for some women to disclose intimate details or subject themselves to examination. Opportunities to address family violence issues are missed, not least because continuity of health care record, carer and thus care is next to impossible in these situations.

- In some areas, people may find it difficult or impossible to register with a GP, certainly with the GP of their choice. Although there is an obligation (currently of the health authority) to find a GP for someone, if necessary by compulsory allocation, patients, particularly if they are difficult or challenging, may find themselves being passed from one GP to another. GPs can choose whom they register (unless they are allocated) and a few unfortunately choose not to register 'difficult' patients. They are also not obliged to keep patients they do not want.

- GP premises, particularly in inner cities, have suffered decades of neglect and under-investment. Their location in converted houses often makes them impossible to adapt for disabled access, or to enlarge them to accommodate an extended team. Practices housed in local authority or trust premises may fare little better.

- Recruitment into general practice and retention of GPs has fluctuated for decades, but the profession's claims of a rapidly worsening situation is now accepted even by government (see below). The failure to recruit and retain adequate numbers is widely seen as a reflection of persistently low morale. GPs in some areas of the country, chiefly deprived inner city and isolated rural areas, have great difficulty in recruiting new partners, and the majority of GPs express a desire to retire early if they can afford to. Many GPs who came to the UK from the Indian subcontinent, often to work in the most deprived areas, are now reaching compulsory retirement age. Two-thirds of the GPs who qualified in South Asian medical schools will have retired by 2007.

- This shortage of GPs is one of a number of factors exacerbating what is possibly the prime weakness of general practice in the UK—lack of time for patients. Time is an essential diagnostic and therapeutic tool for the GP, particularly important when dealing with patients experiencing family violence, and when liaising with colleagues and other agencies in its aftermath. Yet with average list sizes of 1853 in 2000, an average consultation time of about 8 minutes, and ever-increasing externally driven demands to do more (see below), most GPs and many patients are aware that they are only able to offer a suboptimal and sometimes minimal service—a demand-led, reactive, fire-fighting approach to the job which in turn acts as a major drain on morale and retention.

- The long-term relationship that the GP builds with a patient and their family may have certain disadvantages in relation to family violence as well as advantages. The problems of conflicting loyalty towards different family members are discussed below, but there are issues also around being almost too close to a family to see what is really going on. This is particularly likely with neglect, where health professionals' expectations and standards drift downwards with the family's—familiarity breeding complacency. There is also a danger of an unintentionally collusive relationship developing with a family member or members, particularly in close communities where the GP may be part of the same social network as the family.

- GPs do not generally have a culture of sharing their uncertainties and problems, professional or personal, with others. There is currently no system of routine professional supervision as there is for social workers and health visitors, whereby practitioners can discuss difficult cases on a regular basis with a senior colleague. Nor is there at the time of writing more than a vestigial voluntary occupational health service that GPs in difficulties can access. A significant number of GPs, particularly those in single-handed practices, work in relative professional isolation, with potentially serious implications for their practice and well-being.

Opportunities

In this section we will briefly address how general practice might make a difference with regard to family violence: how, using its strengths and minimizing its weaknesses, family violence might be prevented, detected at an early stage, or at least have its consequences mitigated. Specific strategies for each area of abuse are explored elsewhere in this book, but some generally applicable principles with examples are listed here.

Prevention and early detection

Primary prevention

By addressing the prevention of known risk factors, and by facilitating access both to the practice itself and to other resources, the GP and rest of the PHCT can play a part in the primary prevention of family violence.

- Providing contraceptive advice and services as part of a strategy to prevent unwanted pregnancies in very young women is a case in point. The entire team has a role in this: waiting room information and posters explaining methods, access and confidentiality issues; after-school appointment times or walk-in clinics; welcoming reception staff; available practice nurses and doctors of either gender; free condoms; easy access without appointment to emergency contraception (which is too expensive for many girls to buy over the counter); on-site pregnancy testing; and impartial counselling about termination and adoption options. Raising contraception opportunistically and matter of factly in the consultation can also pay dividends.

- Parenting advice, and young pregnant women's and mothers' support groups can be advertised or provided antenatally to help prevent isolation and inappropriate care of children.

- Providing multilingual information about accessing practice services, language classes, the provision of interpreters and health advocates; improving disabled access; screening of older patients for depression and cognitive impairment; and home assessment visits by team members.

- Helping patients and families to access housing, benefits and debt counselling advice.

- Using health education materials, patient health checks, and the consultation opportunistically to raise awareness about the effects of illicit drug and inappropriate alcohol intake.

Identification of vulnerable patients and families

Violence in families rarely comes out of the blue. There are almost always pointers to risk which knowledge of the family as a whole will help identify. Often these will be one or (more often) a number of health-related, relationship or social stressors, but there may also be a history of violence involving one or more members of the family. Although not inevitable, there may be a *cycle* of abuse within families, whereby someone may, from being an abused child, become an abusing sibling or an abusing adult towards a partner, their own children, or a dependent elder who may have abused them in the first place.[21] There may certainly be an *overlap* of violence: violence towards an adult partner is frequently associated with child abuse. In one study, 700 out of 1000 abused women reported that their abuser also abused their children.[22] And finally, there can be a *career* of violence within a family: an abusing father is likely to abuse all his children and to become an abusing grandfather; a violent spouse may become a violent carer in old age. Ongoing relationships with different family members, reviewing the historical medical record, sharing, tagging and cross-referencing the medical record, sharing concerns with other members of the PHCT at team meetings, and home visits can all be employed to advantage here.

Therapeutic interventions

The GP can intervene therapeutically to address physical or emotional health problems that might increase the risk of family violence. They can offer this themselves, or by referral to other team members, or to outside sources of treatment, respite, information and self-help. Examples include treatment and support for: adults who were themselves abused in childhood; siblings of abused children; children with feeding problems or sleep disturbance; parents with disabilities; substance-abusing adults and young people;

and adults with ongoing mental health problems, postnatal depression, early dementia or incontinence.

Early detection of abuse

Repeated abusive incidents are often recognized only in retrospect, after a disclosure or an unequivocal incident raises the alarm. The GP who has an ongoing relationship with family members, a comprehensive, accessible, written historical record, and a team of colleagues with knowledge of the family from different perspectives, is far more likely to make a diagnosis of abuse at an earlier stage.

- Repeated consultations over a period of time can reveal telling changes in a patient's appearance, demeanour, physical and emotional state, or growth. When family connections are known to the practitioner, or flagged in the records, these changes can sometimes be correlated with events or changes occurring elsewhere in the family.

- Good records provide the opportunity to revisit and if necessary re-interpret: minor injuries (the classic 'walking into doors' syndrome, recurrent burns, scalds), neglected injuries, alcohol-related injuries; seemingly trivial symptoms (vaginal discharge, dysuria, recurrent impetiginized lesions); and aggressive, apparently inappropriate or delayed presentations.

- Less tangible, but just as important, are the preparedness of a practitioner to think of abuse or neglect as a possible differential diagnosis; and the collective wisdom, experience and trust that allows a team to have and articulate a 'gut feeling'. If such a feeling, supported by some evidence and preferably backed by knowledge and training, is shared within a team and then appropriately conveyed to others out-side, it can more quickly be either substantiated or scotched. Why has a woman persistently failed to attend antenatal classes; why has a child missed his appoint-ments for immunizations or orthoptic checks; why is a 13 year old who should be at school bringing her younger siblings to frequent emergency appointments; why is an elderly woman with dementia so distressed when she is discharged back to her daughter's care?

'Appropriately conveyed to others outside' begs all sorts of questions: what constitutes a reasonable threshold for disclosure; what is a reasonable and safe timescale; how much information or concern is shared and about whom in the family; and who should those 'others' be—expert colleagues, others who know the family (relatives, neighbours, teachers, carers, home helps) or other agencies? The answers to these questions do, of course, depend on individuals, situations and contexts; even then, there are relatively few, unequivocally right answers. Some attempt is made later in this chapter to address general principles and workable guidelines for particular scenarios are suggested in later chapters.

Damage limitation

If family violence and its aftermath create difficulties, dilemmas and conflicts for the general practitioner and the rest of the practice team, these are, of course, minor as compared with the impact on the abused person/s and their family. Here too though, there are opportunities to make a difference.

Early referral

Once a critical threshold of professional concern has been reached, and an onward referral made, measures to assess need and ensure protection from abuse or further abuse should follow. The practice team's knowledge of the family and its situation can influence the urgency with which a referral is investigated as well as the proportionality and appropriateness of statutory agencies' immediate response.

Involvement in the assessment/investigation

Factual information as well as opinion can be communicated in reports or in person at strategy meetings and case conferences, and is generally valued highly by statutory agencies. A GP's or health visitor's perspective and background knowledge of the strengths and weaknesses of family members, the possible contribution of the extended family to care alternatives and so on, can shape decisions made on child protection registration, removal of children from families, or the sensitivity and extent of police involvement. The appropriateness and extent of services or other interventions offered can also be influenced.

Advocacy role

A decision on offering services or therapeutic interventions may sometimes have to be fought for—getting them delivered will very often have to be fought for. Here, too, the practice team has a role in monitoring, chasing and cajoling if necessary. The GP may also need to promote the needs of a family member whose situation has been ignored or worsened by decisions taken in the interests of another family member. Housing needs, financial problems, educational problems, etc. may be identified by the assessment process, but may also be exacerbated in the aftermath of abuse. Finally, the GP's or team's perspective may lead them to disagree with decisions taken by statutory agencies or hospitals, and to take the side of their patient/s in countering them.

Therapeutic help and support

Continuity of care may be disrupted by family members moving away or choosing to leave the list in the aftermath of abuse. The practice must also frequently have to overcome the damage done to relationships with family members (see below). None the less, there is much that team members may be able to retrieve and to offer both the abused person and the rest of the family.

- Updating records and prompt forwarding of records belonging to practice leavers may itself be important for the future care and protection of those patients.

- Continuing care from trusted and familiar professionals may be critical for people whose lives have been turned upside down by abuse. Needs may be *medical*: care following injury, sexual abuse or neglect; contraception, termination of unwanted pregnancy or treatment of sexually transmitted infections; or treatment of depression, anxiety, traumatic stress or substance misuse. *Emotional* support will certainly be wanted as patients may need to talk about what they have experienced, or may be trying to come to terms with the disruption and loss of important relationships with partners, children or elderly relatives, up to and including bereavement. Some GPs have the expertise to work themselves with abused patients in the immediate aftermath; many more offer treatment and support to adult survivors of child abuse. Sometimes the health visitor, practice counsellor or practice nurse may be a key worker in these situations. Sometimes too, members of the team will find themselves treating or offering support to those in the family responsible for the abuse.

- Onward referral to other agencies and services: specialist medical care; counselling, psychiatric care or substance misuse services; self-help or survivors' groups; carers' or parenting support groups; benefits advice; legal advice about divorce, care proceedings or power of attorney; housing departments; women's refuges; and residential accommodation.

Threats

As we have suggested in our introduction to this chapter, family violence represents a deeply disturbing challenge to our preconceived ideas of what the family and general practice should be. Its ramifications threaten the relationships or GPs with their patients, stretching and sometimes breaking the bond of trust on which these relationships depend.

The GP's position as the family's doctor may force him or her to take action on behalf of a vulnerable patient who is believed to be being abused by other patients of the practice. Almost inevitably, the doctor is brought into conflict with other family members, as the latter may be exposed to accusation, disgrace, loss of their home, their partner and children, their livelihood, or even their liberty. GPs thereby expose themselves to anger and possibly aggression from family members, including sometimes the abused person who, it is hoped, is being helped. Doctors must make judgements about the capacity of the very young, the old or those vulnerable by virtue of disability to make decisions about their own lives, and sometimes, based on those judgements, these decisions must be taken and implemented without their consent.

Conflict is not confined to the GP's relationship with the family. It is internal, as the doctor wrestles with his or her ethical dilemmas about confidentiality and capacity and to try to retain that unconditional positive regard for patients in the face perhaps of some fairly unpalatable truths about them. There is inward conflict in the attempt to reconcile what must be done to protect a child or vulnerable older person with the knowledge that the process they are being exposed to is fallible, often insensitive, certainly under-resourced, and occasionally abusive itself. GPs may also feel compromised by competing demands on their time as well as their loyalty: involvement in a difficult family violence situation can eat up disproportionate amounts of that most precious commodity. Finally, there is the nagging worry, more so than with most clinical situations, of the public opprobrium that might follow if a doctor gets an abuse case wrong.

Family violence cases can generate conflict too within the practice team and with outside agencies. Different perspectives of, and loyalties to, different family members may strain relationships within the team. Other agencies are frequently felt not to deliver on response times, not to understand the family situation adequately, to communicate decisions poorly, and to deliver too little, too late by way of services (feelings sometimes reciprocated towards general practice). Often though, the underlying conflict with outside agencies, particularly social services, has to do with a failure to understand each other's ways of working and ethical constraints. The most contentious areas in this regard are confidentiality and its limits, and decisions about capacity and consent. In the remainder of this section, we shall examine these areas in more detail.

Confidentiality

General practitioners are increasingly concerned about issues of confidentiality within the generality of their work and these issues are compounded when dealing with problems of family violence. In the context of the exponential growth in the electronic transfer of information, the implementation of the Data Protection Act and the new human rights legislation, which guarantees a right of privacy, the longstanding principle of medical confidentiality has appeared ever more vulnerable. From a position of having been the guardians and standard-setters of confidentiality, medicine has now fallen far behind the highest standards, and routine practice now fails to fulfil the basic principles of the data protection legislation:

- that personal data should only be disclosed with the fully informed, voluntary consent of the subject;

- that personal data held should be adequate, relevant, but not excessive, for the purpose;

- that information should only be used for the purpose for which it was disclosed.

All health care professionals and those responsible for the running of the health service have, over recent years, made ever greater assumptions about the legitimacy of what is termed 'implied consent'. This situation is compounded increasingly by the speed and ease of the electronic transfer of data. There has been no public debate and the public, as both citizens and patients, are mostly ignorant of the degree to which information is passed around on the basis of this dubious concept. Implied consent is invoked to allow the use of patient-identifiable information:

- in teaching, at both undergraduate and postgraduate levels;
- in examinations and assessments;
- for health service accounting;
- for audit, both clinical and financial;
- in disease registers;
- in research;
- and, most relevantly for our purposes, to facilitate joint working and shared care by different members of the primary care team or similar multidisciplinary teams in other health care settings.

All theses purposes have undoubted benefits both for individual patients and for the wider public health, but worthy ends do not legitimize the erosion of the fundamental principle of patient confidentiality and the trust that rests on it.

More recently, the government has proposed that patients' records should be transferred electronically to facilitate care in different settings across, and even beyond, the health service. For example, in May 2000, the then Health Minister Gisela Stuart was quoted as saying that 'eventually online patient records will be accessible by family doctors, hospitals, NHS Direct, out-of-hours and ambulance services, mental health trusts and social services'. The government seemed not to have even begun to consider the implications of these, and other proposals, for patient confidentiality.

In response, the Royal College of General Practitioners, among many other organizations, pointed out the urgent need to put the use of implied consent on a firmer ethical and legal footing. In September 2000, the General Medical Council issued new guidance on confidentiality and protecting and providing information to all registered doctors.[23] This clarifies the responsibilities of doctors to:

- seek patients' consent to disclosure of information wherever possible, whether or not they judge that patients can be identified from the disclosure;
- anonymize data where unidentifiable data will serve the purpose;
- keep disclosures to the minimum necessary.

This new guidance was welcome but remains insufficient. By emphasizing the responsibility of the individual doctor, the guidance leaves doctors vulnerable to censure in a situation where the main reasons for the frequent failure of doctors to fulfil their responsibilities arise from the managerial and financial systems of the NHS, or the increasingly frequent encouragement, even exhortation, to joint working with other agencies.

In the face of mounting public concern, instead of taking steps to reassert the importance of the duty of respecting and protecting confidential information, the government took powers to bring the current unsatisfactory situation within the law. Clause 60 of the Health and Social Care Act 2001 gives the Secretary of State for Health powers to make regulations requiring the disclosure of patient-identifiable information without the patient's consent. This seems to have been done primarily to protect the uninterrupted flow of information to cancer registries, and to ensure the continuing completeness of a very important research database. However, the seeking and granting of explicit consent seem much more likely to ensure continuing public support of the work of cancer registries in the longer term. Of even greater concern is the extent of the power to make regulations that allows the Secretary of State to authorize any transfer of confidential patient-identifiable information provided that it is for a medical purpose and is in the interest of patient care or in the public interest. In the context of problems of family violence, this legislation can be seen to be helpful to the extent that it may be used to put joint working and sharing of records on a more secure legal footing; but counterproductive in that it may further erode patient's trust in the system and the health professionals who work within it.

Many general practitioners are already aware of parents who are reluctant to discuss and disclose mental health problems because of fears that their ability to care for their children will be called into question and that they will run the risk of having their children taken away. Research by Carman and Britten[24] demonstrates that patients are very aware that their general practice records are likely to contain more personal and sensitive information than their hospital records and that, as a result, they regard the confidentiality of the GP record as being the more important. The same study showed that patients are also much more wary about computer-held records as opposed to manual records, with a clear understanding of how much more easily computer-held records can pass to a wider audience. On the basis of this evidence, it seems highly probable that if patients were able to believe that their account of their problems would be treated as truly confidential, they would be more likely to present at an early stage.

There is a widespread misunderstanding that a doctor or nurse can freely share any information with any other doctor or nurse on the grounds that they are also accountable to a professional body and will not divulge the information inappropriately. However, in law, the fact that a third party is also bound by a professional duty of confidentiality is only relevant in that the patient is likely to be reassured and therefore more likely to give consent for the transfer of information.[25]

Working Together to Safeguard Children[26] includes the following apparently unequivocal statements:

- Good record keeping ... is essential to working across agency and professional boundaries (para. 7.47).

- Safeguarding children requires information to be brought together from a number of different sources and careful professional judgements to be made on the basis of this information (para. 7.49).

However, it is important for primary health care professionals to understand that this does not legitimize the free sharing of medical records. It is a mistake to confuse 'sharing information' with sharing a full patient record. The data protection legislation requires that the release of information should not be excessive. Providing access to an entire record will inevitably allow information to be shared that is not relevant to the immediate concerns of the professionals involved.

The law underpinning partnership throws further interesting light on this undoubtedly fraught situation. A general practice partnership is regarded as a single legal entity: this may serve to legitimize the sharing of information between partners,[24] and even extend to cover the sharing of information with employees of the partnership. However, any employee of another agency is viewed as part of another legal entity and the release of information to such a person invokes the full authority of the Data Protection Act. It is interesting that this corresponds to the extent of control exerted by the GP to whom the information is first entrusted. Once other agencies are allowed access to the patient's record, actions may ensue which the GP has no power to influence, and of which he or she may even have no knowledge. The GP can no longer provide any assurance to the patient that any undertakings given, or implied, will be honoured.

It may well be that the most useful and pragmatic approach to an extremely complex situation is, wherever possible, to seek explicit verbal consent to the verbal sharing of selected and relevant information with appropriate professional colleagues, supported where necessary by written confirmation of the same information.

Capacity and consent

A clear understanding of issues of consent and capacity are essential when approaching problems of family violence. Whenever a health professional takes action on behalf of a patient by examination, investigation, treatment, referral, sharing personal information about the patient with another agency, or providing personal care, that action should be taken with the agreement and consent of the patient.[27] Patients may indicate consent non-verbally (for example, by holding out an arm to allow blood pressure to be measured), orally or in writing. For the consent to be valid, the patient must:

- be competent (have the capacity) to take the particular decision;
- have received sufficient information to take the decision;
- not be acting under duress.

Legally, there is no difference between consent given in writing, orally or even non-verbally. A signature can be used to record consent but it does not prove that genuine consent has been given. People who have given consent to a particular intervention are entitled to change their mind and withdraw their consent at any point if they have the capacity (are 'competent') to do so. Equally, they can change their minds and consent to an intervention that they have earlier refused. It is important to let the person know this, so that they feel able to tell an appropriate person if they change their mind.

Adults with the capacity to take a particular decision are entitled to refuse any intervention being offered, even if this will be clearly detrimental to their health. The only exception is where treatment is being provided for a mental disorder under the terms of mental health legislation. Even in these circumstances, detention under mental health legislation does not give power to intervene other than directly in relation to the mental disorder without consent.

Adults should always be presumed to have capacity unless the opposite can be demonstrated. For someone to have capacity to take a particular decision, they must be able to:

- comprehend and retain information material to the decision, especially as to the consequences of allowing or not allowing the intervention to occur;
- use and weight this information in the decision-making process.

Methods of assessing comprehension and ability to make an informed choice include:

- exploring the patient's ability to repeat and reword what has been said;
- exploring whether the patient is able to compare alternatives and their probable and possible consequences;
- exploring whether the patient applies relevant information to his or her own case.

Some people may have the capacity to consent to some interventions but not to others. For example, a patient suffering from the early stages of a dementing illness may retain the capacity to make straightforward decisions about accepting personal care but might lack the capacity to take the sort of complex decisions which might arise in cases of family violence.

Capacity should never be confused with the health professional's assessment of the reasonableness of the person's decision. People are entitled to make a decision based their understanding of their own situation, even if that decision is perceived by others to be irrational, provided that they understand the implications of their decision. Seeking consent is about helping someone to make their own informed choice.

Children over the age of 16 are presumed to be competent, unless, as for adults, the opposite can be demonstrated. Under the age of 16, children are not automatically assumed to be legally competent to make decisions in relation to their health care. However, the courts have ruled[28] that under 16s are competent to give valid consent to a particular intervention if they have 'sufficient understanding and intelligence to enable him or her to understand fully what is proposed'. There is no specific age at which a child becomes competent to consent so-called ('Gillick competence') capacity depends both on the child and on the seriousness and complexity of the intervention being proposed.

If a child is not competent to give consent for themselves, consent should normally be sought from a person with 'parental responsibility'. According to the Children Act 1989, these include:

- the child's parents if married to each other at the time of conception or birth;
- the child's mother, but not father, if they were not so married, unless the father has acquired parental responsibility via a court order or a parental responsibility agreement, or he becomes the child's legal guardian, or the couple subsequently marry;
- the child's legally appointed guardian;
- a person in whose favour a court has made a residency order concerning the child;
- a local authority designated in a care order in respect of the child (but not where the child is being looked after under Section 20 of the Children Act, also known as being 'accommodated' or in 'voluntary care');
- a local authority or authorized person who holds an emergency protection order in respect of the child.

Foster parents, step-parents and grandparents do not automatically have parental responsibility.

If the mother is herself under 16, she will only be able to give valid consent for her child's treatment if she is herself competent to take the decision in question. Whether or not she is able to give valid consent on behalf of her child may therefore vary depending on the complexity of the decision to be taken.

Under English law, where an adult lacks capacity to make a decision, no-one can give consent on their behalf and the health professional is required to provide treatment and care that is in the person's 'best interests'.

Adults and older children with learning difficulties should never be automatically assumed to lack capacity and their understanding should be properly and carefully assessed. Again, their capacity is likely to vary according to the complexity of the proposed intervention.

Autonomy, neglect and prevention

In cases of family violence, where the subject of abuse is an autonomous adult with full mental capacity, they are entitled to complete confidentiality and professionals may only intervene or share information with other agencies with the subject's explicit consent. However, where the abuse puts at risk a dependent child or a vulnerable adult, the imperative to protect begins to take precedence over the duty to respect confidentiality and autonomy.

Although the responsibilities of the general practitioner in relation to both child abuse and domestic violence are relatively clearly defined, the correct response to the abuse of vulnerable adults remains elusive.[29] In child abuse, the practitioner must always prioritize the interests and protection of the child; in domestic violence, the prime

Table 3.1 The overlaps and differences between domestic violence and elder abuse.[28]

Domestic violence	Elder abuse
• Physical and sexual violence, emotional abuse	• Also includes financial abuse and neglect
• Violence as criminal behaviour	• Emphasis on protection
• Violence by men towards women	• Violence by men and women towards men and women
• Violence by partners and ex-partners	• Violence by adult children, partners, siblings, friends, neighbours
• Clear victim; clear perpetrator	• Ambiguities over victim

responsibility is to respect and promote the autonomy of the abused women and support her in making her own decisions. In the abuse of vulnerable adults, a delicate balance must be struck depending on the mental competence of the abused person. When the person is fully competent, no matter how physically frail or impaired, the appropriate response parallels that to domestic violence. Indeed, some abuse of vulnerable older people represents the progression of longstanding domestic violence over time so that both the perpetrator and the abused person have become old. In such cases, the abused older person's wishes must be elicited and respected, although much can be achieved by offering extra help within the home, so that the stresses of daily living are minimized and the transactions of care more closely supervised. In situations where the vulnerable adult is rendered incompetent through learning difficulty, mental illness, confusion or dementia, the priority shifts towards the protection of the abused person from both abuse and neglect. However, all these situations can be complicated by relationships in which each party is both a victim and a perpetrator of abuse.

The close relationship between a vulnerable adult and their carer may easily compromise the vulnerable adult's rights to confidentiality, and health care professionals will need to pay very explicit attention to these rights. When the vulnerable adult has severe learning difficulties, significant mental illness or is suffering from confusion or dementia, the situation becomes even more complicated as the imperative to protect begins to override the duty of confidentiality.

McCreadie[30] has usefully tabulated the overlaps and differences in understanding between domestic violence and elder abuse, which can be extended to help our understanding of the abuse of all vulnerable adults (Table 3.1).

New opportunities, new threats?

The NHS may appear to outsiders and many Britons alike as a huge, somewhat neglected, but much loved monolith, a given of postwar Britain that politicians ('the NHS is safe in our hands') meddle with at their peril. In fact, as those of us working within the NHS will attest, it is constantly being improved and reformed, or meddled with, depending on one's point of view. One of the few givens for those working in the NHS—apart from the belief that there is not enough money for it—is that almost nothing will stay the same for long.

British general practice is sometimes regarded as something of an anachronism, seen by some as at the heart of, and yet still an outlier within, the NHS. Its independent contractor status, a compromise solution when the NHS was founded in 1948, has, it has been suggested, made general practice resistant to the changes going on around it. Most GPs would disagree. They would point to the many changes that general practice and general practitioners have undergone, albeit with varying degrees of enthusiasm and effectiveness. These changes have often been driven from within the profession itself, but undoubtedly general practice has not been immune either to the many changes in structure and direction that have characterized (and sometimes convulsed) the NHS over the past fifty-plus years.

Arguably, the reforms under way in the NHS as we write (2001) are having a more profound impact on general practice than anything certainly since 1966, when a new GP contract paved the way for 'modern' general practice as described above. In this last section of the chapter, we shall list some of these changes. The possible impact of these changes on general practice's effectiveness in dealing with family violence will be highlighted. Of necessity, these thoughts will be largely speculative and subjective, as implementation, let alone objective evaluation, of some of these changes is still pending. There may also, of course, be still more changes in the meantime.

The following paragraphs apply primarily to NHS changes in England. The detail of similar legislation in Wales, Scotland and Northern Ireland may differ, but the underlying principles are broadly identical.

The new NHS

The 1997 white paper *The New NHS. Modern, Dependable*[31] set out the then new government's health agenda, their NHS Plan. The NHS Confederation, representing senior management of most NHS organizations, welcomed the plan in that it would, 'embed work on prevention and tackling health inequalities within core NHS functions, as well as developing Local Strategic Partnerships to draw together strands of cross-agency work' (para. 2.2).[32]

The Confederation also welcomed the fact that, 'The PCG/PCT reforms have seen primary care services brought under the managed framework of the NHS for the first time' (para 3.12).[32]

At first sight this would certainly seem to be good news for a consistent and cooperative approach by general practice to family violence. Working within a context of wider health and social reforms addressing prevention and health inequalities, some of the root causes of family violence would be tackled too. There is undoubtedly some good news even on closer examination, although the repercussions for families of some of the changes which will affect general practice may not be so good after all, as we shall suggest below. The ability of general practice to deliver the new agenda without losing some of its core strengths will be tested as never before. And, of course, the wider determinants of poverty, ill health and social exclusion require social, political and economic change, the scale and cost of which dwarfs anything that has been promised for the new NHS.

Various interconnected strands of the NHS Plan can be seen to be of particular relevance.

1. *Primary care trusts (PCTs)*. [Note: PCTs are the English and Welsh version of Primary Care Organization (PCO) envisaged in the new NHS. This term will be used through-out the book, but Northern Irish and Scottish readers will be aware of their own, broadly equivalent, PCOs: Health and Social Services Trusts (HSSTs) in North-ern Ireland; and Local Health Care Cooperatives (LHCCs) in Scotland.] PCTs are becoming the standard organization for the delivery of primary care services, includ-ing general practice. At their highest level they will *inter alia* be responsible for the commissioning, provision and development of primary care and community health services. They will employ the necessary staff and own property. The provision of care will often be devolved to localities covering 'natural communities' of up to 150 000. PCTs will incorporate local authority representation in their management, and some social work services will be PCT-based. Decisions as to whether to base children's and families' services, including child protection services, within the PCT will be taken locally, until a generally acceptable model emerges.

    Localities sound attractive as a way of devolving decision-making and accountab-ility in a way that might increase flexibility according to local needs. On the other hand, concerns have been expressed in some areas that health visitors and district nurses will be pooled at locality level, with greater emphasis on geographical case-loads, and with staff shortages being met by cross-cover and hiring of resources. This could spell the death knell of the primary health care team serving a practice population, with significant impact for the organizational strengths of this unit in dealing with family violence amongst other things.

2. *Care trusts.* PCTs are themselves likely to be transitional organizations. The Health and Social Care Bill[33] envisages the formation of Care Trusts where health and social services will be fully integrated. As Lowton points out (see Chapter 6b), GPs organized within PCTs or Care Trusts will be under the same duty as a member of any other NHS Trust to comply with, for example, a child protection S47 investiga-tion. Trusts will in turn be obliged to ensure interagency working and to set service standards.

3. *Multidisciplinary teams.* Care management, assessment and service delivery will be coordinated by multidisciplinary health and social care teams working with a single budget, joint priorities, a single management structure and one information system. We are likely to see these teams increasingly working to jointly agreed care pathways.

The potential benefits for work around family violence are self-evident, as are the potential difficulties (notably the implications for confidentiality of shared access to the medical record).

4. *Personal medical services (PMS).* GPs are being encouraged to change their working relationship with the NHS: to enter into a PMS contract with their local PCT whereby they sign a service level agreement committing to provide a range of services to a certain standard. This is aimed at improving the quality, consistency and control of GP service provision, based on identified national and local health priorities. Some PMS doctors (working to a PMS Plus contract) will receive extra funds to provide innovative services to particular groups. Another aim of PMS is to simplify the working arrangements for GPs and thereby encourage recruitment and retention. PMS doctors also have the option to become salaried employees of trusts, including PCTs, which may similarly encourage GPs to stay within the NHS or to return part-time to it. The advantages are clear, but the potential change to the individual doctor's relationship with an individual patient, to the continuity of both carer and care, may have significant negative implications. Contractual obligations may also dictate how the GP spends their time, to the detriment of the flexible response that is often required. On the other hand, as with the formation of PCTs, there are opportunities for PMS contracts to set clear service standards for safeguarding children or vulnerable elderly people.

5. *New contracts for other GPs.* Doctors that choose not to enter into PMS contracts, are likely to be subject to sweeping changes in their existing contract anyway. These changes to the so-called general medical services (GMS) contract will bring a welcome emphasis to rewarding quality of provision rather than numbers of patients treated: as with PMS, standards and priorities will be increasingly controlled from the centre and by PCTs. Single-handed practitioners may, if the new GMS contract is not sufficiently to the government's liking or is inadequately fulfilled, be obliged to sign PMS contracts. Whilst the undeniable variability in standards of general practice may be levelled out by these measures, there are concerns at the loss of independence and diversity of UK general practice, that is seen as such a strength by doctors and patients alike.

6. *Premises.* Here too there are pluses and minuses. Long overdue investment in primary care premises is promised, bringing with it the possibility of more purpose-built centres large enough to house extended PHCTs and other resources, including social services, housing, benefits advice, healthy living initiatives, etc. The 'one-stop shop' idea could certainly benefit disadvantaged families in particular. Economies of scale, however, could force many smaller practices into these centres, which are likely to be built in redundant community trust or hospital properties. There are concerns about reduced choice, access and intimacy for patients, and also concerns about the implications of the favoured private finance input (through the LIFT mechanism).

7. *GP workforce.* The recognition that there is a national shortage of GPs and the promise that more will be trained have been welcomed, even if the 2000 extra GPs promised for England by 2004 falls far short of the 10 000 that the BMA thinks are needed. Efforts to improve retention include reductions in paperwork; simplified, more flexible, family-friendly contracts; increased childcare provision; an occupational health service for GPs; and financial incentives. Most GPs identify reduction in list size as the chief prerequisite for improving quality of care by making more time available for each consultation.

8. *Workforce flexibility.* This is seen as a key feature of NHS reforms, addressing (it is hoped) workforce shortages, morale and cost pressures. Skill-mix concepts applied to general practice include: practice nurses or nurse practitioners taking on more of the GP's workload, including, in the case of nurse practitioners, initial consultations, prescribing and referring; health care assistants in turn taking on some of the practice nurse's duties; or nursery nurses taking on some of the health visitor's routine cases. Joint training for community nurses is seen as a precursor to other forms of flexible working, with the distinction between the various types (health visitor, practice nurse and district nurse) disappearing. It is also becoming easier for nurses to train as doctors, again with joint initial training of doctors and nurses seen as a springboard. Undoubtedly, breaking down some of the barriers between disciplines could have a beneficial effect with family violence as elsewhere, and skill mix might well address staff shortages amongst health visitors and others. There is also no question that many of the specific tasks undertaken by a doctor, nurse or health visitor could be performed as well, and at less cost, by someone with less training.

   The concern is, however, that this misses a crucial point about the work of a skilled primary care practitioner. To a significant extent, and nowhere more so than with family violence, GPs depend on their ability to integrate and sift the disparate strands, physical, psychological or social, that make up a patient's story; to use their knowledge of and relationship with that patient, as well as their training and experience, to weigh the uncertainties, to know when a situation is out of the ordinary or changing; and to take responsibility for the decisions then made. This work cannot be easily compartmentalized, parcelled out and performed to protocols, just as the health visitor's or practice nurse's cannot. At the edges of skill mix, at the boundaries of competence and experience, these considerations can be vital.

9. *Accountability.* The NHS is now subject to various quality assurance mechanisms, operating at every level. These include or are soon to include:

   - *Appraisal and revalidation.* Under the auspices of the National Clinical Assessment Authority, a review will be conducted (probably annually) of a GP's clinical practice, educational needs and attainment. This will lead to the production of an agreed personal development plan and, if necessary, further training. Every few years, the doctor's fitness to practice will be revalidated, with the ultimate sanction of removal from the register if compulsory retraining fails.

- *Clinical governance.* Mechanisms for clinical governance (the means by which organizations ensure the provision of quality clinical care by making individuals accountable for setting, maintaining and monitoring performance standards) are required at practice level and above. Components include: clinical audit; clinical risk management; evidence-based approaches to clinical effectiveness; staff and organizational development through 'lifelong learning'; quality assurance with monitoring systems of service provision; and ensuring a learning, blame-free culture.

- *National Institute for Clinical Excellence (NICE).* This body aims to ensure that evidence-based guidelines for best practice are available and applied across England and Wales.

Detailed critiques of these mechanisms are beyond the scope of this book. Whilst the potential benefits in helping educate and guide GPs in the complexities of family violence may be considerable, certain questions arise such as: are issues around family violence given high enough priority educationally or by organizations like NICE; who are those best equipped to define the standards and produce guidelines; do the complexities of family violence scenarios defy useful protocols; are protocols which are to be followed, rather than guidelines which guide, a hindrance rather than a help; are GPs any good at following protocols anyway (history suggests otherwise); are GPs going to be so overwhelmed by all the work involved in appraisals, etc. that they have even less time to devote to patients; are the pressures and implied threats posed by these initiatives going to exacerbate the profession's morale and retention crisis?

10. *National Service Frameworks (NSFs).* National Service Frameworks set national standards and define service models for a specific service or care group, put in place programmes to support implementation and establish performance measures against which progress within an agreed timescale will be measured. Again, undoubted benefits can be envisaged for end users and for practitioners working to them, but the workload and resource implications are huge. It has been estimated that implementing the coronary heart disease NSF alone will add 10 per cent to a GP practice's workload. Obviously it is to be hoped that the NSF for older people and that for mental health will have a beneficial, if indirect, impact on reducing family violence towards older people or that associated with mental health problems. An NSF for children is at the time of writing still in the planning stages.

11. *Access to the NHS.* Improving access to the NHS is one of the big ideas in the NHS Plan. There are several components to this, all of which may have potential significance for family violence.

- *NHS Direct/NHS24.* These nurse-led telephone (and internet) based services aim to provide an information and advice service round the clock. They are seen as gateways and gatekeepers to the rest of the NHS. Advice is strictly pro-tocol guided and may offer self-help, referral to casualty departments, admission by ambulance to hospital, or an appointment with a GP. Benefits for the ser-vice are suggested to include reduced workloads for general practices and less inappropriate casualty attendances. On the other hand, there is no automatic communication with a patient's GP; the operator has no background informa-tion (other than what the patient or carer gives them) on which to interpret the patient's story or base their assessment; and their assessment cannot be visual (discovery of other injuries, demeanour and appearance).

- *Walk-in centres.* The provision of primary care centres staffed by doctors or nurses confers obvious benefits, particularly on working people with minor ill-nesses or injuries. Again, though, there are potential problems with communic-ation with the GP; with access to previous records; and there is also the potential for people with something to hide to use these resources rather than go some-where where knowledge of their background might alert a professional to abuse.

- *Out of hours care.* Increasingly, GPs have formed cooperatives to provide out of hours care, with the provision of primary care centres (PCCs), which patients can attend rather than have a home visit. Telephone advice or attendance at the PCC accounts for about two-thirds of encounters. These have made a great difference to many GPs' working lives: they are less tired, more motivated, less isolated, and more likely to work to evidence-based guidelines for emergency care. The care given by GPs is often more appropriate to patients' needs than that on offer from casualty departments. Patients' own GPs are informed within 24 hours of the encounter. Not visiting can occasionally miss important evid-ence of abuse, however, and cooperatives share with the other systems above a problem of access to previous knowledge of the patient.

- *48-hour access.* The government promise of access to a GP for routine consulta-tion within 48 hours by 2004, or access to another professional within 24 hours may seem to be a huge benefit to patients, and some practices already provide this. Potential problems include: the reversion by GPs to a purely demand-led, non-appointment service, which, whilst possibly of benefit to some patients who find it difficult to use an appointment system, is likely to lead to more hurried, less prevention-based consultations; increased reliance on telephone consultations; and the increased use of deputies, locums, commercial services or cooperatives to provide routine care as well as emergency care to patients they do not know.

12. *Information technology.* Plans include comprehensive computerization of GP sur-geries and hospitals; linking via the NHS Net of health information about patients;

access to records by other agencies working within the same Care Trust (see above); improved access for patients to web-based health information; and the eventual roll-out of patient-held electronic health records (probably a smart card which can be accessed by the patient, and accessed and written on by health professionals). The possible benefits for communication across agencies, for patient education, for continuity at least of record if not of carer, and for audit, are clear. To the extent that the patient has their own record and can access it, patient autonomy may also benefit. On the other hand, the risks of information being more widely available electronically are huge—not merely the risk of hacking by unauthorized persons, but more importantly, and more likely perhaps, the accessing of confidential information by persons or organizations who are authorized, but to whom consent by the patient to view the record has not been given. The belief of some that continuity of record is all that matters for good patient care is also, in our view, dangerously misplaced. The effective functioning of the NHS depends on trust. Over recent years, individual trust in bureaucracies, government and professional authority have all been drastically undermined with a striking increase in the sense of insecurity experienced by individuals. The MMR vaccine debacle demonstrates very clearly how the erosion of trust can undermine the delivery of effective health care. If, through inappropriate enthusiasm for the power and capability of information technology, confidential patient information is passed on without appropriate consent, trust will be lost and vulnerable patients may be deterred from presenting for care and support.

References

1 McWhinney I. The importance of being different. *British Journal of General Practice* 1996; **46**: 433–6.

2 British Medical Association. *The Training of a Doctor*. BMA Report. London: British Medical Association, 1948.

3 Heath I. *The Mystery of General Practice*. London: The Nuffield Provincial Hospitals Trust, 1995.

4 Kleinman A. *The Illness Narratives: Suffering, Healing and the Human Condition*. New York: Basic Books, 1988.

5 Heath I. The future of general practice. In: Lock S, ed. *Eighty-five Not Out: Essays to Honour Sir George Godber*. London: King Edward's Hospital Fund for London, 1993.

6 Berger J, Mohr J. *A Fortunate Man: the Story of a Country Doctor*. Harmondsworth: Allen Lane/Penguin Press, 1967.

7 Rudebeck CE. General practice and the dialogue of clinical practice: on symptoms, symptom presentations and bodily empathy. *Scandinavian Journal of Primary Health Care* 1992; **1** (Suppl.): 1–87.

8 Toombs SK. *The Meaning of Illness: a Phenomenological Account of the Different Perspectives of Physician and Patient*. Dordecht: Kluwer Academic Publishers, 1993.

9 Sabin JE. Fairness as a problem of love and the heart: a clinician's perspective on priority setting. *BMJ* 1998; **317**: 1002–4.

10 Gelles R, Straus M. Violence in the American family. *Journal of Social Issues* 1979; **35** (2): 15–39.

11 Hallett C. Child abuse: an academic overview. In: Kingston P, Penhale B, eds. *Family Violence and the Caring Professions.* Basingstoke: Macmillan Press, 1995: 47.

12 Ferris LE, Norton PG, Dunn EV, Gort EH, Degani N. Guidelines for managing domestic abuse when male and female partners are patients of the same physician. *JAMA* 1997; **278**: 851–7.

13 Heyrman J, Spreeuwenbergh C, eds. *Vocational Training in General Practice.* Leuven: Katholieke Universiteit Leuven, 1987.

14 Olesen F, Dickinson J, Hjortdahl P. General practice—time for a new definition. *BMJ* 2000; **320**: 354–7.

15 Heath I, Evans P. The specialist of the discipline of general practice. *BMJ* 2000; **320**: 326–7.

16 Hart JT, The inverse care law. *Lancet* 1971; **1**: 405–12.

17 Read J. *Royal College of General Practitioners' Reference Book.* London: RCGP, 1990.

18 MORI. *Opinion Poll Conducted on Behalf of the British Medical Association in the Wake of the Shipman, Alder Hey and Bristol Cases.* London: British Medical Association, 2001.

19 General Medical Council. *Confidentiality: Guidance from the General Medical Council.* London: GMC, 1995.

20 Roach JO, Dorling D. Medical schools are still failing to recruit a broad spectrum of students [editorial]. *Student BMJ* 2000; **8**: 178–9.

21 Wynne J. Personal communication, 2001.

22 Bowker LH, Arbitell M, McFerron JR. On the relationship between wife beating and child abuse. In: Yllo K, Bograd M, eds. *Feminist Perspectives on Wife Abuse.* Newbury Park, CA: Sage, 1988.

23 General Medical Council. *Confidentiality: Protecting and Providing Information.* London: General Medical Council, 2000.

24 Carman D, Britten N. Confidentiality of medical records: the patient's perspective. *British Journal of General Practice* 1995; **45**: 485–8.

25 Paul Thornton. Personal communication, 2001.

26 Department of Health, Home Office, Department for Education and Employment. *Working Together to Safeguard Children.* London: Stationary Office, 1999.

27 http://www.doh.gov.uk/consent

28 Gillick V. West Norfolk and Wisbech Area Health Authority. A.C. 150, House of Lords, England, 1986.

29 Heath I. The role of the general practitioner. In: Pritchard J, ed. *Good Practice with Vulnerable Adults.* London: Jessica Kingsley Publishers, 2001: 82–92.

30 McCreadie C. *Elder Abuse: Update on Research.* London: Age Concern Institute of Gerontology, Kings College London, 1996.

31 Department of Health. *The New NHS. Modern, Dependable.* London: Stationery Office, 1997.

32 NHS Confederation. *Memorandum to the Select Committee on Health.* London: Stationery Office, 2000.

33 House of Commons. *Health and Social Care Bill.* London: Stationery Office, 2000.

Part 2

Violence against children

Chapter 4

The context

Wendy Stainton Rogers

Introduction

Something strange happened in the USA in 1875. A little girl called Mary Ellen was presented to a court as an 'animal' in need of protection from the cruel treatment she was suffering from her guardians. You may wonder why she had to be identified as an 'animal' rather than a child. The answer is that, in the USA at that time, while there was legislation to protect animals (such as horses and dogs) from cruelty, there was none to protect children. The reason for that is that there was then—in Britain as well as in the USA—a strong belief that the family was a private sphere in which nobody had any right to intervene. Evidence for this in the British context can be found in a statement made around this period in a parliamentary debate about the high rate of infant mortality among the poorer classes. The question being discussed was whether the government should do something about it. In this debate a noted reformer, Whately Cooke Taylor argued that it should not, stressing: 'I would rather see an even higher rate of infant mortality prevailing . . . then intrude one iota further on the sanctity of the domestic hearth'.

To put this further into context, not long before, historically speaking, children as young as 3 or 4 years worked long hours in factories, and children not much older were employed in mines. Children were also, alongside adults, being hanged for petty crimes. For example, in February 1814 at the Old Bailey, five boys were condemned to death for stealing. The youngest was 8 and the oldest 12.

These draconian conditions did not just affect children from the poorer classes. For middle and upper class families, in both schools and at home, the maxim for childrearing was 'spare the rod and spoil the child'. A good illustration of this can be found in the writings of Susannah Wesley, mother of the religious leader John Wesley, when she recommended in 1872 that parents must:

> Break their will betimes: begin this great work before they can run alone, before they can speak plain, or perhaps speak at all . . . make him do as he is bid, if you whip him ten times running to effect it. . . . Break his will now and his soul will live, and he will probably bless you to all eternity.

In other words, not much more than a hundred years ago, the main concern about children was for their mortal souls—for their spiritual well-being—rather than for their physical, emotional or psychological well-being. The general assumption was that children needed to be taught right from wrong, and it was their parents' duty to instil this in their children, using physical punishment if necessary. Any pain the child might experience was justified, so long as it enabled the child to become 'saved' from sin.

Alongside this was a view that parents knew what was best for their children and had absolute rights over them. The sanctity of the family and, particularly, the father's authority over it, were also generally viewed as far more important than any risks to children from the treatment they received at their parents' hands. Such views go back as far as Roman times, when a father had a legal right to do anything to his children that he believed right, including taking their life.

This historical backcloth is important for our understanding of child abuse in the Britain of today, since these attitudes are far from dead and buried. We can see them, for example, in the current debates about a parent's right to 'smack' a child. While a number of countries (most notably in Scandinavia) have made any physical punishment of children unlawful, this is not (at the time of writing) currently so in Britain. In cases where parents use physical punishments on their children—that is, when they act in ways which would otherwise be legally defined as an assault—there is a defence in law that such action constitutes 'reasonable chastisement'. Currently this position is being challenged, most notably by the Children are Unbeatable Alliance (see Chapter 9a.). Yet the sentiments of Susannah Wesley still prevail, as illustrated by this argument from a professor of paediatrics in the USA:[1]

> When properly applied, loving discipline works! . . . It allows the God of our ancestors to be introduced to our beloved children. It permits teachers to do the kind of job in classrooms for which they are commissioned. It encourages a child to respect other people and to live as a responsible, constructive citizen.

The history of concern about child mistreatment

Some social historians have painted a very bleak picture of child mistreatment in historical times—what Corby[2] has termed 'the barbaric past perspective'. The most influential of these, De Mause,[3] has claimed that:

> The history of childhood is a nightmare from which we have only recently begun to awaken. The further back in history one goes, the lower the level of child care, and the more likely children are to be killed, abandoned, beaten, terrorised and sexually abused.

De Mause divided up the past into what he views as seven 'evolutionary' stages—from what he calls the 'infanticidal mode' which, he claimed, lasted from at least Roman times until the fourth century, up to the present day 'helping mode' which, he suggested, began in about the 1950s. There have, however, been many criticisms of his analysis. De Mause has been accused of reading history in a naive manner, without taking account of social and cultural context. To take just one aspect, Boswell,[4] in an intricately detailed analysis of child abandonment, demonstrated that in Roman times—when abandonment was common—this was not any simple act of callous indifference. It arose out of the legalities of inheritance, wherein, when a man died, his property had to be divided between his sons. In order to avoid the splitting up of property, rich families tended to 'abandon' third and subsequent sons. But, Boswell points out, almost always arrangements were made to ensure that a neighbouring family would take them in and rear them.

Certainly concern about children goes a lot further back than the 1950s. By the Middle Ages in Europe, the Church established homes for foundlings. It also legislated over parental conduct. Hanawalt[5] describes that in the thirteenth century it instructed parents not to sleep with their children or allow them alone near unattended fires. In the sixteenth century infanticide was punished with severe penalties.[6] Cruelty to children was also acted upon much earlier. Pollock[7] reviewed newspaper reports of child cruelty between 1785 and 1860. There were references to 385 tried cases, and in all but 7 per cent the accused was found guilty. Thus even though there was no specific law at that time against cruelty to children, it is clear that prosecutions were pursued. And the newspaper reports were written in terms that make it clear that parents who mistreated their children were generally seen, even at that time, as 'unnatural' and their cruelty 'horrific' or 'barbaric'.

However, child cruelty became a particular concern towards the end of the nineteenth century. In part in response to Mary Ellen's case, in 1871 the Society for the Prevention of Cruelty to Children was established in New York in the USA, and in 1883 a Society for the Prevention of Cruelty to Children (SPCC) was set up in Liverpool in Britain. Soon others followed in a number of British cities including London. Members of these societies lobbied to introduce laws specifically to protect children from parental mistreatment. In England and Wales this led to the Prevention of Cruelty Act in 1889. Among other provisions, this gave courts the power to issue a warrant for the police to enter a home if there were suspicions that a child was being ill-treated, to arrest those suspected and to remove the child.

State provision for children's welfare

The Prevention of Cruelty Act 1889 was an important turning point in English legal history. It reflected a change in thinking about children, in particular an emerging view that the state should take responsibility for children's *welfare*. This view had, briefly, been adopted in the eighteenth century when the philanthropist Thomas Coram, distressed by the numbers of abandoned babies to be found by roadsides and in churchyards, persuaded parliament to set up and fund an institution—the Infant Foundling Hospital.[8] It opened in 1741 and soon afterwards parliament granted £10 000 (a very significant sum in those days) to pay for the wet-nursing in infancy and institutional care in childhood of every baby presented to the authorities 'in need of care'. But parliamentary support did not last long. Nineteen years later it decreed that no more state money should be provided, and it was not until the end of the nineteenth century that children's welfare came to be the focus of state concern.

Corby[2] suggests that up until the 1860s the state's predominant preoccupations were the dangers and demands that children posed. The state was concerned about street children, children who were vagabonds and beggars; child delinquency; child workers; and destitute children who had to be supported by the Poor Law authorities. But in the 1860s the perception of children changed from them being seen merely as nuisances and immediate threats to social order, to being viewed as 'adults in the making'. Emerging understandings began to concentrate upon childhood experiences as formative. Religious opinion had long taken this stance—remember the words of Susannah Wesley. Now this became overlaid with psychoanalytic ideas, which had begun to enter into professional if not popular consciousness. The concern was still about social order, but now the focus shifted to the *potential* threat that deprived, uneducated and damaged children would, without intervention, pose when they grew up.

This era was characterized by a belief in reform: that 'the poor' could be rehabilitated to become respectable and decent citizens who contributed to the common good rather than being a drain and a menace to people of superior character. And improving children's welfare came to be seen as the most effective strategy for reforming society. This, it was believed, could be achieved through education—the 1880 Education Act introduced compulsory education for all children up to the age of 10—and through improving the standard of parental care among the poorer classes.

Protecting children by intervening in the family

Whereas earlier 'child savers' like Dr Barnardo sought to rescue destitute street children, the SPCCs that were set up in the 1880s and 1890s and the national society—the NSPCC—that was founded from them sought to rescue children who were being mistreated within their families. They appointed inspectors to actively seek out cases of child cruelty and report them to the police. And although these inspectors became popularly known as 'the cruelty men', they also did a great deal of what would now be called 'family support work', helping poor parents who were struggling to raise their children in extremely deprived conditions. This approach was partially influenced by their ultimate aim—to make parents more responsible—and partly by the very practical need to gain the respect and support of local communities if they were to be able to do their jobs. That they were successful in this is evidenced by the fact that between 1896 and 1897, of the 23 124 reported cases, 58 per cent arose from referrals by neighbours and relatives. Indeed, Ferguson[9] argues that NSPCC inspectors were grappling, in the late nineteenth century, with much the same issues and problems facing social workers today: how to keep children safe without undermining parents and alienating local communities.

It is worth mentioning that even from their beginnings, the NSPCC and its forerunners the SPCCs also dealt with what we would now call 'sexual abuse'. For example, the London SPCC in its first year of operation pursued 12 cases of what it rather coyly, to our sensibilities, termed 'an evil which is altogether too unmentionable', but which later came to be called 'moral danger'. At that time there were no specific laws against incest—this was not achieved until the 1908 Incest Act. The 1880s and 1890s also saw action beginning to be taken against child prostitution,[10] and against 'baby farming'—the practice by which impoverished parents (especially lone mothers) placed their children to be nursed and reared outside the home in order to be able to work. These 'baby farms' were typically overcrowded and unhygienic, and large numbers of the babies died. This action was led by the medical profession, which, in 1870, set up the Life Protection Society. It established systems to regulate and inspect the practice and lobbied parliament to introduce the Infant Protection Act in 1872. This required adults who looked after more than one child (what we would now call 'foster parents') to register with the local authority and to meet set standards of care. In time such moves led to more comprehensive child welfare legislation: the 1908 Children Act and the 1933 Children and Young Person's Act. Dingwall[11] claims that by this point the main components of child protection law, as it now operates, had been put in place.

Child protection in a cultural context

If you remember, De Mause identified infanticide as the most barbaric mode of child mistreatment. Commentators like Corby[2] have pointed out that to regard infanticide in this light is to ignore the very different material conditions of historical times, when contraception and abortion were not freely available, and abortion, at least, posed significant health risks to women.

Scheper-Hughes[12] has made much the same case in respect to the practice of infanticide in the poorest countries in the world. She writes of the affluent countries being 'feticidal'—one of its main means of dealing with unwanted pregnancies is to kill fetuses. Is this actually morally superior, she asks, to infanticide? In countries and communities where abortion is not available, infanticide may be the only practical option. She describes how, in some communities in South America, sickly babies come to be called 'children of God'. They are treated tenderly but not fed, and soon enough they weaken and die. In pragmatic terms this means that the very limited food available to the family is reserved for those children who have a real chance of surviving.

Cultural relativism

This example highlights the need to treat cultural differences with great caution. Certainly we need to avoid the kind of ill-informed moral superiority that runs through De Mause's work. At the same time there is a potential trap in 'cultural relativism'. The dilemma is neatly exposed in Turnbull's[13] description of what childhood is like for indigenous ('pygmy') children growing up in the Ituri forest: '. . . life is one long frolic interspersed with a healthy sprinkle of spankings and slappings. Sometimes these seem unduly severe but it is all part of their training.'

Turnbull's use of words like 'frolic' and 'a healthy sprinkle' imply approval, albeit rather patronizingly put. The impression given is that in such 'primitive' societies physical punishment is acceptable since it is seen as 'normal' and 'all part of their training'.

Dingwall cautions against such assumptions, especially when applied to minority ethnic cultures living in Britain. He criticizes professionals like social workers and health visitors who justify not taking action in cases where black British children are beaten by their parents 'by seeing such treatment as the reflection of a traditional use of physical punishment in that community'.[11] He argues that we cannot assume that just because a practice may be more socially acceptable in a particular group, community or culture, that it is therefore not abusive to children.

The most extreme example usually offered is female circumcision—or, to use a more emotive term, 'female genital mutilation'. This practice is now proscribed in English law by the Prohibition of Female Circumcision Act 1985. Katz[14] points out that male circumcision is almost universally regarded as 'normal' and acceptable, across a range of cultures. In some (notably Jewish and Muslim) it is an essential rite of passage. Yet female circumcision is almost universally seen as 'barbaric' and totally unacceptable except in those cultures where it is practised. Katz argues that this is mainly because the physical consequences and risks are different. Female circumcision varies in its form, but it usually involves the excision of the clitoris and may include the 'surgical' closure (e.g. with thorns) of the vagina in a way that leaves only a very small opening. There is a high risk of infection, both from the practise itself, and from its aftermath (for example, where the vagina has been closed, it has to be 'opened'—often with a knife—to allow sexual intercourse).

But Katz also comments that female circumcision is also much more 'other' to Western sensibilities, and those who seek to practise it in the West (mainly rural African refugees) are a less powerful group to 'take on' than the Jewish and Muslim communities. And crucially, he observes, female circumcision 'has become part of the global struggle for women's rights', not surprising given both its symbolic meaning and its strategic use (i.e. to de-sex women and to forcibly impose virginity and fidelity upon them). This raises an important point: that simply because a practice appears to be acceptable within a particular community, this does not mean that all members of that community have an equal stake in its continuance. Action against female circumcision has been led by the resistance of women from the very communities in which it is 'part of the culture'. Dorkenoo and Elsworthy,[15] for example, argue that it is part of a more general patriarchal system and they are seeking to challenge the ways in which male power is operated against the interests of women and children.

Similar arguments have been put forward in relation to incest. Some anthropologists have claimed that father–daughter incest is viewed as 'normal' in some cultures. Equally, it was not at all unusual up until the 1980s for some professionals to assume that incest was acceptable among some social classes: 'It is a way of life in some families, you know. They just seem to accept it and don't feel horrified like we would' (quoted in [16]).

In large part as the result of feminist criticisms of these preconceptions (see, for example, [17]), such attitudes are much less viable today.

It is salutary to recognize that in many cultures it is Britain that is regarded as 'barbaric'. There was, for example, considerable outcry in the press across much of the rest of Europe, as well as criticism from the European court, about our treatment of the two 10-year-old boys who murdered James Bulger (see [18] for a detailed analysis). More generally, Britain is seen as unusually punitive towards children in its tolerance of the use of physical violence in the name of 'discipline', and the practice of its upper class of sending 7-year-olds into institutional care (i.e. to boarding school).

Child abuse as socially constructed

The historical and cultural differences in concerns about children show that what is considered as mistreatment of children at one period of time or in one culture may not be considered in the same way during another period or in another cultural location. Our contemporary understanding of 'child abuse' is socially constructed.[19,20] It is meaningful only within a particular time and sociocultural location—the one we are in here and now. Definitions are not static but change over time with new knowledge, awareness and understanding. Child abuse is a dynamic, changing concept.

A recent example is that of domestic violence. This has only recently been recognized as harming children either directly or indirectly. Humphries[21] outlines increasing evidence that children can be significantly harmed by exposure to domestic violence. This includes children being directly injured—in the womb, following assaults on the mother while she is pregnant, or, for instance, if they try to intervene in the assault. Children are also often abused within an overall context of violence and aggression within the household. This can include physical, emotional, psychological and sexual abuse. Domestic violence may also result in a failure on the part of the child's mother to care for the child properly because of the impact of the violence upon her. Witnessing violence is itself damaging: children are often terrified and traumatized by the experience and, where the violence is chronic and severe, they may go on to exhibit features of post-traumatic stress disorder and other emotional disturbances.

Defining child abuse

Thus it is clear that there is no single, consensual definition of child abuse, and this contributes to making the subject area a complex one, both to theorize and to deal with professionally. For example, compare these two definitions of child abuse, by Gil[22] and in a leaflet provided by the National Society for the Prevention of Cruelty to Children:[23]

> ... any act of commission or omission by individuals, institutions or the whole society, together with their resultant conditions which deprive children of equal rights and liberties, and/or interfere with their optimal development.[22]

> Child abuse/cruelty is neglect, physical injury, sexual abuse, and emotional abuse inflicted or knowingly not prevented which causes significant harm. Cruelty can be inflicted or knowingly not prevented by the person having care of the child, a person known to the child but not a carer, and by someone not known to the child.[23]

The first is nothing if not inclusive—by this definition almost all children would fall, at some time, into its remit. The second is much more focused, and, many would argue, is therefore more practical.

Over the last few years the government has commissioned research to explore how the child protection system works and whether it is doing the job effectively that it was intended to do, namely to prevent and protect children from harm. *Messages from Research*[24] has been a particularly influential summary of 16 research studies that looked at different aspects of the child protection system. The researchers identified that professionals view parenting behaviour on a continuum from 'good' to 'abusive', and that they have to decide whether to intervene and, if so, how. To do this they must draw a threshold; this involves deciding both the point beyond which behaviour (or parenting style) can be considered maltreatment, and the point beyond which it becomes necessary for the state to take action. Thus, decisions about what is abusive are, in practice, usually closely tied to decisions about whether the state should intervene.

Working definitions

The government document *Working Together to Safeguard Children*[25] identifies four main categories of child abuse and neglect:

1. *Physical abuse* constitutes a physically harmful action directed against a child. It may involve hitting, shaking, throwing, poisoning, burning or scalding, drowning, or suffocating. Illness by proxy (also known as Munchausen's syndrome by proxy or factitious illness by proxy—see Chapter 5a), whereby a parent or carer feigns the impression of, or deliberately brings about, ill health in a child, also constitutes physical abuse.

2. *Emotional abuse* is the persistent emotional ill-treatment of a child such as to cause actual or potential harm to the child's emotional development. It may involve conveying to children they are worthless or unloved, inadequate, or valued only in so far as they meet the needs of another person. It may involve causing children frequently to feel frightened or in danger, or the exploitation or corruption of children. Some form of emotional abuse is usually involved in all types of child maltreatment, though it may occur alone.

3. *Sexual abuse* entails forcing or enticing a child to take part in sexual activities. The activities may involve physical contact, including penetrative or non-penetrative acts. They may include non-contact activities such as involving children in looking

at pornographic material or watching sexual activities, or encouraging children to have sex together.

4. *Neglect* is the persistent failure to meet a child's basic physical and psychological needs, likely to result in the serious impairment of the child's health or development. It may involve a parent or carer failing to provide adequate food, shelter and clothing, or failure to protect a child from physical harm or danger. It may also include neglect of a child's basic emotional needs.

The same four categories are identified in Northern Ireland (Garda Siochana and the Department of Health 1995) and Scotland (the Children (Scotland) Act 1995) although the wording of each of the definitions is slightly different.

Assessing prevalence

Given the difficulty in arriving at a consensual definition of child abuse, it is hardly surprising that it has proved virtually impossible to arrive at any accurate estimate of its prevalence. Taylor[26] also points out that prevalence is difficult to estimate because of under-reporting, and because some families (notably the poorest and most disadvantaged) are generally exposed to more scrutiny than affluent, middle class families. This means that some forms of abuse are more 'visible' than others, and hence tend to be included in the data collected about prevalence.

Some attempt at estimating it can, however, be made. One of the main sources for doing this is to use data on the number of children recorded on child protection registers. These data should not be interpreted as a record of all child abuse, since registers are not intended to be a list of children who have been abused, but of those for whom there are currently unresolved child protection issues. In England and Wales there were 31 600 children on child protection registers at 31 March 1998, 2 per cent less than a year earlier. This figure represents 28 children per 10 000 population aged under 18 years.[27]

Neglect is the most commonly used category, accounting for 39 per cent of children registered during 1997–98. There were slightly more boys than girls on the register at the end of the year. However, there are different age and gender patterns within each category of abuse. Girls predominate in the over 10s and sexual abuse category. Boys were more likely to be placed on the register because of physical abuse, particularly between the ages of 1 and 10 years. Younger children were more likely to be on the registers than older children. Of the children on the registers at 31 March 1998, 9 per cent were aged under 1, 30 per cent aged 1–4 and 31 per cent aged 5–9 years. Children aged under 1 had the highest registration rate at 64 per 10 000 children in that age group.

Criminal convictions against adults are another way of gaining information about the scale of child abuse: 110 000 men aged 20 and over in 1993 had a previous conviction for a sexual offence against children.[28] In view of the low reporting and even lower conviction rate for such offences, this suggests a significant level of sexual offences against children by men. Women also commit sexual offences against children but in much smaller numbers.

As already mentioned, the actual prevalence of child abuse in any given area will be higher than the reported incidents, as cases will either not be recognized as abuse or, if recognized, often not be reported as such. One way of trying to estimate the true extent of the problem is to conduct research with adults who report on their childhood experiences. Creighton and Russell[29] studied the abusive childhood experiences of a representative sample of over 1000 adults aged between 18 and 45 living in England, Scotland and Wales. Some 12 per cent of the respondents had experienced physical punishments during childhood that would now be considered abusive, and 16 per cent had experienced sexual abuse. Over half the sexually abused respondents did not tell anyone about the abuse at the time, and they were less likely to tell if the abuser was a relative. Just over a third had still not told anyone. However, the implication of this is that the statistics available about the prevalence of abuse under-represent the true scale of the problem.

The National Commission of Inquiry into the Prevention of Child Abuse[30] estimates that:

- at least 150 000 children annually suffer severe physical punishment;

- up to 100 000 each year have a potentially harmful sexual experience;

- 350 000–400 000 live in an environment low in warmth and high in criticism;

- 450 000 are bullied at school at least once a week.

More recently still, the NSPCC's 2000 survey of 18–24 year olds[31] revealed experience of physical abuse in 20 per cent of respondents, sexual abuse in 14 per cent, moderate to severe emotional abuse in 16 per cent, and neglect in 18 per cent (see also Chapter 5a).

Finally, while child abuse covers a wide spectrum of behaviours that are harmful to children, it is worth recognizing that in its most extreme form child abuse can result in death. In the period 1992–96 there were 446 homicides of children aged 16 or under in the UK, an average of 89 per year.

References

1 Dobson J. *The New Dare to Discipline*, 2nd edn. Eastbourne, UK: Kingsway, 1993.

2 Corby B. *Child Abuse: Towards a Knowledge Base*. Buckingham, UK: Open University Press, 1995.

3 De Mause L, ed. *The History of Childhood*. London: Souvenir Press, 1976.

4 Boswell J. *The Kindness of Strangers: the Abandonment of Children in Western Europe from Late Antiquity to the Renaissance*. Harmonsworth: Penguin, 1988.

5 Hanawalt B. Childrearing among the lower classes of late medieval England. *Journal of Interdisciplinary History* 1977; **8**: 1–22.

6 Sharpe J. *Crime in Early Modern England 1550–1750*. London: Longmans, 1984.

7 Pollock L. *Forgotten Children: Parent–Child Relations from 1500 to 1900*. Cambridge: Cambridge University Press, 1983.

8 **McClure R.** *Coram's Children: The London Foundling Hospital in the Eighteenth Century.* New Haven, CT: Yale University Press, 1981.

9 **Ferguson H.** Rethinking child protection practices: a case history. In: Violence Against Children Study Group, eds. *Taking Child Abuse Seriously.* London: Unwin Hyman, 1990: 29–48.

10 **Goreham D.** The maiden tribute of Babylon re-examined: child prostitution and the idea of childhood in late-Victorian England. *Victorian Studies* 1978; **21**: 354–79.

11 **Dingwall R.** Labelling children as abused or neglected. In: Stainton Rogers W, Hevey D, Roche J, Ash E, eds. *Child Abuse and Neglect: Facing the Challenge.* London: Batsford, 1992: 158–64.

12 **Scheper-Hughes N**, ed. *Child Survival: Anthropological Perspectives on the Treatment and Maltreatment of Children.* Dortrecht: Reidel, 1987.

13 **Turnbull CM.** *The Forest People.* London: Pan, 1976.

14 **Katz I.** Is male circumcision morally defensible? In: King M, ed. *Moral Agendas for Children's Welfare.* London: Routledge, 1999: 90–104.

15 **Dorkenoo E, Elworthy S.** *Female Genital Mutilation: Proposals for Change.* London: Minority Rights Group International, 1992.

16 **Nelson S.** *Incest Fact and Myth.* Edinburgh: Stradmullion, 1987.

17 **Bell V.** *Interrogating Incest: Feminism, Foucault and the Law.* London: Routledge, 1993.

18 **Davis H, Bourhill M.** The demonisation of children and young people. In: Scraton P, ed. *Childhood in 'Crisis'.* London: UCL Press, 1997: 143–72.

19 **Parton N, Thorpe J, Wattam C.** *Child Protection: Risk and Moral Order.* London: Macmillan, 1997.

20 **Worrell M.** *The discursive construction of child sexual abuse.* Doctoral dissertation: The Open University, Milton Keynes.

21 **Humphries C.** The impact of domestic violence upon children. In: Tucker S, Roche J, Foley P, eds. *Working with Children and their Families.* Basingstoke: Macmillan, 2000: 142–50.

22 **Gil D.** *Violence Against Children.* Cambridge, MA: Harvard University Press, 1970.

23 **National Society for the Prevention of Cruelty to Children (NSPCC).** *Leaflet on child abuse.* London: NSPCC, 1999.

24 **Department of Health.** *Child Protection: Messages From Research.* London: HMSO, 1995.

25 **Department of Health, Home Office, Department for Education and Employment.** *Working Together to Safeguard Children: a Guide to Inter-agency Working to Safeguard and Promote the Welfare of Children.* London: HMSO, 1999.

26 **Taylor S.** How prevalent is it? In: Stainton Rogers W, Hevey D, Roche J, Ash E, eds. *Child Abuse and Neglect: Facing the Challenge.* London: Batsford, 1992: 40–9.

27 **Department of Health** (1998). Quality Protects: Framework for Action. London, Dott.

28 **Utting W.** *People Like Us: the Report of the Review of the Safeguards for Children Living Away from Home.* Stationery Office: London, 1997.

29 **Creighton SJ, Russell N.** *Voices from Childhood: a Survey of Childhood Experiences and Attitudes to Child Rearing Among Adults in the United Kingdom.* London: NSPCC, 1995.

30 **National Commission of Inquiry into the Prevention of Child Abuse.** *Childhood Matters*, Vol. 1. London: Stationery Office, 1997.

31 **National Society for the Prevention of Cruelty to Children (NSPCC).** *Child Maltreatment in the United Kingdom: a Study of the Prevalence of Child Abuse and Neglect.* London: NSPCC, 2000.

Chapter 5

The presentation and diagnosis of child abuse

Chapter 5a

Physical symptoms and signs of child abuse

Jane Wynne

Introduction

The primary care team has the opportunity to work with families towards prevention of all types of child abuse. However, as the causes of abuse, especially child sexual abuse (CSA), are not well understood, often the most professionals may do is to constantly be vigilant and have good networks of communication, both between team members and also with local organizations such as nurseries.

Members of the primary care team should also have the skills to recognize abuse at an early stage. If a family has been known to the practice for some time, knowledge and understanding of the family members are invaluable in recognizing when things begin to go wrong at a stage where intervention may avert or minimize abusive behaviour.

Unfortunately many families with young children are particularly mobile: as many as one in seven families in the inner city are not registered with a GP. This is compounded by the fact that most health visitors are GP-attached and unless the family registers with a GP practice this support is lost too. Health surveillance, immunization and family planning advice are not taken up and other childrearing problems are not discussed. The child, who may be disadvantaged in a variety of ways, is at additional risk with incomplete immunization and unrecognized failure to thrive.

Case

A child of 18 months died of pneumonia, the complication of measles following whooping cough. She had been seen in infancy because of failure to thrive and neglect but the family moved several times and were 'lost' to follow-up. When the ambulance arrived at the house the child was moribund. The parents and 10–15 adults were milling around the house—high on drugs and alcohol. The family was visiting from a neighbouring town 10 miles away. They were apparently regular attenders of the accident and emergency departments in both towns, and they received some primary care there. Immunizations, although commenced, were never completed. The A and E health visitor offered support but the family were uncooperative with all professionals and relationships were also weak with friends and family as they were so mobile and their use of drugs made them unpredictable. The resulting social isolation and inability to make use of professional support systems made the children even more vulnerable.

In circumstances like this, professional involvement will appear threatening, as inevitably crises will occur and intervention will be imposed with expectation of cooperation and change.

The aetiology of child abuse

Factors which have been found to be important in the aetiology of child abuse are summarized in Table 5.1

The prevalence of child abuse

For a National Society for the Prevention of Cruelty to Children (NSPCC) survey[6] almost 3000 18–24 year olds (15 per cent of whom had had children of their own) were interviewed after being randomly selected by postcode. The results are important as they reflect relatively recent parenting and cover all forms of abuse.

- *Physical abuse* within the home was reported by 20 per cent of the sample; 7 per cent met the criteria for severe physical abuse.

- *Neglect* involving lack of care was reported by 18 per cent; 6 per cent were subjected to severe neglect at home.

- *Sexual abuse* by a parent/step-parent or other relative was reported by 4 per cent of respondents; 10 per cent reported unwanted sexual behaviour (penetrative or oral sex, actual or attempted) by non-relatives; a fifth of this was by parents' or siblings' friends, neighbours, babysitters or strangers.

- *Emotional abuse* was reported by up to a third of respondents; 10 per cent reported 'loveless childhoods' and 6 per cent were found to meet the criteria for severe emotional maltreatment.

(See also p. 79)

Table 5.1 Common factors in family violence (after Browne[1]).

Socialization experiences of carers	Abuse and neglect as a child, especially prolonged emotional deprivation Role model of violence—conflicts resolved by the use of violence Aggressive interactions as means of communicating Partner violence
Situational stress	Difficult relationship with partner: *domestic violence is common** Poverty: poor education, few work skills Poor housing/frequent or recent moves Unrealistic expectations of child Child-produced stress: ex-premature; cries too much; does not sleep; illnesses such as vomiting, cough Mother tired; puerperal depression; physical illness Mother too young; too many babies too fast; ?too old Family illness/bereavement New baby
Psychological traits	Personality and learned family characteristics Poor impulse control Psychological disorder (although major psychiatric disorder is rare) Drug and alcohol misuse†
Community	Values regarding violence—'subculture of violence' Poor community resources, e.g. playing areas. Note high levels of RTAs Poor housing stock, inadequate heating and safety checks, etc. Note high incidence of accidents and house fires‡
Immediate precipitating situation	Child 'misbehaves': naughty, bad, insolent, answers back, defiant, greedy, lies, steals, violent towards sibs, carers, etc. Infant cries incessantly

RTA, road traffic accident.

* *Domestic violence* is now recognized to be common within all sections of society: women (and a few men) are physically, sexually and emotionally abused. Recently it has been recognized[2] that in violent households children are not only emotionally abused but are commonly physically abused, and as many as one in three are victims of child sexual abuse (CSA). Domestic violence resulting in *fetal abuse* is increasingly recognized and is said to occur in 1–20 per cent of pregnancies. Fetal abuse may be part of ongoing violence toward the woman or the violence may begin in pregnancy. Sixty per cent of women in a refuge reported violence during pregnancy, 13 per cent described miscarriage after violence and 22 per cent threatened abortion.[3] Blows and kicks to the abdomen may lead to placental separation or even uterine rupture.[4] Occasionally, the fetus may be stabbed.

† *Illicit drugs and alcohol misuse* by parents/carers adversely affect child health, as may tobacco smoking. Children born to drug and alcohol misusers may be brain damaged, difficult to feed and may cry a lot and sleep poorly. Childcare is often sub-optimal and increased levels of violence and neglect are noted. Deaths from methadone administration or self-ingestion causing respiratory arrest and overlying due to parental intoxication have been recorded. HIV infection may be transmitted vertically to the infant: illness and premature death in parents may leave children neglected and orphaned. Opinion is currently divided as to whether an informed choice to breastfeed a child where there is a risk of HIV constitutes a child protection issue.[5]

‡ *Fatal accidents* are five times as common, and drownings 10 times as common in the lowest social class as in the highest. *House fires* are 17 times more common in privately rented houses than in owner-occupied accommodation.

Assessment of families

The medical record of family members often provides invaluable information as to specific *background factors* that may assist in the assessment of the risk or recurrence of abuse. The noting and collation of such background factors by the practice team (with due regard to issues of confidentiality, see Chapters 3 and 5c) will certainly help in the identification of children in need and children in need of protection. Some of these factors are summarized in Table 5.2.

In some cases, even background information found in the records of members of the extended family (e.g. history of sexual abuse or convictions for abuse), may be relevant to the index child.

In certain types of abuse, such as factitious illness, the practice records and frequently those of the mother too will be pivotal in making the diagnosis. As eating disorders are common in mothers who have infants who fail to thrive, so is Munchausen syndrome in mothers who present their infant or child with a factitious illness (previously known as Munchausen syndrome by proxy). Factitious illness is discussed further below (p. 92).

Table 5.2 The medical records of the family.

Medical records of mother	A history of childhood abuse
	Mental health problems
	Eating disorder
	Poor physical health
	Alcohol/drug abuse
	Learning problems
	Previous childrearing problems, e.g. unrealistic expectations in terms of child's behaviour and development (toilet training, tidiness, etc.)
	Many children, too closely spaced, started having children at very young age
Medical records of father	A history of childhood abuse
	Mental health problems
	Poor physical health
	Alcohol/ drug abuse
	Learning problems
	Convictions for violence
	Previous childrearing problems
	Poor employment record, low expectations/self-esteem
Medical records of index child	Unwanted pregnancy
	Abortion or adoption considered
	'Difficult' pregnancy or birth
	'Difficult' or ill neonatally (crying, sleeping, feeding problem)
	Failure to thrive
	Repeated minor illness
	Repeated minor injury; child 'bruises easily'
	History of child abuse
	History of behavioural/emotional problems
	Learning difficulties
	Repeated failures to attend appointments, e.g. immunization, ENT, squint
Siblings' medical records	As index child, including previous or current abuse

Physical abuse

Physical abuse is defined as occurring when a child suffers physical injury (or injuries) as a result of acts (or omissions) on the part of his parents or guardians. This definition also includes failure to protect from injury and other deliberate acts like suffocation or poisoning.

Whilst most physical abuse is recognized in children under the age of 10 years, and most 'serious' abuse in children under 5 years, teenagers too are physically assaulted by their carers. Retaliation by the older child or initiation of violence by them may result in an escalation of violence with the parent or carer, and may precipitate the child running away.

Creighton and Noyes[7] found that, by the age of 18 years, 2 per cent of young people will have been physically abused. A 1995 study by Smith et al.[8] looked at 403 London families from varied social backgrounds, with a child aged 1, 4, 7 or 11 years. This found that:

- 90 per cent of the children had been hit, three-quarters of them by the age of 1;
- 50 per cent of carers 'hit to hurt' the child, although few were bruised;
- 15 per cent were bitten, kicked or punched;
- most smacking was an angry rather than a controlled response;
- 3 per cent of children lived in 'situations of low warmth and high criticism'.

The NSPCC study[6] asked for experience of specific acts of violence:

- being hit on the bottom or another part of the body with a hard implement such as a stick;
- being hit with a fist or kicked hard;
- being shaken;
- being thrown or knocked down;
- being beaten up (hit over and over again);
- being grabbed around the neck and choked;
- being burned or scalded on purpose;
- being threatened with a knife or a gun.

Of the quarter of respondents who had experienced at least one of these violent acts, four-fifths had experienced them at home. The study considered the abuse to be serious where the violent treatment either caused injury or carried a high risk of injury if continued over time or throughout childhood: 7 per cent of respondents fulfilled this criterion.

In the UK the law allows parents to punish their children by hitting (and hurting) them, as long as they only use 'reasonable force'. The rule of thumb has been that if the child is bruised then this is not reasonable force but physical assault or abuse. In 1995, John Bowis, the then Junior Health Minister, defending the law on hitting, said all that was acceptable was a 'gentle smack on the wrist'. Only parents and registered childminders with parental approval may hit children. This too is under review, with the government (as at 2000) carrying out a widespread consultation exercise on hitting and the law. Most professionals working in the field of child abuse support a 'zero tolerance' position towards hitting children but it appears likely that the law will remain unchanged (see Chapter 9a).

Considerable force is needed to bruise a child and physical abuse covers the spectrum from a bruise to fracture to brain injury and death. Most parents do not intend to cause severe injury but a few are sadistic and cause, for example, cigarette burns and scalds. Sadistic injury is associated with CSA.

Parents or parent figures are responsible for over 90 per cent of physical abuse, and although mothers and fathers both injure children, men are more likely to cause the serious injuries. Families may be very convincing in their denial of the causation of the injury and it may be very difficult for the professional who has known the family well, to challenge the history.

The challenge for the primary care team is then to recognize the family which is struggling, to offer appropriate support, but if the carers' behaviour becomes abusive, to name the abuse. It is not possible to prevent all abuse, but it is possible to recognize injuries as abuse.

History

Injuries may come to the health professional's attention in different ways (Table 5.3). Many pointers in the background history may help alert the professional to the possibility of abuse (see also Tables 5.1 and 5.2 above). Hobbs et al.[9] draw attention to:

- *discrepancies in history*, e.g. changes in a story with repeat telling, vague as to who was there and what they did;

- *unreasonable delay*, e.g. pain from trauma denied by the carer; fractures or scalds presenting with signs of healing; a baby left fitting for 24 hours;

- *trigger factors*, e.g. baby crying all night; a toddler refusing to feed; a 5 year old who wets the bed; a teenager who steals or comes in late;

- *family problems* in addition to current mental health, alcohol and drug misuse: carers' relationship difficulties; bereavement; illness; redundancy; housing problems; debt; lack of family's or friends' support;

- *unrealistic expectations* of the child in terms of his or her behaviour and development, e.g. to eat tidily, to sit quietly, to achieve early toilet training;

Table 5.3 Recognizing physical abuse.

Someone tells	• the child • the parent • a neighbour • a teacher
A carer seeks advice	• for the injury • for the child about another medical problem and injury is found incidentally
The health professional has concerns	• injuries are inconsistent with history (too severe, too many, wrong distribution) • injuries have been inflicted at different times • 'accident' inconsistent with child's developmental abilities • repeated minor injuries • poor weight gain • developmental delay • signs of neglect • concern about parent's care, e.g. delay in seeking medical help; refusal of appropriate treatment; previous neglect • mother shows signs of recent domestic violence

- *past history of child*: preterm; illness as neonate; frequent minor illnesses, attendances at accident and emergency departments, or admissions to hospital; a history of accidents; 'bruises easily'.

Case

The health visitor asks the GP to see Amy, aged 3 months, who has an unexplained 1 cm bruise on both cheeks, a healed tear of the frenulum and her weight gain is poor. The 2-year-old sister has been seen before because of breath holding attacks and has had 'too many bruises'. Their mother was depressed after the birth of Amy. Her partner is known to have been violent to his partner on occasions in the past.

The GP talks to the mother, examines Amy and discusses the problem with the health visitor and the local community paediatrician, who sees Amy that afternoon. She is admitted the same day, and a skeletal survey reveals rib fractures. Her mother, resident on the ward, tells of her fear that her partner will kill someone when he has a drunken rage. Social services and the police are involved and the baby, her sister and mother go home to the maternal grandmother whilst an investigation takes place.

Examination

Certain injuries are particularly associated with abuse.[10]

1. Some *bruises* are more worrying than others:

   - any bruising in infancy;
   - bruising of the ears, face (other than forehead and chin in toddlers), upper arms, thighs, back, buttocks, abdomen and genitalia;

- particular patterns of bruising, e.g. hand or finger-tip bruising; implement (strap, stick); kick; bite.

2. Accidental *fractures* usually occur after ambulation; thus *any fracture in infancy* is of particular concern; others of particular concern include:

   - skull fracture(s), especially multiple, wide, long, depressed;

   - spiral/oblique/transverse fracture of humerus or femur (the 'toddler fracture' is an exception: this is a spiral fracture with no displacement at the lower end of the tibia and occurs when the running toddler falls awkwardly and twists);

   - rib fracture(s)—may be associated with a shaking injury or direct impact;

   - metaphyseal fracture(s)—usually distal ends of long bones are a 'pull and twist' fracture;

   - multiple fractures which may be at different stages of healing.[11]

3. *Head injury*: an infant or young child presenting with fits, coma or 'near-miss cot death' and on further investigation has:

   - retinal haemorrhages;

   - skull fracture(s);

   - cerebral contusion;

   - subdural haematoma.

4. *Burns and scalds*: may present acutely, as a neglected injury or, if old, as a scar. Particularly worrying are:

   - forced immersion injury (glove and stocking distribution, buttocks);

   - splash or thrown hot fluid scald;

   - contact burn (shape of iron, grill, radiator);

   - cigarette burn (round, deep, cratered);

   - particularly significant sites are the buttocks, back of hands/feet, and genitalia.

5. *Poisoning*: ingestions are commonly due to accident or neglect and often involve toddlers, but in deliberate poisoning:

   - the age at poisoning may vary from infancy through childhood;

   - there may be no history of drug ingestion but the child presents with repeated unexplained illness;

   - the child may present with seizures, drowsiness, vomiting, diarrhoea or sudden death;

   - there may be a history of previous unexplained death in the family;

   - there may be a history of other abuse in the family.

The diagnosis of deliberate poisoning is difficult: there are often symptoms at variance with the history and the clinical picture as a whole does not make sense. Advice from a toxicologist is often very helpful once the diagnosis of poisoning is considered.

Drugs more commonly used in deliberate poisoning are analgesics, anticonvulsants, antihistamines or household substances such as salt. More recently, there have been deaths from methadone when carers may deliberately 'sedate' a child, or the neglected toddler ingests the drug which has been left accessible. Other drug/substance deaths have occurred when the carer is intoxicated and 'overlies' the young child or infant. Overlying does not (in my experience) occur in normal sleep.

6. *Suffocation* in childhood.[12] Attempts should be made to differentiate this from sudden infant death syndrome (SIDS) but this may not be possible. Suffocation should be considered:

   - at all ages, including infancy, but especially over 6 months;
   - when the infant has had previous episodes of floppiness or cyanosis, but investigations are all negative;
   - when there is a previous history of unexplained deaths of infants or children in the family.

   At post-mortem there may be no sign to differentiate suffocation from SIDS but there may be petechiae around the neck, upper eye lids and face; subconjunctival haemorrhages and other bruising, including retinal haemorrhages; the skeletal survey may show bony injury; and a CT brain scan may show cerebral contusion or subdural haematoma.

7. There is a clear association between physical abuse and *child sexual abuse*.[13] An anogenital examination in cases of suspected physical abuse is thus indicated, although in practice is not always possible. Suitable training, experience, surroundings and equipment are particularly important when this is contemplated (see p. 101).

Further investigation

From the information given in the presenting history, past medical history, family and social history, followed by a thorough examination, which includes looking at the child's injury(ies), growth and development as well as full physical examination, the physician will often be in a position to decide whether further medical investigations (Table 5.4) are needed to evaluate the injuries and to think about any differential diagnosis.

The general practitioner's role

The general practitioner's role in the recognition and management of physical abuse varies. For some it will be limited to recognizing a child with worrying injuries and making an appropriate referral to a paediatrician, but other practitioners will take on

Table 5.4 Clinical investigations in physical abuse.

Injury	Medical investigation
Bruises	Photograph—all injuries Haemoglobin/FBC Clotting screen: platelets/PT/PTT* NB ageing of bruises is difficult
Bites	Paediatric orthodontologist/photo/dental impression ?Saliva for DNA
Fracture in child <3 years old	Skeletal survey[†‡]
Bruised child <3 years old	Skeletal survey
Retinal haemorrhages	Confirmation by ophthalmologist CT brain scan ?MRI scan Cranial ultrasound
Burns	Microbiology
Poisoning	Toxicology
Apnoea	Monitoring of episodes

CT, computed tomography; FBC, full blood count; MRI, magnetic resonance imaging; PT, prothrombin time; PTT, prothromboplasmin time.

* More detailed clotting/bleeding investigations should be done on advice of haematologist. The ageing of bruising should be circumspect—recent research suggests that all that can be said is that yellowing in not seen before 18 hours. All the other colour changes are inconsistent.[9]

[†] A skeletal survey is essential if there is unexplained bruising or an unusual fracture in a child <2 years old; some authorities suggest <3 years. The ageing of fractures is well described by Klineman[14] with periosteal new bone seen at 10 days—this is important, especially in infancy when rib fractures are difficult to see but are highly significant in the diagnosis of a shaking injury.

[‡] In the differential diagnosis of fractures, the following should be noted:

- *neonatal rickets* may be seen in ex-preterm infants, usually about aged 3 months but the bones then strengthen quickly;
- *copper deficiency* is no longer seen in the UK;
- *osteogenesis imperfecta* (OI) is a rare, usually dominantly inherited disorder associated with a positive family history, blue sclerae, dentinogenesis imperfecta, fractures and early-onset deafness. There are several types of OI of variable severity: not all have blue sclerae or dominant inheritance. The diagnosis is not usually difficult clinically—a skin biopsy shows a constitutional abnormality but this does not equate with fragile bones. Type IVA OI is very rare: there is no family history, there are white sclerae, normal teeth and a history of fractures, making this variant more difficult to distinguish from abuse—a careful history with detail of every fracture usually makes for clarity.

the clinical responsibility for the management of the child. Butler-Sloss[15] set out the medical tasks in child abuse (Table 5.5). Those pertinent to most GPs are highlighted. (see also Chapters 6c and 7c.)

The diagnosis of abuse by any clinician should be built up following the usual clinical method of history-taking, examination and investigations, leading to a differential diagnosis and probable diagnosis based on the whole picture. There has been a tendency

Table 5.5 Medical tasks in child abuse (after Butler-Sloss[15]).

1. *Take a full medical history*
2. Make a thorough medical examination
3. Arrange appropriate investigations for: • sexually transmitted diseases • forensic tests • pregnancy • bruising • bony injury
4. *Complete full and accurate records (at the time of examination)—always sign and date clinical notes*
5. Prepare a medical report for GP, SSD or community, child health
6. *Prepare a statement for the police on request*
7. *Ensure results of investigation are recorded*
8. *Arrange referral for psychiatric, psychological or paediatric follow-up*
9. *Attend child protection conference or court hearing*
10. *If there are differences of medical opinion endeavour to resolve these differences or at least to identify the area of dispute*

SSD, Social Services Department.

in abuse for this method to be by-passed and 'spot diagnoses' to be made. Given the enormity of the diagnosis of child abuse, which may finally be evaluated in the wider context of a police and social services investigation (and possibly the criminal and civil courts too), a thorough medical assessment, with as robust a diagnosis as possible, is mandatory.

The pieces of information making the whole may be evaluated individually, but finally it is their relevance to the whole picture which makes the diagnosis.

Factitious illness in childhood/Munchausen syndrome by proxy

Nowhere is the above advice more appropriate than in the consideration and diagnosis of factitious illness in childhood or Munchausen syndrome by proxy (MSBP). Even the nomenclature of this complex form of abuse reflects the difficulties in defining and characterizing it, with the same scenario variously being described as factitious (i.e. artificially produced) illness in childhood, factitious illness by proxy and Munchausen syndrome by proxy. Munchausen syndrome describes behaviour in adults who fabricate symptoms and signs of illness in themselves: it too is now sometimes described as factitious illness.

P00I09P8V
AMANDA MINNS

Ship To: 22595003 F

AMANDA MINNS
HAIRNYRES HOSPITAL
EAGLESHAM ROAD
GLASGOW
STRATHCLYDE
G75 8RG

Bill To: 22595000

LANARKSHIRE ACUTE HOSPITA
MONKLANDS HOSPITAL
MONKSCOURT AVENUE
AIRDRIE
STRATHCLYDE
ML6 0JS

Sales Order
F 8983716 1

Cust P/O List
43.00 GBP

ISBN 9780192628282   **Qty** 1

Customer P/O No E27822

Fund:

Title: Family violence in primary care / edited by Stephen

Format: Paperback

Author:

Publisher: Oxford University Press.

Volume:

Edition:

Year: 2003.

Order Specific Instructions
CUST CONTACT AMANDA MINNS
TEL:01355 585488

COUTTS LIBRARY SERVICES: UK 032157253 LGUK001R001 UKRWLG14

Factitious illness by proxy is rare: according to one estimate of non-accidental poisoning and suffocation in the British Isles,[16] there is an expected combined annual incidence in children under 16 years of at least 0.5 per 100 000, and for children under 1 year of at least 2.8 per 100 000. This translates as an estimated one child per million head of the population per year, although this is widely thought to be an under-estimate, because of difficulties in identification and recording. International research findings suggest that up to 10 per cent of affected children will die, with approximately 50 per cent experiencing long-term morbidity. Siblings are frequently affected: McClure[16] found that, amongst 83 affected children with siblings, 15 had had siblings who had died previously (18 siblings in all): five of these had been classified as sudden infant deaths (cot deaths).

Attempts to clarify the essence of factitious illness in childhood may lead to over-simplification, but it can perhaps most usefully be regarded as child abuse which results from 'the fabrication or induction of illness in a child by a carer'.[17]

Parents are expected to respond to their child's needs and distinguish them from their own needs. In factitious illness by proxy, they are unable to do so; indeed, the child's needs are ignored. Certain behaviours in the carer/abuser include:

- 'mothering to death' by an apparently loving mother, in constant contact with her 'sick' child, and his increasingly severe illness(es);
- 'doctor shopping' as she seeks more and more medical opinions from an ever-widening spectrum of specialisms;
- 'overanxious parents'; whilst most parents are understandably anxious when their child is unwell, there is no possibility of reassuring these carers.

As a consequence the carer gains attention, care for themselves as the parent of a sick child and status with friends and family. Other gains might be financial (disability allowances, etc.) or social (hospital staff, other parents). Some abusers become involved with the media or lawyers (although usually they remain appreciative, despite the elusive diagnosis and cure), or become active in parent support groups.

The harm to the child from factitious illness by proxy is diverse and results from:

- the physical effects of the illness (poisoning, near suffocation, etc.);
- the effects of repeated investigations and treatment;
- time at or in hospital and undergoing treatment, restricting aspects of the child's social life and education;
- the betrayal of trust by the adult of the child;
- associated pervasive emotional abuse: lack of empathy, cruelty, dishonesty and deception, and disregard of the child's needs, in the context of a 'caring' façade.

For factitious illness in childhood to be recognized, it is necessary to understand the dynamics between the carer (the abuser) who takes on the sick role by proxy; the child who is dependent and unable to prevent the deception; and the doctor or other professional who is deceived. *Diagnosis then can be seen to depend largely on whether the professionals consider the possibility of parental deception.*

Illness can be fabricated or induced by a carer in three main ways:

1. Fabrication of signs and symptoms, including past medical history.

2. Falsification of hospital charts and records, letters or documents, or specimens of body fluids.

3. Induction of illness by a variety of means.

The following list gives examples of behaviours that may be exhibited (from supplementary guidance to *Working Together*[17]):

- inducing symptoms by administering medicines or other substances (e.g. salt), or by means of suffocation;

- interfering with treatments, e.g. by overdosing, withholding medication or interfering with infusion lines;

- exaggerating symptoms, causing professionals to undertake unnecessary investigations and treatments which may be invasive and therefore harmful or dangerous;

- claiming the child has symptoms that are unverifiable unless observed directly, e.g. pain, frequency of micturition, fits or vomiting;

- alleging psychological illness in a child.

A significant number of such children have an illness 'career' from birth. They may have been seriously ill as a result of prematurity (possibly itself due to the mother interfering with her pregnancy). They may go on to have multiple minor illnesses in the first few months of life; non-organic failure to thrive (attributed often to alleged allergies or feeding problems); as well as genuine organic problems which may pre-date or be a consequence of the abuse.

Those children who do not die as a result of the abuse face a number of long-term consequences, including impairment of their physical, emotional, educational and psychological development.[18]

Child sexual abuse (CSA)

The *Report of Inquiry into Child Sexual Abuse in Cleveland 1987*[15] began its conclusion thus:

> We have learned during the Inquiry that sexual abuse occurs in children of all ages, including the very young, to boys as well as girls, in all classes of society and frequently within the privacy of the family.

This statement reflects the current position in the UK. Although most media attention is focused on the activities of paedophiles preying on strangers, and on organized paedophile rings, the vast majority of child sexual abuse occurs in the home and, in nearly all cases, the abuser is known to the child.

A widely used definition of CSA is the one of Schechter and Roberge:[19]

> The sexual exploitation of children is referred to as the involvement of dependent, developmentally immature children in sexual activities they do not fully comprehend, are unable to give informed consent to and that (socially) violate the social taboos of family roles.

More directly, CSA is the use of children for sex.

Men and older boys are responsible for most CSA but women and girls may also abuse. Adults, teenagers and older children misuse their power to derive sexual gratification from the sexual abuse and this behaviour may become very addictive. It is this addictive quality of the abusers' behaviour which makes intervention so difficult. Being 'found out' rarely stops the abuse.

The abusive behaviour usually begins during adolescence but the abuser may be as young as 7 years. The younger the abuser the more likely it is that he too is a victim of CSA. Treatment programmes are likely to be most effective when targeted at these young abusers and the hope is that they will be diverted from a lifetime of abuse. The treatment of young abusers is discussed by Eileen Vizard in Chapter 9b.

Some abusers will abuse girls and boys of any age and also adults, whereas others only abuse prepubertal children. Clinical practice shows that it is rare for an abuser to abuse only one child. Some abusers abuse many children, their own and others, for example as a teacher or scout leader who has access to many children.

Abuse is now widely recognized in any residential setting: schools (especially schools for the 'maladjusted' or children with learning problems); children's homes; detention centres and secure units; and even foster or adoptive homes. Children who have been abused once are at greater risk of further abuse. Children with any disability (physical, learning or sensory) are also at particular risk from sexual abuse, but also other maltreatment (neglect, failure to thrive, physical and emotional abuse).

There are a large number of papers now looking at the prevalence of abuse. The variations in the different studies are probably due to different methodology, i.e. questionnaires or interviews (telephonic or face to face) and the detail of the questioning. In the more developed world, 15–30 per cent of women and 10–15 per cent of men will give a history of some sexual abuse during childhood, and in over 30 per cent of these this will have been repeated abuse.[6,20–22]

In the 2000 NSPCC survey,[6] the following points about sexual abuse emerged:

- Of the 1 per cent of respondents sexually abused by a (virtually always male) *parent or step-parent*, male and female respondents were equally likely to have suffered.

- Girls made up the majority of the 3 per cent of respondents abused by *other relatives*. Most commonly the abusers were brothers or step-brothers, but uncles, grandfathers and cousins were also mentioned.

- Most sexual abuse occurs in the abused's *home* or that of the abuser.

- In only 7 per cent of those abused by non-family members was the abuser a *stranger*.

- Very few reported sexual activity involving *professionals* responsible for their care, and none involving *care workers.*

In the Leeds Child Protection Clinic:

- twice as many girls as boys are seen;

- the average age at referral is 7 years (range 1 month to 19 years);

- the type of abuse varies from exposure to pornography to touching to penetration;

- in the abuse of very young children oral and anal abuse is common;

- intracrural intercourse is also common in the abuse of younger girls;

- vaginal penetration is more frequent in girls of 7 years or more.

Presentation of CSA (see also Table 5.7)

Disclosure

The child may tell of the abuse; disclosure by the child is the usual way by which those caring for the child learn of his plight, accounting for around 60 per cent of recognized cases. An older child may be explicit but a younger child may, for example, complain using age-appropriate language ('I don't like it when Grand-dad puts his sausage in my bum'), or disclose obliquely, for example during play with another child ('Shall I suck your cock like I do for Daddy?').

Children rarely make false allegations, although clearly their testimony requires careful scrutiny, and they do not exaggerate: in fact the usual disclosure is an understatement. False allegations, even of further abuse are in the order of 1–2 per cent, although higher figures have been described in adolescence.[22]

The child may tell of the abuse only when she feels safe from the abuser, who frequently will have used threats to ensure secrecy. Fear of escalating abuse or concern for younger siblings may give the child courage to talk of the abuse.

Sex education lessons at school may precipitate disclosure as the child realizes that what is happening to them is not what every child endures. Conversely, the child may discover as a result of media publicity and the high profile of organizations such as Child Line that many others are suffering abuse as they are, and find the means or the courage to disclose.

A difficult situation arises when carers separate and the child discloses to his mother about her previous partner abusing him. The timing of the disclosure at this time is usually because the child now feels safe but there are, exceptionally, women who will fabricate disclosures.

Children tell their story to someone they trust: their parents, teacher, aunt or, for older children, it may be their GP. The listener should accept the story at face value initially; disbelief at this stage may stop any further disclosure. Later the allegation will be scrutinized in the context of the whole picture and its probity assessed.

Physical symptoms associated with CSA

- *Vaginal bleeding* prepubertally usually signifies trauma and, in the absence of an appropriate history, think of CSA. Straddle injuries are common but on examination the injury is anterior or unilateral and the hymen is not involved.

- *Vaginal discharge* is seen most often in the 3–5-year age group. Microbiological investigations are usually unhelpful: candidal infection is often presumed and 'treated' but is in fact rare. Reassurance and the avoidance of bubble-bath is often all that is needed. Some mothers clean their daughters overzealously and this may itself become abusive.[23] Management may be difficult but it is the mother who needs help: she may be a compulsive 'washer' having a past history of CSA herself.

  Prepubertal vaginal bleeding and *vaginal foreign bodies* have greater specificity for CSA than other physical presenting symptoms. With vaginal foreign bodies, which are rare,[24] there may be an offensive discharge which may also be blood-stained.

  A proportion of children with non-specific discharges will have been abused. Mothers nowadays seem to expect to be asked about the possibility of CSA and may even present the child in the expectation of the question, which will then allow her to express her fears.

- *Sexually transmissible disease* (STD) in childhood is usually sexually acquired. There are, however, cases of vertical transmission, usually manifest during the neonatal period. Table 5.6 illustrates the range, mode of transmission and principal manifestations of perinatally acquired infection. Table 5.7 shows the range of sexually transmissible infections seen in childhood, indicating their incubation periods. It also attempts to weight the probability of CSA being the likely origin of the infection.

- *Dysuria* and 'soreness' not associated with a urinary tract infection is a worry: has the child been rubbed vigorously as in masturbation?

- *Rectal bleeding* is uncommon after infancy (when it is usually associated with fissures caused by constipation) and requires careful investigation. Anal abuse should be in the differential diagnosis.

- *Female genital mutilation*, also (wrongly) called female circumcision, is still practised in some minority ethnic communities in the UK, despite being against the law in this country. It is a mutilation which may have serious consequences, ranging from emotional trauma, to difficulties with micturition, menstruation, intercourse and childbearing, to death. Some girls, usually between the ages of 6 and 12 years, are mutilated by illegal practitioners in the UK: others are sent to their parents' country

Table 5.6 Perinatally acquired infections.

Infective agent	Mode of transmission	Signs/symptoms
Gonorrhoea	Birth canal	Ophthalmia; vaginal discharge (rare)
Trichomonas	Birth canal	Vaginal discharge
Chlamydia	Birth canal	Ophthalmia; pneumonia
Human papilloma virus (warts)	*In utero*; birth canal	Localized lesions, may manifest up to 2 years later (e.g. laryngeal warts)
Herpes simplex 1 and 2	*In utero*; birth canal	Localized lesions; rarely disseminated disease
Bacterial vaginosis	Birth canal	Vaginal discharge
Hepatitis B	*In utero*; birth canal	Hepatitis
HIV	*In utero*; birth canal	AIDS-related infections
Syphilis	*In utero*; birth canal	FTT; signs of secondary syphilis; keratitis; deafness, etc.

FTT, failure to thrive.

of origin for 'a holiday' and are mutilated there. Specialist gynaecological clinics have been set up in parts of the UK to help treat these girls, who may not present until late in their first pregnancy.

Psychological symptoms

- *Psychosomatic symptoms* are common in childhood and the cause of the stress should be sought. Whilst commonly due to family tensions (parental discord; family illness; arrival of a new baby, etc.) or school difficulties (bullying; a new school, class or teacher; performance anxiety, etc.), CSA should be considered.

- *Sexualized play* in preschool children, for example demonstrating oral or anal sex, always requires investigation. Skilled professionals can distinguish between behaviours learned by observation or by involvement in sexual activity.

- *Masturbation.* All children masturbate, but by the age of 3–4 years most have learned to be discreet in the presence of adults: if a child compulsively masturbates a reason should be sought. The reason may be that for whatever reason the child requires this emotional comfort or that he has been masturbated by another and seeks further gratification.

- Distressed children for whatever reason may become *depressed and withdrawn.*

- *Behavioural disturbance* like self-mutilation, repeated overdoses, eating disorders (especially bulimia) are particularly associated with CSA in girls. Boys are more

Table 5.7 Sexually transmissible infections in childhood.

Infective agent	Average incubation period	Signs/symptoms	Probability of CSA
Gonorrhoea	3–4 days	Discharge	+ + +
Trichomonas	1–4 weeks	Discharge	+ + +
Chlamydia	7–14 days	Nil	+ + +
Human papilloma virus	2–3 months	Visible warts, may be sore, itchy or bleed	+
Herpes simplex 1 and 2	2–14 days	Painful sores/ulcers	+ +
Bacterial vaginosis	2–14 days	Discharge	?
Hepatitis B	<3 months	Systemic illness	+ + +
HIV	3 months to convert (majority)	Systemic illness	+ + +
Syphilis	<3 months	Systemic illness	+ + +

1. In infections marked + + +, sexual abuse is highly likely, and consideration of CSA up to and including comprehensive assessment to exclude it should occur in all cases. The diagnosis of a STD prepubertally would in general lead to a child protection investigation.
2. When children or teenagers present with one STD, others should always screened for.
3. Remember to look for oral or anal infection too.

likely to 'act out' and present with conduct disorders. All abused children are at greater risk of early sexual activity with peers and alcohol and substance abuse.[25]

The psychological and emotional presentations of child abuse are discussed in detail in the next chapter. Table 5.8 summarizes the presentation of CSA.

Physical signs of CSA

The physical signs of child sexual abuse depend on the type of abuse, the age of the child, the frequency of the abuse, the time passed since the last assault and the presence of any infection.[10]

Sexual abuse may lead to recognizable patterns of injury. The signs are listed in Table 5.9 and the differential diagnoses in Table 5.10. It is acknowledged that many, if not most, GPs will examine too few children with suspected CSA to feel confident in distinguishing the abnormal from the normal.

Labial fusion is common in infancy and whilst the girl is in nappies. Minor trauma (nappy rash) may cause the surface epithelium to be rubbed off: adjacent denuded tissue is sticky and forms a superficial fusion (or agglutination). If there is more trauma (such as friction) in some forms of CSA, a thicker fusion may be formed, reflecting the greater insult. Tears following forcible rape may result in a thick, long, irregular fusion.

Table 5.8 The presentation of CSA.

1. *The child tells* of the abuse (about 60 per cent of recognized cases)

2. *Physical symptoms*
   - vaginal bleeding prepubertally
   - vaginal discharge
   - vaginal foreign body
   - 'Soreness' +/− dysuria, frequency
   - rectal bleeding

3. *Psychosomatic illness*, e.g. abdominal pain, headache

4. *Behavioural problems*
   - Specific, e.g. sexualized play; obsessive masturbation; sexual precocity; prostitution
   - Non-specific, e.g. anxiety; depression; conduct disorder
   - Substance abuse

Table 5.9 Physical signs associated with CSA.

Injury to penis/scrotum, e.g. bruise, burn, laceration, torn frenulum
Injury to labia, e.g. bruise, burn, laceration
Swelling, erythema of labia minora, hymen
Signs of STD, e.g. discharge, warts
Wide hymenal opening (stretched, attenuated)
Hymenal tears, notches, scars
Widened vagina
Injury to posterior fourchette, e.g. abrasion, tear
Labial fusion (more significance at 3+ years and longer, thicker fusion)
Perianal injury, e.g. bruise, burn, laceration, erythema
Injury to anal margin, e.g. swelling, fissure, scars, laxity
Dilatation of perianal veins
'Reflex' anal dilatation
Signs of physical or emotional abuse or neglect

Some signs such as posterior hymenal tears or the presence of gonorrhoea are diagnostic of abuse; other signs such as erythema, whilst consistent with rubbing, are not more specific than this. Masturbation is a universal phenomenon and may cause some erythema, but not damage to the hymen in prepubertal girls. The use of tampons may cause minimal stretching.

Changing signs following trauma may be due to resolution, i.e. healing; further trauma, i.e. further abuse; or occasionally an evolving disorder, for example, lichen sclerosis.

Injuries to the penis and testes are relatively uncommon, although tears of the foreskin frenulum will occasionally be seen.

Table 5.10 Differential diagnoses of CSA.

Straddle injury
Skin disorder, e.g. lichen sclerosis
Infection, e.g. streptococcal, threadworms
Poor hygiene, e.g. causing erythema
Neurological disorder, e.g. spina bifida causing lax anus
Rarities, e.g. Crohn's disease; haemolytic uraemic syndrome; sacral tumour

In older girls, the breasts must also be examined for injury and bite marks.

Reflex anal dilatation (RAD) is a sign described in all the early forensic textbooks from the time when buggery was illegal. To elicit the sign the child is examined in the left lateral position and the buttocks are gently separated: the examiner observes over 20–30 seconds. In RAD the external sphincter relaxes after 10 seconds or so (which is normal), followed in positive cases by the internal sphincter, which gives a view up to the rectum. When the abuse ceases the sign goes unless the child learns . . . 'to make my bottom big'.

RAD is a dynamic sign, i.e. the sphincter opens and shuts, as compared with severe constipation when large stools may load the rectum and anus and are visible on examination as the external sphincter is stretched around large masses. Acute anal dilatation has also been described in inflammatory bowel disease. Most GPs will not have seen the sign and the same applies to paediatricians. The Cleveland Inquiry found that RAD was abnormal but not proof (i.e. not diagnostic) of abuse.

The physical examination in cases of suspected CSA in prepubertal children is relatively non-invasive, as it chiefly comprises careful visual inspection. Sometimes swabs need to be taken, and some experts make use of graduated glass rods to evaluate hymenal opening dimensions (which may be of use in recognizing minor signs of CSA). There is rarely a case for the digital vaginal examination of prepubertal children; if it is considered essential (after, for example, an acute rape), this may be performed under anaesthetic. After puberty the hymen under the influence of oestrogen becomes thick and redundant. An internal examination is then obligatory in order to see hymenal tears, dilatation, scars, etc.

Examination in cases of suspected CSA is a delicate and sometimes fraught task, which runs the risk of appearing to the child and non-abusing parent as further abuse. The following points should be borne in mind:

- The number of times a child is subjected to examination should be kept to an absolute minimum.

- Building up a relationship with the child and attending parent prior to examination will reduce the distress of the examination and may help in further disclosure (although children disclose when they are ready and not when professionals want them to).

- Anogenital examination should be part of, and be preceded by, a general physical examination and an evaluation of growth and development.

- The examiner requires some expertise in normal/abnormal appearances and findings.

- There should be suitable facilities and equipment for the taking of photographs, screening for STDs and collection of forensic specimens.

- The environment should be child-friendly and the atmosphere quiet and unhurried.

- The child should be accompanied at all times by a suitable chaperone.

- Informed consent is mandatory for examination, photography and investigations: this may be given by a Gillick-competent child or adult with parental responsibility (*see Chapters 3 and 5c*).

- No physical sign can be regarded as uniquely diagnostic of child sexual abuse.

- On the other hand, a normal exam does not prove that no CSA occurred.

The general practitioner's role

From the information given on the presenting history, the past history, family and social history and a general examination, the practitioner will normally in cases of possible CSA seek further advice from a consultant community paediatrician or other paediatrician with a special interest in CSA. This is further discussed in Chapter 5c.

Neglect and failure to thrive (FTT)

Neglect is the most common form of abuse in the UK but often goes unrecognized.[26] The Department of Health defines neglect as 'The persistent failure to meet a child's basic physical and/or psychological needs, likely to result in the serious impairment of the child's health or development. It may involve a parent or carer failing to provide adequate food, shelter and clothing, failing to protect a child from physical harm or danger, or the failure to ensure access to appropriate medical care or treatment. It may also include neglect of, or unresponsiveness to, a child's basic emotional needs'. (para. 2.7)[27]

If the physical needs of a child are not met it is likely that there is, in addition, emotional deprivation and a lack of learning opportunities. The history and examination of a neglected child are listed in Tables 5.11 and 5.12.

Failure to thrive is present when an infant or child fails to achieve the expected growth as assessed by measurements of weight and height. *Only 5 percent of all FTT seen in the UK is due to organic disease* (for example coeliac disease, cystic fibrosis or cyanotic heart disease). A careful history and examination will establish which children require clinical investigations. It is worth checking for iron deficiency anaemia once children are on mixed diets as it is so common and treatment is said to improve the appetite.

Table 5.11 The history of neglect.

Poor antenatal care; preterm; small baby
Substance abuse by carers
Repeated failure to attend child health clinic for health surveillance or immunization
Repeated failure to attend hospital appointments, e.g. for squint; audiology
History of repeated emergency admissions to hospital for, e.g., feeding problems; upper respiratory tract infections; ingestion of drugs; accidents; RTA
Recurrent colds, wheeze, gastroenteritis; cigarettes (passive smoking) are associated with upper respiratory infections and wheeze, and poor hygiene with 'tummy upsets'
Poor growth rate (FTT)
Delayed development, especially speech, social skills
Behavioural problems, e.g. aggressive; withdrawn; poor concentration

Table 5.12 The physical signs of neglect.

Dirty child with poor hair, cradle-cap, yellow nails
Chronic nappy rash
Small stature
Malnourished
Skin infection, conjunctivitis, purulent nasal discharge

However, over 90 per cent of infants who have FTT have non-organic FTT. To thrive optimally a child needs to be loved as well as have an adequate number of calories. FTT frequently occurs in the context of parenting difficulties and there are often attachment problems between the child and his or her carers. The carers become very anxious with their whole lives focused, or so it seems, on feeding. Indeed, the carers may also have a history of eating problems of one sort or another.

FTT and neglect often occur together in the context of poverty and social disadvantage. FTT and emotional deprivation, however, may be seen in socially advantaged families.

Failure to thrive may begin with breastfeeding difficulties in some or weaning problems in others, and the role of a good midwife or health visitor in addressing these early difficulties, and in picking up the attachment difficulties that may underlie them, is vital. Children with difficult, emotionally based feeding problems are best referred early, with their parent(s) to a specialist team.

Uncommonly, food is willfully withheld from children, or adulterated with, for example, salt to make them reject it or vomit. Sometimes, food is simply not available, as a result of poverty or parental incapacity.

More than with any other form of child abuse, there is a strong association between social deprivation and poverty, and neglect. We know that for a child to grow optimally, they need love and attention, as well as the right food. The impact of emotional deprivation and abuse can be devastating in many ways, as Judith Trowell discusses in Chapter 5b. But poverty undoubtedly makes the already difficult task of parenting much more so. Children may already be disadvantaged if their parents' capacity to care for them is limited by physical or mental illness, by disability or substance abuse. The commonly impoverishing consequences of this further limits the opportunities for these children to develop to anything like their full potential.

Adequate parental income; access to nurseries and quality schooling; safe play areas; dry, warm and safe housing; affordable healthy food; an accessible, proactive health service: these are some of the needs that every child has. These needs are the responsibility of a caring society.

References

1 **Browne KD.** Child abuse: defining, understanding, and intervening. In: Wilson K, James A, eds. *The Child Protection Handbook.* London: Balliere Tindall, 1995: 43–64.

2 **NCH Action for Children.** *The Hidden Victims: Children and Domestic Violence.* London: National Children's Home (NCH), 1994.

3 **Casey M.** *Domestic Violence Against Women: the Women's Perspective.* Dublin: Social Psychology Research Unit, UCD, 1989.

4 **Morgan D,** ed. *Domestic Violence: a Health Care Issue?* London: British Medical Association, 1998.

5 **Department of Health.** *HIV and Infant Feeding.* Revised guidance from the Expert Advisory Group on AIDS. London: DOH, 2001.

6 **National Society for the Prevention of Cruelty to Children (NSPCC).** *Child Maltreatment in the United Kingdom: a Study of the Prevalence of Child Abuse and Neglect.* London: NSPCC, 2000.

7 **Creighton SJ, Noyes P.** *Child Abuse Trends in England and Wales 1983–87.* London: NSPCC, 1989.

8 **Smith M, Bee P, Heverin A, Nobes G.** *Parental Control Within the Family: the Nature and Extent of Parental Violence to Children.* London: Thomas Coram Research Unit, 1995. (Quoted in *Child Protection: Messages from Research.* London: HMSO, 1995.)

9 **Hobbs CJ, Hanks HGI, Wynne JM.** *Child Abuse and Neglect: a Clinician's Handbook,* 2nd edn. London: Churchill Livingstone, 1999.

10 **Hobbs CJ, Wynne JM.** *Physical Signs of Child Abuse: a Colour Atlas,* 2nd edn. London: Saunders, 2001.

11 **Chapman S.** Recent Advances in the Radiology of Child Abuse. In: Hobbs CJ, Wynne JM, eds. *Child Abuse.* London: Balliere Tindall, 1993: 1063–5.

12 **Emery JL.** Cot death and child abuse. In: Hobbs CJ, Wynne JM, eds. *Child Abuse.* London: Balliere Tindall, 1993: Chapter 12.

13 **Hobbs CJ, Wynne JM.** The sexually abused battered child. *Archive of Disease in Childhood* 1990; **65:** 423–7.

14 **Klineman PK.** *Diagnostic Imaging of Child Abuse.* Baltimore: Williams & Wilkins, 1987.

15 **Butler-Sloss E.** *Report of the Inquiry into Child Abuse in Cleveland 1987.* London: HMSO, 1988.

16 **McClure RJ, Davis PM, Meadow SR, Sibert JR.** Epidemiology of Munchausen syndrome by proxy: non-accidental poisoning and non-accidental suffocation. *Archives of Disease in Childhood* 1996; **75:** 57–61.

17 **Department of Health, Home Office, Department for Education and Skills.** Safeguarding Children in Whom Illness is Induced or Fabricated by Carers with Parenting Responsibilities. *Supplementary Guidance to Working Together to Safeguard Children.* London: Stationery Office, 2001.

18 **Jones DPH, Bools CN.** Factitious illness by proxy. In: David TJ, ed. *Recent Advances in Paediatrics,* vol. 17. London: Churchill Livingstone, 1999: 57–71.

19 Schechter MD, Roberge L. Sexual exploitation. In: Helfer RE, Kempe CH, eds. *Child Abuse and Neglect: the Family and the Community*. Cambridge, MA: Ballinger, 1976: 102–10.

20 Baker A, Duncan S. Child sexual abuse: a study of prevalence in Great Britain. *Child Abuse and Neglect*, 1985; **9**: 457–67.

21 Kelly L, Regan L, Burton S. *An exploratory Study of the Prevalence of Child Sexual Abuse in a Sample of 18–21 year olds*. London: University of North London, 1991.

22 Jones PH, *Child Sexual Abuse: Informing Practice from Research*. Oxford: Radcliffe Medical Press, 1999.

23 Herman Giddens ME. Harmful genital practices in children. *JAMA* 1989; **261** (4): 577–9.

24 Herman Giddens ME. Vaginal foreign bodies and child sexual abuse. *Archives of Paediatric and Adolescent Medicine* 1994; **148**: 195–200.

25 Hanks H, Stratton P. Family perspectives on early sexual abuse. In: Browne KD, ed. *Early Prediction and Prevention of Child Abuse*. Chichester: Wiley, 1988: 244–64.

26 Wynne JM, ed. Failure to thrive. *Child* 22 (4) (Suppl.): 219–82.

27 Department of Health, Home Office, Department of Education and Employment, the National Assembly for Wales. *Working Together to Safeguard Children: A Guide for Interagency Working to Safeguard and Promote the Welfare of Children*. London: Department of Health, 1999.

Chapter 5b

Psychological and emotional presentations of child abuse

Judith Trowell

Introduction

Uncertainty, muddle and confusion continue to surround this subject. Although mental health or mental well-being are acknowledged as important, the question has to be asked: does society have a commitment to the psychological and emotional health of its children?

Officially, the answer would be in the affirmative. The UK government is a signatory to the UN Convention on the Rights of the Child, including the right (Article 3) to 'such protection and care as is necessary for his or her well being'. There is also the Children Act (1989) which states clearly (Part 1.1) that, 'The child's welfare shall be the Court's paramount consideration' and (Part 3) 'a court shall have regard, in particular, to (a) the ascertainable wishes and feelings of the child concerned (considered in the light of his age and understanding) and (b) his physical, emotional and educational needs'.

Why then the scepticism? In recent years, rising expectations and rising living standards have led to a recognition that children are different from adults and that they need their childhood. They need the time to grow and develop physically, socially, emotionally, psychologically and educationally. At the same time, there is a wish not to know about, not to recognize that there are many distressed and troubled children and that some of these children are in this state because of abuse. Family life and growing up are stressful: life events, physical and mental illness in parent or child, poverty and deprivation can make it more so. But, in addition, some of our children are struggling to survive what Gabarino[1] uses as his definition of child abuse: 'Acts of omission or commission (of parent or guardian) that are judged by a mixture of community values and professional expertise to be inappropriate or damaging'.

Thus defined, child abuse is a matter of judgement, requiring professionals to make value judgements on behalf of society. Hence, it follows that the threshold of what constitutes abuse varies and so the level of acceptable distress varies. This explains the uncertainty and the problems over recognition, assessment and diagnosis, particularly of emotional and psychological aspects of abuse.

What is child abuse?

Child abuse covers a broad spectrum of child maltreatment: physical abuse and physical neglect; sexual abuse; emotional abuse and neglect; psychological abuse and neglect; parent-induced illness (Munchausen syndrome/factitious illness by proxy) and deliberate child poisoning. I would suggest that, unless life threatening, the damage inflicted by these abusive events inheres not so much in what happens to the child's physical body but what happens in the child's mind, to the child's emotional, psychological and social development.

And yet as professionals, we are swept along by the child protection process, the legal process, the need to prove or disprove that 'abuse' has occurred. Even if we avoid total preoccupation by this all too often fruitless pursuit, 'partnership with parents' and now 'family support' become other diversions to blind us from seeing the distress of the child. Of course, most children rightly grow up in their families and, when there are difficulties, working with parents to help and support them in their difficult task is vital, *but it must not blind us to the child.* After the Jasmine Beckford inquiry[2], Louis Blom-Cooper wrote in his report:

> Throughout the three years of social work with the Beckfords, Ms Walstrom totally misconceived her role as the field worker enforcing care orders in respect of two very young children at risk. Her gaze focused on Beverly Lorrington and Morris Beckford; she averted her eyes from the children to be aware of them only as and when they were with their parents, hardly even to observe their development, and never to communicate with Jasmine on her own.

This could all too easily be written about any of us as we hurry through our daily work routine. After all, it is so much easier not to see, particularly as there are no clear nationally agreed definitions, no specific tests or criteria that can assist us. Concerns usually arise because there are a number of symptoms and behaviours that come together, like pieces of a jigsaw. If they make a certain picture, if there is a certain pattern, then it is appropriate to think seriously about child abuse.

It is vital to bear in mind during this process issues of race, culture and religion. Child development is a universal process but most research has been conducted with specific racial and cultural groups and the implications for children in terms of what is acceptable behaviour and how emotions are expressed in their culture or religion must be understood before judgements can be made.

In order to think about the emotional and psychological consequences of abuse, it may be helpful to start by considering emotional and psychological abuse themselves. O'Hagen[3] made a good attempt to define these. Emotion is about feelings and expressing feeling adequately and appropriately, hence, O'Hagen defines emotional abuse as:

> the sustained, repetitive, inappropriate emotional response to the child's expression of emotion, and its accompanying expressive behaviour.

Psychological development is about cognition and intelligence, about memory, about perception and attention, language development, and the development of a moral code. Hence, O'Hagen[3] defines psychological abuse as:

> sustained, repetitive, inappropriate behaviour which damages or substantially reduces, the creative and developmental potential of crucially important mental faculties and mental process of the child. These include intelligence, memory recognition, perception, attention, language and moral development.

When confronted by a particular child or young person, these definitions can perhaps serve to alert us and may be helpful in reminding us of the areas that need to be considered when, for example, writing a report for a case conference or court. What is clearly needed for a more comprehensive assessment is a perspective that bears these definitions in mind but that can also incorporate child development, attachment, parenting capacity, physical development, issues of disability and contextual issues (the child in his/her family, in their social setting paying attention to race, culture, gender and religion).

Assessment

An assessment needs to consider the pervasiveness of the problems, the persistence and inflexibility of parenting patterns and the evidence of damage to the child—that is, significant harm.

There has been recent recognition of the problems and concerns over the complexity of assessing children and their families and this has lead to further guidance from the Department of Health (DOH). *Working Together to Safeguard Children*[4] acknowledges more strongly than before the multidisciplinary, multiagency roles in the assessment process. The role of health professionals has been stressed much more strongly, and there is more clarity about the collaboration required from health professionals with the police and social services. There are general instructions (paras 3.18, 3.19) and then the specific requirements for each sector, such as 'Primary Care Groups and Primary Care Trusts', 'General Practitioners and the Primary Health Care Teams', 'Mental Health' and 'Child' and 'Family Mental Health'. The crucial role of GPs and the primary care team in recognizing possible abuse and alerting other agencies is stressed, as is attendance by general practitioners at case conferences and involvement in child protection training. Issues of confidentiality are explored, and also the implication of the introduction of the Human Rights Act in October 2000. Disclosure of information to safeguard children is considered to be exempt from the right to privacy for the individual and his family provided the concerns are appropriate.

The DOH has also produced the *Framework for the Assessment of Children in Need and their Families*[5]. This is a well written, helpful document outlining the areas that need to be covered, Child development is emphasized, and also the importance of *attachments*. It encourages professionals to look at education, emotional and behavioural development, identity, family and social relationships, social presentation, emotional warmth, stimulation, stability and family functioning. However, it does not set out how these assessments are to be conducted and given the broad areas outlined, the social workers who are likely to be undertaking or commissioning the assessments do not have much guidance on how to proceed. There is an assumption that the assessing team are highly trained, highly skilled staff who have a thorough grasp of all the concepts. Supplementary assessment forms are likely to be essential for the implementation of this excellent framework and implementation will depend on the quality of these forms and the level of training and skills of the professionals involved.

One model for looking at the emotional environment of children is that which has evolved out of the Expressed Emotion test. This looked at the interaction, verbal and non-verbal, between family members as recorded on videotape. More recently, it has proved possible to obtain almost comparable data by asking a family member, such as the mother, to talk for 5 minutes about the child in question. This account is audiotaped. The video or audiotapes are rated for expressed emotions; the dimensions rated are high or low warmth, and high or low criticism. Low warmth and high criticism were found to predict recurrent breakdown in young schizophrenics. These dimensions are found to be very helpful in looking at the parent–child relationship, particularly alerting professionals to the possibility of emotional or psychological abuse.

Harm can also be defined[6] as seen in Figure 5.1.

When looking at the individual child, the factors listed in Table 5.13 need to be assessed and explored. Those in the left column are highlighted because we all too easily make instant judgements about individuals (the 30 second assessment!) and unless we thoughtfully and carefully check all initial perceptions, our decision-making can become

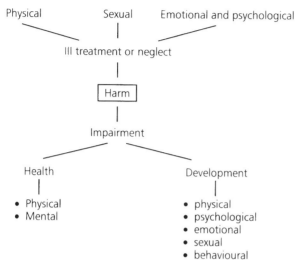

Fig. 5.1 'Significance Harm' causes and outcome.[6]

Table 5.13 Assessment factors.

Race	Physical health
Culture	Medical history
Class	Mental state
Language	Communication capacity
Disability	Behaviour
Intellectual capacity	Family composition
	Attachments
	Social relationships
	School issues
	Life events
	Religion

biased or distorted. The right-hand column we usually recognize takes more time, but the length highlights the complexity, all the strands that need to come together as we begin to consider if child abuse is a possibility.

Attachment theory and understanding of attachment is particularly helpful in making sense of a child's behaviour. Children come into the world seeking relationships, emotional interaction and proximity. By their behaviour such as smiling, crying, eye contact, babbling and seeking physical contact they elicit caregiving, usually from the mother or father—their primary attachment figure. They may also have secondary attachment figures. These attachments are separate from the need for food, warmth, shelter, etc.

The majority of children (about 63 per cent[7]) develop secure attachments. Insecure attachments are shown by most of the remainder, These are in two forms—*anxious insecure* where the child clings to the adult on separation and becomes very distressed, or *avoidant insecure* where on separation from a primary attachment figure the child appears externally to be indifferent but, in reality, is distressed, emotionally, as shown by physiological measures such as the galvanic skin response (GSR) which measures the extent of sweating in different situations. If the key figure really has left the child, then the child's distress is overwhelming. There is another group of insecurely attached children who show what is called *disorganized attachment,* who on separation show episodes of behaviour such as freezing, or engage in some repetitive activity, e.g. flapping their hands. A small group of children have a form of attachment—*reactive attachment disorder* (DSM-IV[8])—where they do not respond appropriately to interaction and stimuli or are indiscriminately responsive.

Exploratory behaviour is a component of attachment behaviour. Securely attached children play and explore with toys and are creative; securely attached older children and young people play with ideas and their imagination. Insecurely attached children engage in more concrete repetitive play, have limited creativity and take fewer risks in their exploration.

Assessment of a child's attachment can, therefore, be very helpful. A securely attached child may become distressed if the attachment figure leaves the room, but when the person returns, the child's distress quickly settles and the child will play using the toys creatively and continue to explore. An insecure child may use the toys provided but often there is a repetitive quality to the play or it may be quite sterile, picking things up or putting them down. When the attachment figure leaves, the child may be distressed or not (anxious or avoidant) and when the person returns the distress persists, the anxious child tending to cling, an avoidant child watchful and preoccupied with the attachment figure, neither able to resume their own spontaneous play.

Children who have been abused are more likely to show forms of insecure or disorganized attachments, although such attachment behaviours are not diagnostic. Paradoxically (and often confusingly for the professionals involved), these same children may cling frantically to their abuser, or may be desperate to return home from care. If this is seen as a manifestation of an insecure or disorganized attachment, then the child's behaviour is more easily understood.

Emotional and psychological consequences

So what are the important consequences that need to be taken seriously? They tend to group together in certain clusters, some children showing them all, some one specific cluster.

Psychological consequences

Many children who are being abused, by whatever means, lose the capacity to think, to make links. Perhaps it can be understood as a way of reducing the mental pain; the child stops thinking about what is happening, perhaps by denial or dissociation. But the consequence of this is that other thinking and memory is damaged. These children and young people have considerable problems in concentrating and their attention span is limited. All this leads to problems in school, an inability to learn or a fall-off in school performance. Memory, language and academic performance are poor. This may be in children of average or above average capacities. Children with disabilities are more likely to be abused than able-bodied children and in children with pre-existing learning difficulties where abuse is occurring, there can be a further decline in their level of functioning.

Emotional consequences

Where children are being abused, they can display a range of emotional responses. The child may present as flat and depressed, withdrawn and unresponsive, cut off and avoidant, or the child or young person may be defiant, rude, angry and aggressive.

Younger children may have suicidal thoughts and may make attempts to injure themselves, e.g. with plastic bags over their heads or skipping ropes around their necks. *But many of these children do not tell anyone about these thoughts and feelings unless they are asked directly.* Asking does not put the thoughts into their minds, they are there already and probably have been for some time.

Older children may self-harm by cutting or overdosing: many of these young people, if asked, will talk about the abuse they are experiencing. Older children may also run away from home or may take alcohol or illegal substances, presumably to escape from the abusive situation.

Many abused children have symptoms that come within the diagnosis of *post-traumatic stress disorder* (PTSD). This includes *flashbacks* where the child feels as though the abuse is happening all over again, right now. A child being interviewed by me suddenly became distraught and started screaming at me 'you hit me, you hit me, why did you hit me, don't hit me'. I felt very shaken and shocked and realized, alone in the room with this child, I was in a vulnerable position. With her foster mother in the room with us, we were able to establish that it had at that moment felt as though I had actually hit her, although now she knew I had not. She added that at that moment I looked just like her mother.

Re-experiencing can also happen. The child or young person goes over and over the abuse in their mind, unable to push the thoughts, feelings and sensations out of their mind. These preoccupying experiences may explain some of the child's inability to concentrate as well as their difficulties in responding appropriately to friends, teachers and others.

Abused children may be *hypervigilant* and watchful, constantly on the alert to monitor both the emotional environment in case tension is building up in their carers and also needing to judge when they may need to take avoiding action. This alertness results in *hyperarousal*: the child or young person is easily startled, easily becomes very distressed in response to small problems or when anything reminds them of the abuse.

Abused children may be very *anxious*—this may be shown as anxiety itself where the child is fearful and apprehensive or the child may be *phobic* or *obsessional*. Many abused child experience panic attacks when suddenly, for no obvious reason, they develop a tachycardia, sweating, tremor, breathlessness and may feel faint.

Many abused children lack energy and are very tired. This may be because they are having insufficient sleep because of the actual abuse, but it may be because of sleep problems. Many lie awake for hours, others wake early in the mornings and may be afraid to fall asleep either because they might then be abused (sexual abuse) or because of the terrifying dreams they may have. These may be nightmares or they may be repeats of the abuse (part of PTSD) that recur as dreams.

But, perhaps, the most painful and difficult consequences are their feeling of betrayal and rage with their abuser and also their feeling about the non-abusing parent who did not protect them or did not realize what was happening. The rage and the hate are powerful, the underlying pain excruciating. The child is left with enormous doubt, with low self-esteem, seeing themselves as bad, as damaged, as rubbish and often guilty, blaming themselves—did they bring it on themselves, was it their fault?

Mental health consequences

A small number of children and young people may develop mental health problems. *Anorexia nervosa* and *bulimia* may occur. Some of the young people presenting with these conditions have been sexually abused, whilst some of the others have been abused in other ways. Welch and Fairbairn[9] discuss the link between anorexia, bulimia and childhood sexual and physical abuse. They suggest that earlier reports[10] of a quarter of eating disordered children having experienced sexual abuse may be excessive and that the causation is multifactorial. The overall conclusion is that family variables, and emotional and psychological factors play a significant part in the complex etiological relationship that leads to eating disorders.

Some children become profoundly *depressed* so that they are clinically depressed. Many children develop *dysthymia* (low mood) even where there is no clinical depression and many experience anxiety, particularly *separation anxiety*. Other children and young people may, perhaps because of innate vulnerability, develop some features of *psychosis*, but usually these can be understood as aspects of PTSD such as, 'flashbacks' and 're-experiencing phenomena'. It must be remembered that for the child and those around, these can be very frightening and the fear of 'madness' can exacerbate the problem.

Some abused children also develop *gender identity* problems, perhaps with confusion about their own gender or the gender of the partner they might choose to select. Many of these children and young people need help because they are left uncertain if their sexual orientation is theirs from choice or if the abuse influenced it.

Physical consequences

The body is not separate from the psyche or from feelings, so there are also physical consequences. The most obvious is *non-organic failure to thrive* in babies and small children or psychological dwarfism. But there are other physical consequences worth noting: the child who is inappropriately dressed or whose clothes somehow do not seem to fit; the child whose hair or skin looks scruffy or uncared for; the child with dark rings under their eyes; or the child who is inappropriately instantly familiar (this may involve touching, coming very close, seeking affection or sexualized behaviour).

It also needs to be remembered that children with physical disabilities are more likely to be abused and this needs sensitive exploration. Deaf children who may have language difficulties are particularly vulnerable, and it is important to arrange for an interpreter who can sign to be present.

Conclusion

All of these presentations can lead one to the view that abuse is everywhere. This is not so. What is important is to remember that some children and young people are being abused and if there are a number of these problems or symptoms, then abuse must be considered as part of the differential diagnosis. The child or young person themself may be able to talk about what is happening or may show it in their play. At other times there may be a need for a multidisciplinary team assessment to look at the whole child to try and understand.

As part of this, it is essential to clarify the child's race, culture and religion, in order to make sure the context is understood. It is often very helpful to have an advisor as part of the team who is familiar with the cultural and religious issues.

The psychological and emotional consequences persist long after the abuse may have ceased. It is important not only to recognize these consequences but also to ensure that those children that need help receive it. The children and young people who cause society problems often demand help from one agency or another—the angry, antisocial, aggressive ones, the anorexics or parasuicides. But the sad, depressed, anxious, tearful, underfunctioning children are often left sitting silently in their classrooms. No one is aware of their pain, their suffering, and no one questions why they are not learning. These are the parents of tomorrow who will have relationship problems and who are likely to lack parenting skills and who may well go on to abuse or fail to protect their children.

References

1 Gabarino J. The elusive crime of emotional abuse. *Child Abuse and Neglect* 1978; 2: 89–99.

2 Blom-Cooper L. *The Jasmine Beckford Inquiry.* London: Borough of Brent, 1985.

3 O'Hagen K. *Emotional and Psychological Abuse of Children.* Buckingham: Open University Press, 1993.

4 Department of Health, Home Office, Department of Education and Employment and the National Assembly for Wales. *Working Together to Safeguard Children: a Guide for Interagency Working to Safeguard and Promote the Welfare of Children.* London: Department of Health, 1999.

5 Department of Health. *Framework for the Assessment of Children in Need and their Families.* London: Stationery Office, American Psychiatric Association, Washington DC, 1999.

6 White R, Adcock M, Hollows A. *Significant Harm.* Significant Press, Croydon, UK, 1991.

7 Bretherton I, Waters E. *Growing Points of Attachment.* Monograph of the Society for Research in the Child Development, Vol. 50, University of Chicago Press, Chicago, USA, 1985.

8 American Psychiatric Association. *Diagnostic Criteria from DSM-IV.* Diagnostic and Statistical Manual of Mental Disorders. 1994.

9 Welch S, Fairbairn C. Childhood Sexual and Physical Abuse as Risk Factors for the Development of Bulimia Nervosa: a Community-based Case Control Study. *Child Abuse and Neglect* 1996; 20 (7): 633–42.

10 Oppenheimer R, Howells K, Palmer R, Chaloner D. Adverse sexual experiences in childhood and clinical eating disorders: a preliminary description. *Journal of Psychiatric Research* 1985; 19: 357–61.

Chapter 5c

Child abuse and general practice 1: prevention and presentation

Stephen Amiel

Introduction

In Chapters 5a and 5b, Wynne and Trowell have emphasized the many ways in which child abuse may come to be suspected by, or may present to, the general practitioner and the primary health care team. As well as evaluating the significance of various symptoms and signs, and the *context* of the presentation (appropriateness, timeliness, affect of the child and carer, etc.), they stress the importance of assessing the *background* to a presenting event (past history, family history, social circumstances, etc.). Few cases of child abuse within the family occur in isolation as a one-off act of violence or neglect, and they make clear that the early detection of abuse and often its prevention depend crucially on an awareness of an individual child's background and an understanding of the clinical and social pointers which may indicate increased risk.

In Chapter 3, we argued that the general practitioner and the primary health care team are in many ways ideally placed to identify all forms of family violence and neglect at an early stage, as well as to play an important role in their prevention. We also, on the other hand, identified weaknesses and threats that could, and often do, get in the way of this. In this chapter and Chapter 5d, I will try to set what Wynne and Trowell have written in the context of the realities of general practice, and in so doing attempt to set out an approach that is proactive, safe and practicable. These chapters will address:

- the *prevention* and *early identification* of abuse and potentially abusive situations that may present in general practice;

- appropriate *initial action* commensurate with the nature and severity of the suspected abuse or risk of abuse.

I will draw on and hopefully adequately reflect current thinking on best practice, but attention is drawn to the fact that there are often local guidelines and protocols that may interpret certain things somewhat differently. *General practitioners and primary health care teams should be in possession of current local child protection guidelines and are urged to consult these.* These guidelines are produced by the local Area Child Protection Committee (ACPC) and can normally be obtained from relevant officers in social service departments, or sometimes through the Primary Care Trust (PCT) or equivalent locality organization. In addition, some health authorities/boards have themselves produced guides for their area's primary health care teams (PHCTs) that both reflect local practice and inform of local resources. With the changing status of health authorities in 2002, these responsibilities are likely to be devolved to PCT level.

Whatever local variations might apply, however, there are basic principles that cannot be reiterated too often. These principles should underpin any involvement in child protection matters, at any level of engagement, by any member of the PHCT. They are:

- The child's interests come first.

- Relevant information should be shared with other authorized childcare professionals.

- Concerns about possible abuse must be acted on: no action is not an option.

None of these principles is easy to apply in practice. They all have ramifications for the child, family and the health professional that may seem to conflict with other obligations, duties, rights and relationships. And how can one reliably ascertain what is in a child's best interests, especially when the outcome for a family sucked into the child protection process (including the child themselves) may be so poor? How much information about a child or family member can legitimately be considered relevant, and should it be offered unsolicited, or only given when specifically asked for? What constitutes a sufficient level of concern to trigger a referral?

Whilst no-one can pretend that interpretation of anything is easy in child protection, the practitioner does at least have some guiding principles to measure the consequences of their actions or non-actions against. And, whilst most general practitioners are, at the time of writing, still independent contractors, bound by a national contract that does not specify particular procedures with regard to child protection, it would be difficult in practice to justify actions that are counter to those principles.

The joint commissioning and provision of primary health and social care by PCTs and their likely successor organizations, Care Trusts, will inevitably lead to the work of all primary care practitioners being more informed by considerations previously the exclusive preserve of social services. With the advent of clinical governance procedures applying to all practitioners and PHCT members, child protection guidelines and protocols are likely to be more rigorously drawn and expected to be applied. They will certainly be in place sooner rather than later for salaried GPs employed by PCTs and for GPs who have agreed contracts with PCTs to provide personal medical services (PMS) to their local population.

Many GPs may welcome increased guidance and it would be natural in an area as difficult as this to want to take shelter behind a protocol that could not be strayed from. There will always be grey areas, though, around the edges of any protocol, however well drawn up, and the thoughtful practitioner will often still worry if they have got it wrong, in one of several respects:

- Failing to recognize abuse—the false negative diagnosis.

- Wrongly identifying something as abuse—the false positive diagnosis.

- Recognizing a risk of abuse but failing to do enough about it.

- Recognizing abuse or a risk of abuse and acting on it inappropriately, causing more damage.

Failing to recognize abuse—the false negative diagnosis

At the risk of being provocative, I would suggest that all of us fail to recognize abuse more often than not. Abuse is often prolonged over months or even years by the time it comes to the notice of a statutory agency. Most abused children, and/or their carers, will have been seen on a number of occasions over that period by members of the PCHT as well as by other professionals. Often they will have presented in ways similar to those described by Wynne and Trowell; presentations that are clearly—in retrospect—warning signs or early indicators of abuse or neglect. Yet GP practices are infrequent initiators of child protection referrals, and when they are it is almost always after a disclosure by a child or carer.[1] No-one is suggesting that every single warning sign justifies a referral: as has been emphasized above and elsewhere, the judgement that abuse has occurred or is likely to occur is usually a cumulative one. Undoubtedly, however, there could and should be in general practice, as well as in other organizations in regular contact with children, a significant left shift towards earlier diagnosis.

Wrongly identifying something as abuse—the false positive diagnosis

Child abuse must be one of the few conditions (death is perhaps another) where doctors worry more about making a false positive diagnosis than a false negative one. This is hardly surprising given the publicity around the Cleveland and Orkney inquiries, the 'false memory syndrome' controversy, etc. The fear of public opprobrium, let alone the increasing fear of private litigation, is a real and powerful one. At the very least, no GP wishes to jeopardize the well-being of a family and his or her relationship with that family by subjecting them to an unjustified child protection inquiry. I suggest that this view, though understandable, can cloud the practitioner's judgement to the detriment of a child genuinely at risk.

First, it does not adequately take into account the changing nature of child protection enquiries, where greater efforts than before are being made by social services departments to focus on meeting what may be a multiplicity of needs rather than on exposing and punishing a perpetrator of an abusive incident. Even the change in terminology, from child protection 'investigations' to 'inquiries', is indicative of this attempt to stigmatize less and support more.

Secondly, as I shall discuss further below, referring a child to social services because a child is deemed to be suffering or at risk of suffering abuse need not necessarily result in a breakdown in the relationship between general practitioner and family, even if those suspicions are not substantiated.

Thirdly, just because abuse is not substantiated, it does not mean that abuse has not occurred. The practitioner may be right, but like the abused children themselves, may not be heard or believed at first.

And finally, as Meadow observes,[2] 'All doctors make errors in their diagnoses, and if one never made a false positive diagnosis of a common condition one would certainly be failing on many occasions to diagnose it.'

Recognizing a risk of abuse but failing to do enough about it

The challenge for the PHCT is, as Wynne says, 'to recognize the family which is struggling, to offer appropriate support but, if the carers' behaviour becomes abusive, *to name the abuse*' (p. 87). Naming implies acknowledgement both to oneself and to others that abuse is a possibility, and then following through the process and the consequences until, at the very least, one is satisfied that the child is safe. Public inquiry after inquiry has shown how often this does not happen, and I am painfully aware from my own practice how easily a child, even where an abusive situation is predicted or recognized as actually occurring, can still slip through the net.

In some ways, the inaction of the professional stems from responses that seem to mirror those of the abused child who does not tell of their own abuse:

- a misguided sense of loyalty or fear of breaking a confidence;
- learned helplessness and hopelessness ('there's no point in telling social services, they never do anything about it');
- frozen watchfulness (the fear that abuse is occurring or might occur is cancelled out by the fear of exposing it);
- accepting the situation as somehow normal. A particular family or even a subsection of society is seen as beyond redemption or alternatively, as 'dirty, smelly but happy',[3] in the face of obvious and sometimes gross emotional abuse and neglect. (The professional's desire not to impose their own often middle class standards on their patients/clients can result in the most extraordinary, albeit well-intentioned, distortions of perception);
- the sense that, however bad the situation might be, the alternatives are worse (sentiments which find uncomfortable echoes in the children's homes scandals uncovered in North Wales and elsewhere[4]).

Recognizing abuse or a risk of abuse and acting on it inappropriately

Compared with what follows, getting to the stage of recognizing a risk situation or abuse itself may seem like the easy bit, especially when, as has been said above, the child or carer usually presents the practitioner with a diagnosis or allegation. The fresh abysses that then open up include:

- saying the wrong thing or saying too much, too soon to the child or accompanying carer;
- saying too much to the right people—exceeding guidelines on the limits of confidentiality;
- saying anything to the wrong people—insufficient regard to the 'need to know' principle, or misunderstanding of parental responsibility;
- doing too little or too much in terms of physical examination or investigation;
- doing things too quickly: making a referral to a statutory agency when a more informal approach or period of observation or reflection might be more appropriate;
- keeping inadequate records.

These pitfalls—and how to avoid them—will be looked at further in this section and the next, as the prevention, early identification and initial responses to child abuse are considered.

Prevention and early identification of abuse

The skills, techniques and procedures that the GP deploys every day in the diagnosis and initial management of any illness also form the cornerstone for the identification of child abuse or a potentially abusive situation.

In making any diagnosis some or all of the following processes will occur (not necessarily in this order, and not necessarily consecutively). In reality, the listening, thinking, examination and supplementary questioning often overlap, as the patient and practitioner circle around a problem, returning, clarifying, beginning again after a false start, and so on:

1. Listening to the patient.
2. Thinking the thought—could this story mean x or y?
3. Asking supplementary questions.
4. Performing an examination.
5. Initiating relevant investigations.
6. Reviewing the previous medical history.
7. Considering relevant social/family circumstances.

When applying this familiar framework to child abuse or potential child abuse, there are some particular points for the GP or team member to consider (see also Chapters 5a, 5b and 8a).

Listening to the patient

The story that a child or carer tells is always important and may be the most powerful indicator of abuse. There will be an opportunity for questions later, but allowing time for an uninterrupted account may be crucial. It also allows for a statement to be made by the child or carer that can be taken down verbatim: this may be very important at a later stage. The listener should encourage openness by their manner, which should be calm, unhurried and non-judgemental. This is one of those occasions where the rest of the waiting room may have to be forgotten for a while: disclosures or allegations are often made only after a long period of agonizing and are difficult and distressing to put into words. The child or carer may well test the listener with oblique remarks or apparently trivial calling card complaints before feeling safe enough to disclose. Children and non-abusing carers may be intimidated by an unsympathetic manner to the point of staying silent again for months or years.

Unsustainable promises of secrecy should not, however, be made to encourage a disclosure of abuse. Someone wishing to reveal or allege abuse may well preface their remarks by saying something like, 'This won't go any further, will it?' They have to be told that any information they give may have to be shared with other professionals on a need to know basis in the interests of the child. With careful explanation of what might ensue, the limits of confidentiality will often be accepted.

Listening to *what* is said in the consultation should also include paying attention to the *way* things are said (accompanying affect and demeanour, whether they sound rehearsed or coerced, interaction with accompanying adult, etc.); and to the things that are left *unsaid*. Spaces between words and silences can be every bit as eloquent. Where appropriate these non-verbal aspects too should be recorded.

Thinking the thought—could there be abuse?

The kind of holistic listening described above itself becomes a diagnostic tool when a presentation falls short of a disclosure or allegation. Equally important is the willingness to include child abuse or a potentially abusive situation as part of a differential diagnosis. The many physical and emotional symptoms with which abuse may present can easily be passed off innocently and treated at face value. The dissembling account or behaviour of a carer or child may combine with the unwillingness of the listener to confront the possibility of abuse: an unintentionally collusive relationship results and an opportunity is missed.

The possibility of an abusive situation existing for a child should also always be considered whenever a vulnerable adult who is also a carer is seen. It should be routine for the practitioner to be aware if an adult with any significant risk factor (see pp. 86–87) has dependent children and, where necessary, to know what support systems might be in place for those children. Adult mental health services, accident and emergency departments, drug dependency units, etc. are not always as thorough as they might be in making these connections. It can be a vital preventative measure to communicate concerns within the practice team and with other agencies when a vulnerable adult who is also a carer deteriorates or is exposed to new stresses (such as a new pregnancy, relationship breakdown, homelessness, etc.). Consideration should be given within the practice to a system of tagging the notes, not just of the vulnerable child, but also of the vulnerable adult carers. The implementation and implications of a tagged notes system will be discussed later in this chapter.

Much has been made in this book and elsewhere of the background to abuse and how it may often occur within a context of multiple disadvantage and need. As will be further discussed below, appropriate consideration of this context, and intervention to ameliorate it, may be crucial in the prevention, early detection and secondary mitigation of abuse and neglect. It should none the less be borne in mind that abuse of all kinds can and does occur in families ostensibly with *none* of these risk factors. The practitioner should be alert to the natural prejudices that tend to make us all less suspicious of people who we think we know well, who we like, or who are more like ourselves.

Finally, it should be acknowledged that for some practitioners, the thought that a child may be being abused, let alone confronting that abuse openly, raises difficult emotional issues, possibly relating to their own backgrounds. General practitioners are notoriously badly supported in their working lives and tend to neglect their own health and emotional needs. One possibly beneficial outcome of the clinical governance process in primary care could be the setting up of small support groups where the emotional toll on the practitioner of child protection work can be addressed.

Asking supplementary questions

A distinction needs to be made between asking supplementary questions to support a diagnosis as a guide for what to do next, and a comprehensive initial interview that may form the basis for action by a statutory agency.

Where there is an initial unambiguous disclosure from a child, especially of sexual abuse, further questioning should be kept to a minimum, although the child who wishes to have a full discussion should clearly be allowed to do so. In child sexual abuse, the clinical interview might be the most important investigation, and will often also be extremely distressing for the child. Current guidance stresses the importance of the full interview being performed by social workers and police who are experienced in interviewing children of different ages, and who have the right equipment to record the interview for possible use in later court proceedings.[5]

The issue of whether a child should be questioned alone or with their parent or other accompanying adult is a difficult one and official guidance tends to leave this to the doctor's judgement. The child's age, level of understanding and wishes should obviously be taken into consideration, as at this stage must be the accompanying adult's (see Chapter 3). It is tempting but unwise to use some pretext to take a child into another room in order to question them without the carer being present. Openly offering an older child or adolescent the opportunity to come back and talk to you on their own may give a strong message of support to the suspected victim but an equally strong message of another kind to the accompanying carer. This may occasionally expose the young person to later intimidation and is obviously not an option when the practitioner suspects that there is immediate danger and immediate protection of the child is imperative. In cases of suspicion of lesser severity, however, an open, low-key invitation to the young person to come back soon, on their own if they would like to, may be a possibility. Waiting room notices, leaflets and posters, advertising organizations such as Child Line and assuring young people that their confidentiality will be respected except in the most extreme situations of risk, may also help to encourage an abused young person to come back to the practice or to seek help elsewhere.

As with physical examination (see below), direct questioning of a child or carer about suspicious physical injuries, or symptoms and signs suggestive of sexual abuse, should be done in as non-threatening a manner as possible, with the emphasis at first on clarifying the initial story (again recording the words used by the child and/or accompanying adult). Where symptoms and signs suggestive of physical or possible sexual abuse are presented, more searching questions may seem more natural to a small child and their accompanying adult when they are asked during the examination ('I've not seen a bruise like that before—how did that happen?' 'That looks really sore—did somebody hurt you down there?'). Sometimes questions about general health, development and well-being may serve not only to elicit useful information but also to put child and carer more at ease before particular attention is paid to supplementary questions about previous injuries or other suspicious symptoms; emotional/behavioural health; and, in the case of older girls, menstrual, sexual and contraceptive history. The older child and accompanying adult should also be asked about similar or related symptoms occurring in other members of the family.

The GP or PCHT member should also question (if only inwardly) the *context* of the presentation. Concerns about the appropriateness of the presentation, the consistency of the story being told, the timeliness of the presentation, the appropriateness of the accompanying adult's behaviour and so on should be clarified (see also Table 5.3, p. 88). The child and/or adult may be questioned directly about these points, or their stories checked against previous versions (perhaps told at an accident and emergency department or to the practice nurse). Sometimes the receptionists may have observed or been on the receiving end of inappropriate help-seeking behaviour and their observations too may need to be noted.

Finally, the point has already been made that child abuse and neglect are conditions that are often diagnosed on cumulative evidence over what may be a long period of time. Even when the practitioner begins to suspect abuse, it is often impossible and may even be undesirable to try to dot all the 'i's and cross all the 't's at the first attempt. In many cases of abuse seen in general practice, the situation is not so time critical: there is time to bring a reluctant child, young person or hesitant parent back, and to leave some questions unanswered for the time being at least. The offer to come back may be all that is needed (or indeed all that can be done) for an abused child or frightened adult to disclose eventually, or at least to feel that there is someone who wants to listen and who recognizes their distress.

Performing an examination

Observation should be the first part of any examination and this is no less important in cases of suspected or alleged child abuse or neglect: demeanour (clingy, agitated, wary, inappropriately friendly or sexualized), appropriateness of dress, hygiene, etc. should all be noted. Accompanying siblings should also be observed (rapport with each other, is the presented child the real patient, are there discrepancies between the children?) and the accompanying adult(s) too (is the adult the real patient?, signs of domestic violence, smell of alcohol, affect, a new boyfriend in the waiting room, etc.).

A physical examination may serve several purposes:

- Clarifying the nature of an injury or symptom to help establish a working *diagnosis*, where the presentation is ambiguous, or injuries or neglect are observed by chance.

- As a *general examination* for accompanying physical illness, growth and development.

- *Assessing the severity* of an injury and the need for immediate action (medical or social).

- *Documenting other injuries* or physical signs. This may be helpful for injuries which may be short-lived; to help other professionals gauge the urgency or severity of a case; to justify the appropriateness of the practitioner's referral.

- Documenting significant *negative findings*. This is similarly important for other professionals to gauge urgency and severity; to reassure child, adult and practitioner; to use in support of the family if necessary; to justify lesser action or inaction by the practitioner if called upon to do so.

To a greater or lesser extent, it is appropriate for the general practitioner to conduct a physical examination for all of these reasons. Indeed, it could be considered negligent for a practitioner *not* to examine a patient where a decision about immediate necessary treatment or action to ensure the patient's safety depends on it, or where more generally, by failing to examine the patient sufficiently, the practitioner is unable to put themselves in a reasonable position to determine an appropriate course of action in the best interests of that patient. The extent of the examination that the practitioner should perform does, however, depend on a number of factors relating to the *patient*, the suspected *condition* and the *doctor*.

Factors to consider with regard to the *patient* include:

- *Consent and cooperation*. It is difficult and often counterproductive to try and examine a distressed child of whatever age. In these situations, examination can usually be deferred unless there are urgent medical reasons. For Gillick-competent children (see Chapter 3) informed and freely given consent should be sought and, where necessary, this consent may be deemed to override the wishes of a parent (such an antagonistic situation, though feasible, should rarely be allowed to develop in a general practice setting. Where such a conflict arises, advice about referral for examination should be urgently sought).

- Where a competent child *refuses* consent to examination, however, an adult with parental responsibility, or the court, can override the child. This does not apply in Scotland, where those with parental responsibility cannot authorize procedures a competent child has refused. Again, the general practitioner would rarely, if ever, be justified (or sensible) in forcing such an examination on a reluctant, competent child.

- For a child over 16, only the child's consent is required.

- Consent to examination is implied when an *adult with parental responsibility* consults alleging abuse, but should always be sought more formally when examination of a child is indicated because the doctor suspects abuse. The doctor should always clarify whether the accompanying adult has parental responsibility (PR). A mother will automatically have PR unless it is removed by the court, but it should not be assumed that a father does, especially if he is not married to the mother. Conversely, a grandparent or another adult given authority by the court may have PR and therefore be able to give consent to an examination.

- When an *adult without PR* (e.g. a nursery worker, teacher or male partner) presents a child for examination and that child is unable to give informed consent themselves, the examination should be delayed until someone with PR can be present. Such a course is preferable even if the child is competent, provided they are willing for the adult to be contacted. Adolescents should also be given the option of having a trusted adult present.

- In an *emergency*, where examination and/or treatment is deemed urgent and essential, and attempts to obtain consent have failed or cannot be made within an acceptable timeframe, the doctor should proceed in the interests of child.

- Ideally, *siblings* who may be brought to the surgery should also be examined, with the same provisos as above. If a referral to a statutory agency is made, this will normally be arranged by that agency, and will be performed by a community-based paediatrician. The immediate safety of siblings who are not present may occasionally also need to be ascertained (see below).

Factors to consider with regard to the *condition* include:

- *When abuse is not suspected.* The general practitioner is usually expert at making a diagnosis by taking a short, targeted history and performing a focused examination of whichever system or part of the body seems to be at the centre of the patient's presenting complaint. With small or disabled children, who are unable to give an account for themselves, and where illness presentation is often non-specific, falling back on basic training and performing a full physical examination is more often called for. An ill or unhappy child, especially a baby, with no localizing signs in the obvious systems (ENT, respiratory, abdomen) should be systematically examined from top to toe. Apart from revealing important innocent causes (e.g. an isolated meningococcal purpura) or probably innocent trauma (e.g. a pulled elbow), occasionally unsuspected abuse may be revealed. I had a particularly salutary experience when I was called at night to see a 6-month-old baby who would not stop crying. I examined her thoroughly (I thought) but found no explanation. Eventually

I plucked up courage to take off her large and rather unsavoury-looking terry-towel nappy, not looking for abuse but to take a rectal temperature. The cause of her crying was immediately apparent: she had a mid-shaft fracture of the femur that the nappy had hidden and splinted.

- *When abuse is alleged or suspected* it is desirable for a physical examination to be as comprehensive as is feasible, particularly bearing in mind the frequent cooccurrence of some or even all types of abuse and neglect in the same child. However, the nature, severity and timing of the alleged or suspected abuse will partly determine the extent of the physical examination. The examination should in any case include plotting of height (or head circumference in babies) and weight centiles as well as a general examination of the ears, throat, eyes, chest and abdomen. For a detailed consideration of the physical and emotional signs with which abuse and neglect may present, see Chapters 5a and 5b.

- Many doctors are particularly wary of examining for signs of *sexual abuse*. This has variously to do with worries about their competence (see below), spoiling forensic evidence, or perpetrating a further assault on the child. These worries are well founded, but there are some general principles that may help the GP strike a reasonable balance.

- If recent *sexual abuse is disclosed or is highly probable* (e.g. recent unexplained genital or anal injury), the GP should *not* examine the child other than to rule out the need for emergency treatment and should instead arrange for urgent examination by a specialist paediatrician. Where sexual abuse is disclosed or is alleged to have occurred some time ago, specialist examination is still required (although it may often be non-contributory other than as reassurance for the child) within a reasonable timeframe.

- In cases where *sexual abuse is possible* (e.g. an ambiguous statement from a child, genital or anal soreness, behavioural changes, etc.) an inspection at least of the external genital and anal area is a natural and expected part of the general examination and, if the child and parent are agreeable (see consent discussion above), should be done. Overwillingness to be examined, or apparent nonchalance and disconnection from the process on the part of the child should be noted, as this may be more significant than reluctance or distress at the prospect. Any comments made by the child during the examination should be noted. I usually ask the mother to hold a younger child and part the thighs, and sometimes, in cases of vaginal discharge, to gently part the labia. Occasionally, with persistent discharge in a child with an otherwise low index of suspicion, it is reasonable to take an introital swab, although as Wynne points out, microbiological investigations are usually unhelpful and thrush, although often treated for, is in fact rare. Again, the mother may be instructed how to take the swab, or an older child may be happier to do it herself. In this way, further trauma to the child is minimized.

Factors to consider with regard to the *doctor* include:

- *Time available.* This is a perennial problem for most GPs, but I suspect (having been guilty of it myself) that some of us use our lack of time as an excuse for avoiding things we do not want or feel able to do. Child protection issues are occasionally an emergency in general practice and like any other emergency, have to be found time for there and then. Even when immediate action is clearly not imperative, an examination at the time may be important and will of necessity be time-consuming. There may be many situations of lesser severity, however, where a more detailed examination by the GP can be deferred, even if only to the end of surgery or later in the day. (In any case, this sometimes gives the GP an important opportunity to collect their thoughts, to check the records, or to consult informally with colleagues or other team members.) As with history-taking, everything in child protection does not always have to be done straight away.

- *Competence.* Expertise and confidence are generally the product of training and experience, and in the field of examination for suspected child sexual abuse in particular, most GPs have neither. The normal range of appearances of a child's vagina and anus are disputed even by experts, and it would be wholly inappropriate to expect an average GP to have this knowledge in any depth. As set out above, however, with the important exception of probable sexual abuse, there is much the GP can do without specific training or experience in the field.

- Occasionally, a family who are the subject of *formal child protection enquiries,* where a medical examination is required, will request that their GP carry out the examination. Social services will actively discourage this course unless the doctor has adequate training and expertise; has been fully briefed on the circumstances and objectives of the examination; has agreed to attend a child protection conference and to provide a statement for social services; agrees to attend court if required; and agrees to a social worker accompanying the child to the surgery for the medical examination. The lack of training and expertise alone should dictate in the majority of cases that the GP strongly advises the family to cooperate in having the child examined by a specialist.

- The *gender* of the doctor may be important to some children, although the manner of the examination is thought to matter more: where feasible, however, a child should be offered examination by a doctor of the same gender.

- As with any distressing and/or intimate examination, the *facilities* for an examination in cases of suspected abuse must be appropriate, with privacy assured in an environment that is reassuring for the child. If a full examination is being carried out in the surgery, facilities should exist for taking forensic swabs, swabs for sexually acquired infections and for pregnancy testing. Some surgeries have facilities for taking photographs and these may sometimes be a useful way of recording bruises or other injuries, but only as part of a full, 'official' examination.

Initiating relevant investigations

Wynne (see Chapter 5a) discusses the differential diagnosis of different types of abuse and neglect and appropriate investigations are suggested that may help to exclude other conditions. Some are entirely appropriate for the GP to perform; some investigations in cases of suspected sexual abuse, although well within the normal remit of the GP, are best left to specialists, for the reasons discussed above; others are obviously only available to hospital specialists. The following points are worth noting:

- The *interpretation* of results may not be straightforward, and their sensitivity and specificity for diagnosing child abuse is often poor. A full blood count, for example, may indicate iron deficiency anaemia as a cause of poor appetite and failure to thrive, but does the anaemia itself result from poor appetite as an emotional response to abuse or neglect? A plain abdominal film may show faecal loading in a child with abdominal pain, but is the constipation an indirect consequence of sexual abuse? A urinary tract infection may seem to explain secondary enuresis in a girl with no previous history, but could sexual abuse have precipitated the infection in the first place?

- With *sexual abuse* in particular, there are very few unequivocal clinical signs and even fewer unequivocal investigations. The presence of semen, blood of a different type, lubricants or pubic hairs in the rectum, vagina or perineum of a small child is generally conclusive, but very little else is. The identification of sexually transmissible diseases from swabs may make a diagnosis of sexual abuse highly probable, but is not necessarily considered strong enough evidence on its own, even if the adult suspected of perpetrating the abuse is found to have the same infection. Even gonorrhoea is deemed to have less than 100 per cent specificity, as defence lawyers have successfully argued. The GP who has been persuaded to do a low vaginal swab on a child may occasionally identify gonorrhoea or chlamydia, but is more likely to be confronted with genital warts or genital herpes. These infections should certainly raise strong suspicions of sexual abuse, especially if virology shows the infective agent to be of a genitally transmitted type, but accidental transmission of both genital and non-genital types to the child's genital area can and does occur.[6] (See Table 5.6, p. 98.)

- The GP's investigative role in the detection and diagnosis of child abuse does not end, or often even begin with, blood tests, swabs and the like. Rather, it is the enquiries that a GP makes around a worrying clinical presentation that could be seen as the investigations of choice and are more the ones that may really make a difference to early diagnosis. The nature and scope of these enquiries will be discussed further below.

- Finally, abuse is usually diagnosed as occurring on the balance of probabilities, rather than being proved beyond all reasonable doubt. *Proof* that abuse has occurred, let alone proof of who has perpetrated that abuse, is frustratingly difficult to obtain. The doctor as a scientifically orientated diagnostician, the doctor (or social worker, lawyer, policeman, non-abusing parent or society itself) as protector and avenger of the abused child, and certainly the child itself may well find this conclusion unpalatable. The fact remains though that in child abuse, particularly sexual abuse, the best one can often achieve is the protection of that child from further abuse. The GP, who is used anyway to thinking in terms of probability rather than diagnostic certainty, may need to be content with this and, more important, may also need to help the child and their family to come to terms with it (see Chapter 7c). On the positive side, the diagnostic uncertainty surrounding abuse has, amongst other factors, contributed to the reorientation of child protection work towards investing more effort and resources in supporting struggling families to help prevent abuse.

Reviewing the previous medical history

Asking a new patient or their parent about previous medical history is a routine part of any 'clerking'. This may be done by a self-administered questionnaire on registering, by a trained lay member of staff, by the practice nurse or by the GP. Many practices will summarize onto cards or the computer important details from a patient's past notes from the previous practice (if and when they eventually arrive). In addition, when evaluating a problem for the first time, an obvious question to the patient or parent is, 'Has this, or anything similar, ever happened before?' If the patient is unable to give this information, the doctor might look in the previous notes. Increasingly, clinical notes are entered onto GP computer systems, but the majority are still handwritten, sometimes on A4 sheets but more often on the small 'Lloyd George' cards that have been in use since the First World War.

Given the generally cumulative nature of abusive incidents, and the many background risk factors that may predispose to abuse in families, it follows that building up a detailed history of a child and their family may be critical in the evaluation of a clinical picture that may be due to abuse or indicate the risk of abuse. However, certain problems of reliability and accessibility are immediately apparent from the description above and the following points should be noted:

- A patient or parent may reveal only what they choose in a self-administered questionnaire. Those administered by a trained member of staff, nurse or doctor may elicit slightly more accurate information, but little reliance can be placed on them. In any case, standard practice questionnaires rarely contain questions relevant to child protection issues.

- Summarizing previous records when they arrive is good practice and should certainly identify serious previous incidents, hospital admissions and some background risk factors. However, it is unlikely that episodes of, for example, repeated minor trauma or apparently minor genital irritation, will be seen as important enough to summarize, and there is therefore a risk that if the summary is relied on too heavily important clues may be missed.

- Asking the child or the parent about previous or related episodes is, of course, appropriate, but where abuse is being concealed the answers cannot be relied upon.

- *Looking through previous notes, letters, casualty department discharge summaries, etc. is then crucial in worrying cases.* Families with risk factors for abuse and those with abuse to hide are more likely to be highly mobile and medical records are often slow to follow them. GPs should have a low threshold for submitting urgent requests for medical records when there are grounds for suspicion. Sometimes a telephone call to the previous GP, if known, can be enormously informative and in complicated cases they might be able to send on the contents of the medical record envelope, thus bypassing the official system and saving possibly weeks of delay.

- Conversely, if a child who has been abused or for whom there are serious concerns leaves a GP's list, their records should be sent back as soon as requested by the health authority/PCT and requests from the new GP for information or for the notes to be sent on directly should be treated promptly and sympathetically. The outgoing GP can, of course, be proactive in this by telephoning the new GP (if known) and imparting any urgent information. Occasionally, if things have gone badly wrong, a family will leave a GP's list precipitately, or disappear altogether without re-registering with another GP. In these situations, a GP who suspects a child to be at risk of significant harm or who knows a child to be already known to the statutory agencies, should inform social services urgently. If the child has a health visitor, they should also be made aware whenever a child for whom there are concerns leaves the list, as they will be able to hand over information to their opposite number in the child's new area, even if the family do not immediately register with a new GP.

- The accessibility of the clinical record can be improved greatly if Lloyd George cards and/or A4 sheets are kept bound together in date order. The doctor with a 'paperless' record, who may well not have the old written records in front of them during the consultation, should have a low threshold for getting them in cases of even a slightly suspicious nature.

- The *tagging and cross-referencing of notes* where concerns exist about a child, their siblings or a vulnerable adult who is also a carer, may alert members of the PHCT when a household member presents at the surgery. This may be particularly important when locums, GP registrars or agency nurses who do not know the background are seeing patients. The tagging can take the form of a coloured flash on the manual record or a computer entry that is clearly visible on entering the patient's record.

Several points need to be emphasized here:

- First, the tagging, whilst a clear signal to team members, *should in no way be explicit to the casual onlooker.* A computer entry may, for example, merely state 'Significant personal/family history'.

- In almost all cases, however, the carers of the child, and older children themselves, should be informed that their notes are being marked discretely. Usually, if it is made clear that the tagging allows team members to be especially sensitive to the well-being of the child, and especially responsive to the family's needs, this will be accepted and sometimes even welcomed (even when it is made clear that the tagging is also on occasions a trigger to sharing necessary information with other agencies).

- Secondly, a flash or note entry like the above, whilst alerting the practitioner, should generally be supplemented by enough information to guide them in the right direction. However, this needs to be done *without unnecessarily compromising the confidentiality of other household members.* For example, a child whose mother has serious mental health problems should have their notes tagged, as should the mother and any other child in the household. But that child should not be able, when old enough to demand access to their medical record, to read of their mother's illness without her consent. There are provisions in law for such information to be withheld if it breaches a third party's confidentiality, but obviously the best solution is for practitioners to seek the mother's consent to record this information in the child's record. It would though be acceptable to enter a supplementary note advising the practitioner of other household members, identified by name, relationship to the child and/or practice number. Certain clinical computer systems have means of linking members of the same family or household, by use of a common computer number, or by displaying a family genogram.

- Thirdly, tagging *should not be seen as an alternative to vigilance.* Whilst its presence should certainly alert the team member, its absence is not of itself cause for reassurance.

- Fourthly, if concerns for a child or family are found genuinely to be unfounded (as opposed to unproved), or the risk disappears for whatever reason, the *tagging should be removed.* As with child protection registration, however, removal should not be an excuse for removing extra support from families who continue to need it.

- Tagging, if used sensitively as a means of identifying *children and families in need* (rather than merely as a surveillance tool for children where there is a suspicion of abuse), can make a significant difference to the *prevention and early detection* of child abuse. Health visitors are used to having a semiformal 'worry list': their records are often specifically marked when families are of concern, with these records being singled out for periodic review with their supervisors. Tagged medical records can be used within the practice on a similar basis, with perhaps quarterly meetings of the practice team to review those families who are causing concern, to consider additions and removals, to audit practice policies and so on.

- Tagged notes can be used to improve the care of these families in other ways too, by increasing the *responsiveness* and *continuity* of care as well as vigilance when a child or vulnerable adult carer is seen. These can be seen as the 'selling points' that may help to make such a system more acceptable to sceptical or suspicious carers. For example:

  - The threshold for asking to see such patients or visiting them at home if necessary, rather than giving telephone advice, should be set much lower than normal.

  - Reception staff should be more flexible in squeezing them in as extras and should be instructed not to turn them away if they arrive late for an appointment without checking first with the person they are due to see.

  - Wherever possible, they should be seen by the same practitioner. In larger group practices, especially those with GP registrars and/or nurse practitioners, continuity of care is a potential problem, particularly as these families are more likely to present in an unpredictable and disorganized way and may even deliberately avoid seeing the same person on successive occasions. In practices that do not operate a firm personal list system, team meetings can be used to identify the responsible doctor and, where possible, the whole family should be encouraged to see that doctor.

  - When a patient with tagged notes consults another team member, that patient's own doctor should generally be informed. Similarly, a doctor or practice nurse should let a child's health visitor know of attendances, hospital reports, etc., and vice versa.

  - This two-way communication is possibly even more important for *non-attendances*.

  - At-risk children often come from multiply disadvantaged families and these measures will go some way towards redressing the inverse care law (the quality of care received is inversely proportional to need) to which these families are often subject. Ideally, this responsiveness, continuity and internal communication should be the norm for all child patients, whether tagged or not, as these measures will significantly improve the chances of identifying potentially abusive situations and families in need. It is appreciated, however, that the effort involved, particularly when health visitors are not practice attached, may make this impracticable.

- The workload implications for the practice of a tagged notes system like this are considerable in any event. They need to be taken into account when setting up such a system, over and above the ethical considerations of labelling certain families. Practices should therefore give careful thought to the *criteria* to be used for inclusion. As with any sieve or safety net, the mesh size setting will determine the number of cases that will come into the system, but also the number that may slip through it. At best, the system should include all those children who meet the criteria for *'children in need'* (discussed further below), plus those whose pattern of consultations gives rise to concern.

- Finally, as well as helping with *clinical audit*, a systematic review of the records of all children in the practice and the tagging of those which meet the 'in need' criteria can be a valuable component of a *needs assessment* exercise. This may be important at both practice and locality level in terms of demonstrating *unmet need* and attracting/retaining *resources*.

This part of the chapter has dwelt at some length on the importance of the medical record in the prevention and early detection of child abuse. Indeed, dull though this may sound, I would argue that knowing how to use the medical record to its full potential, and organizing the practice team around it, are far more important for the general practitioner than having detailed knowledge of what a perineum should look like, or how bruises of different ages should be evaluated, important as this may be. Clearly, certain changes in the delivery of primary care may mitigate against this. As discussed in Chapter 3, out of hours co-operatives, NHS Direct and walk-in centres will have a significant impact on the assessment and delivery of emergency and out of hours primary care. Rather than the continuity of care traditionally provided by the cradle to grave family doctor, 'continuity of the electronic medical record' is seen by some as the standard to be aspired to. This may eventually be a reality, enabling professionals wherever they may see or speak to a patient to access their complete medical record, but such a system will lag some years behind the changes in clinical care delivery, with significant dangers for potentially at-risk children. Moves towards less practice-based delivery of normal daytime primary care (e.g. by salaried doctors working from trust premises) may be less worrying in that a clinical record may be more comprehensive and easily accessible if such services are operated on a list system, but there remain problems of continuity of carer, as staff turnover will inevitably be higher than in the traditional general practice setting.

Considering relevant social/family circumstances: children in need and the assessment framework

The general practitioner is faced every day with patients whose illnesses or feelings of illness have adverse social and/or family circumstances at their root. In many illnesses, the patient's (and the doctor's) behaviour, as well as the course and severity of the illness are in part determined by social and family circumstances; and the success or otherwise of medical interventions is partly determined by them too. Often indeed, the intervention required may not seem to be medical at all: the occasional sick certificate to give a stressed working mother a short breathing space; the housing letter that may occasionally tip the balance in favour of a struggling family; the benefits agency appeal report that convinces a sceptical assessor to give a few.more pounds in benefit. At other times it is quite clear that the real problem lies with someone else in the family; an alcohol-abusing partner; a dementing elderly relative; a married daughter going through a divorce.

Nowhere is this more true than in child abuse: in its prevention, in its early detection, in the secondary prevention of further abuse, and in the mitigation of some of its consequences. In this part of the chapter, the consideration of social and family circumstances will be seen to be an essential part of the *Framework for the Assessment of Children in Need*,[7] from which stems the assessment of risk and the planning of interventions for those children who are in need and their families. As has been stressed time and again, child abuse rarely comes completely out of the blue: children suffering or at risk of suffering significant harm are invariably children in need.

Determining that a child is 'in need' is more than an academic exercise and more even than a predictor of risk. Under Part III of the Children Act 1989, a child is deemed to be in need if:

- he is unlikely to achieve or maintain, or to have the opportunity of achieving or maintaining, a reasonable standard of health or development without the provision for him of services by a local authority;

- his health and development is likely to be significantly impaired, or further impaired, without the provision of such services, or;

- he is disabled (Section 17(10)).

The local authority has a *duty* (my emphasis) to respond to children in need in the following ways:

- To provide services to children in need in their area (Section 17).

- To provide such day care for children in need within their area as appropriate (Section 18).

- To provide accommodation and maintenance to any child in need in their area (Sections 20 and 23).

- To advise, assist and befriend a child when he ceases to be looked after by the authority (Section 2).

- To provide services to minimize the effect of disabilities (Schedule 2, para. 6).

- To take steps to prevent neglect or ill-treatment (Schedule 2, para. 6).

- To provide family centres.

The general practitioner and the PHCT may thus additionally use the 'in need' categorization as a useful lever for change, a means of pressuring a local authority to provide services irrespective of whether a child is on a child protection register or not. Of course, local authorities are if anything even more short of resources than the health services and this will still be a major limiting factor in practice. Notwithstanding this, many families where a child is considered to be at risk or potentially at risk of significant harm will concede that they have needs within the meaning of the Act: the 'in need' concept, with the beneficial outcomes that are supposed to flow from it, may help the GP and team to work constructively rather than adversarily with the family, as their advocate rather than as merely as some kind of policing agency.

The revised government interagency guide *Working Together*[8] and its companion volume on the assessment framework set out for social services departments the framework they are to use for the assessment of all children in need, including those where there are concerns that a child may be suffering significant harm. This framework 'provides a systematic basis for collecting and analysing information to support professional judgements about how to help children and families in the best interests of the child'.[8] It is worth examining in more detail, both so the GP knows the criteria by which social services departments will be judging the needs of their patients, and as a useful basis on which the GP and the PCHT can themselves build up a comprehensive picture of a child's needs, including their risk of suffering significant harm. For there is also a clear expectation in *Working Together* (para. 3.19) that health professionals will play their full part in all stages of the child protection process, including:

- recognising children in need of support and/or safeguarding, and parents who may need extra help in bringing up their children;
- assessing the needs of children and the capacity of parents to meet their children's needs;
- planning and providing support to vulnerable children and families.[8]

The framework's three main dimensions—the child's *developmental needs*, and the *capacity of the parents* to respond appropriately to those needs within a wider *family and environmental context*—are set out in Figure 5.2, with a more detailed outline of each dimension in Tables 5.14–5.16. They should be viewed as three 'interrelated systems or domains', interacting with and influencing each other in how they affect the child.

This framework by which to judge need is of necessity broad and will rarely be appropriate in its entirety to the GP and rest of the PHCT. It also goes without saying that few if any of our patients (or ourselves) could possibly measure up in all ways at all times in parenting capacity or in providing the optimal family and social environment set out in it. There are, nevertheless, in this framework many factors that the GP and others in the team will be in a position to observe during their routine professional relationships

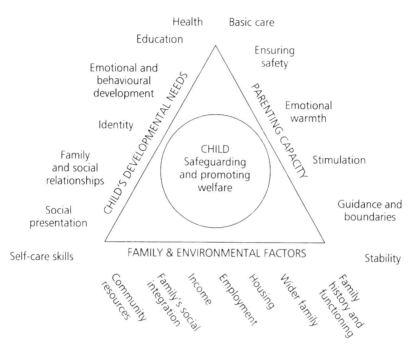

Fig. 5.2 The assessment framework (from [8]).

with child patients and their adult carers. Considerable benefits may follow:

- It provides in my view a particularly useful basis for assessing risk of significant harm due to *neglect* and *emotional abuse*, which tend to more insidious and diffuse in their presentation and therefore tend to be more underdiagnosed than physical and sexual abuse.

- Having *standards* by which to measure parenting capacity and to set them against the particular developmental needs of say, a disabled child, and then also to look at the social support network for that family enables the team to be more discriminating in the development of a *tagged notes* system.

- It helps the team to identify *interventions* that they might themselves undertake or ask others to undertake on the child's behalf, irrespective of whether significant harm or risk of significant harm is present, up to and including referring the child to social services as a child in need. (See also Chapter 9a.)

- It provides a valuable tool for *needs assessment* of, and *resource allocation* to, a practice *population*, a process already required at PCT (or equivalent) level. If nothing else, the practice will be able to use the framework (which, as well as its legislative foundation has an extensive research and practice base to underpin it) as the basis

Table 5.14 Dimensions of child's developmental needs (from [8]).

Health
Includes growth and development as well as physical and mental well-being. The impact of genetic factors and of any impairment may also need to be considered. Involves receiving appropriate health care when ill, an adequate and nutritious diet, exercise, immunizations where appropriate and developmental checks, dental and optical care and, for older children, appropriate advice and information on issues that have an impact on health, including sex education and substance misuse

Education
Covers all areas of a child's cognitive development which begins from birth. Includes opportunities: for play and interaction with other children; access to books; to acquire a range of skills and interests; to experience success and achievement. Involves an adult interested in educational activities, progress and achievements, who takes account of the child's starting point and any special educational needs

Emotional and behavioural development
Concerns the appropriateness of response demonstrated in feelings and actions by a child, initially to parents and caregivers and, as the child grows older, to others beyond the family. Includes nature and quality of early attachments, characteristics of temperament, adaptation to change, response to stress and degree of appropriate self-control

Identity
Concerns the child's growing sense of self as a separate and valued person. Includes the child's view of self and abilities, self-image and self-esteem, and having a positive sense of individuality. Race, religion, age, gender, sexuality and individuality may all contribute to this. Feelings of belonging and acceptance by family, peer group and wider society, including other cultural groups

Family and social relationships
Development of empathy and the capacity to place self in someone else's shoes. Includes a stable and affectionate relationship with parents or caregivers, good relationships with siblings, increasing importance of age-appropriate friendships with peers and other significant persons in the child's life and response of family to these relationships

Social presentation
Concerns child's growing understanding of the way in which appearance, behaviour and any impairment are perceived by the outside world and the impression being created. Includes appropriateness of dress for age, gender, culture and religion, cleanliness and personal hygiene and availability of advice from parents or caregivers about presentation in different settings

Self-care skills
Concerns the acquisition by a child of both practical and emotional competencies required for increasing independence. Includes early practical skills of dressing and feeding, opportunities to gain confidence and practical skills to undertake activities away from the family and independent living skills as older children. Includes encouragement to acquire social problem-solving approaches. Special attention should be given to the impact of a child's impairment and other vulnerabilities, and on social circumstances affecting these in the development of self-care skills

for highlighting *unmet need* and, arguably, as a basis for seeking equitable and adequate resources for families, the practice or the community.

Extrapolating from the framework parameters, the PHCT might consider identifying the following children and their siblings as *possibly* being children 'in need'. Such children

Table 5.15 Dimensions of parenting capacity (from [8]).

Basic care

Providing for the child's physical needs, and appropriate medical and dental care. Includes provision of food, liquid, warmth, shelter, clean and appropriate clothing and adequate personal hygiene

Ensuring safety

Ensuring the child is adequately protected from harm or danger. Includes protection from significant harm or danger, and from contact with unsafe adults/other children and from self-harm. Recognition of hazards and danger both in the home and elsewhere

Emotional warmth

Ensuring the child's emotional needs are met and giving the child a sense of being specially valued and a positive sense of own racial and cultural identity. Includes ensuring the child's requirements for secure, stable and affectionate relationships with significant adults, with appropriate sensitivity and responsiveness to the child's needs. Appropriate physical contact, comfort and cuddling sufficient to demonstrate warm regard, praise and encouragement

Stimulation

Promoting child's learning and intellectual development through encouragement and cognitive stimulation and promoting social opportunities. Includes facilitating the child's cognitive development and potential through interaction, communication, talking and responding to the child's language and questions, encouraging and joining the child's play, and promoting educational opportunities. Enabling the child to experience success and ensuring school attendance or equivalent opportunity. Facilitating child to meet challenges of life

Guidance and boundaries

Enabling the child to regulate their own emotions and behaviour. The key parental tasks are demonstrating and modelling appropriate behaviour and control of emotions and interactions with others, and guidance which involves setting boundaries, so that the child is able to develop an internal model of moral values and conscience, and social behaviour appropriate for the society within which they will grow up. The aim is to enable the child to grow into an autonomous adult, holding their own values, and able to demonstrate appropriate behaviour with others rather than having to be dependent on rules outside themselves. This includes not overprotecting children from exploratory and learning experiences. Includes social problem-solving, anger management, consideration for others, and effective discipline and shaping of behaviour

Stability

Providing a sufficiently stable family environment to enable a child to develop and maintain a secure attachment to the primary caregiver(s) in order to ensure optimal development. Includes ensuring secure attachments are not disrupted, providing consistency of emotional warmth over time and responding in a similar manner to the same behaviour. The above dimensions of parenting to operate reasonably consistently. Parental responses change and develop according to child's developmental progress. In addition, ensuring children keep in contact with important family members and significant others

---

will fall into the following broad categories (there is obviously considerable overlap, i.e. more than one category will often apply):

- Child protection concerns (category a).
- Physical illness/disability/learning difficulties (category b).

Table 5.16 Family and environmental factors (from [8]).

Family history and functioning
Family history includes both genetic and psychosocial factors. Family functioning is influenced by who is living in the household and how they are related to the child; significant changes in family/household composition; history of childhood experiences of parents; chronology of significant life events and their meaning to family members; nature of family functioning, including sibling relationships, and its impact on the child; parental strengths and difficulties, including those of an absent parent; the relationship between separated parents

Wider family
Who are considered to be members of the wider family by the child and the parents? This includes related and non-related persons and absent wider family. What is their role and importance to the child and parents and in precisely what way?

Housing
Does the accommodation have basic amenities and facilities appropriate to the age and development of the child and other resident members? Is the housing accessible and suitable to the needs of disabled family members? Includes the interior and exterior of the accommodation and immediate surroundings. Basic amenities include water, heating, sanitation, cooking facilities, sleeping arrangements and cleanliness, hygiene and safety and their impact on the child's upbringing

Employment
Who is working in the household, their pattern of work and any changes? What impact does this have on the child? How is work or absence of work viewed by family members? How does it affect their relationship with the child? This includes children's experience of work and its impact on them

Income
Income available over a sustained period of time. Is the family in receipt of its benefits entitlements? Is there a sufficiency of income to meet the family's needs? The way resources available to the family are used. Are there financial difficulties which affect the child?

Family's social integration
Exploration of the wider context of the local neighbourhood and community and its impact on the child and parents. Includes the degree of the family's integration or isolation, their peer groups, friendship and social networks and the importance attached to them

Community resources
Describes all facilities and services in a neighbourhood, including universal services of primary health care, day care and schools, includes availability, accessibility and standard of resources and impact on the family, including disabled members

- Emotional/behavioural difficulties (category c).
- Concerns re parental health/capacity (category d).
- Severe environmental concerns (category e).

Examples (with the category to which they are most applicable in brackets) include:

1. Children placed on, or who may be placed on, the *child protection register*, because they have suffered, or are at risk of suffering, *significant harm*, including *failure to thrive* (a).

2. Children with a *disability* (b).

3. Children who are, or have been, *looked after* by the local authority or accommodated by other agencies, or are subject to a care order, supervision order, emergency protection order, child assessment order or police powers of protection (a).

4. Children with serious/complex *special educational needs* (b).

5. Children with a *chronic and/or terminal illness,* or who are HIV positive (b).

6. Children who have committed a serious or several less serious *offences* (c).

7. Children with serious *emotional or behavioural difficulties,* or with drug, alcohol or solvent *dependency* problems (c).

8. Children *excluded* from mainstream, full-time education (c).

9. Children who are *primary carers* of other people (d).

10. Children of *parents whose ability or circumstances seriously limits their capacity* to provide care, and who are unlikely to achieve and maintain reasonable standards of health and development as a result, without the provision of services. Consider children of parents with:

- Chronic mental health problems (d).

- Substance abuse problems (d).

- Severe postnatal depression (d).

- History of domestic violence (a).

- Severe physical illness or disability (d).

- Learning difficulties (d).

- History of abuse in their own childhood (d).

- History of being accommodated ('in care') in their own childhood (d).

- History of early (<18 years) unplanned pregnancy (d).

- Persistently poor compliance/attendance with child (d).

- Homelessness, hostel or refuge accommodation, or severe housing inadequacy (e).

This list is not meant to be prescriptive, in that by no means all the children who fall into these categories will prove to be in need of social services provision, let alone to be at risk of abuse. Nor, on the other hand, is it exhaustive: children may be identified as being temporarily more vulnerable and in need where there is a history of extreme prematurity or recent bereavement; where there is extreme social isolation, e.g. recently arrived asylum seekers; where serious relationship problems or recent separation of parents are identified; or where the child is one of an unusually large, chaotic and/or materially deprived family. It should also be emphasized that a child may still be in need, at risk of suffering, or indeed actually suffering significant harm when none of these factors is suspected or recorded.

There is one final, important caveat. The resources available to social services, as with health, are finite. They are manifestly insufficient to deal effectively with the volume of need that exists. There will undoubtedly be attempts to redefine need to fit available resources. (I call this the Humpty Dumpty position—'When I use a word' . . . 'it means just what I choose it to mean').[9] This may lead, as it did with previous community care legislation, to social workers not being allowed to record unmet need at all: need that is unmet is, by definition, unlawful. GPs are realists, but they are also often the best (if not the only) advocate a vulnerable family can have. They will have to balance their desire not to raise patients' expectations falsely with their desire to strive for the best outcomes for them.

Enquiries from other agencies

I hope the above discussion has demonstrated some of the potential for general practice to be proactive in its approach to promoting and safeguarding the welfare of children. The PHCT can do a good deal to prevent child abuse and, by increasing the team's awareness of the needs of its child patients, to recognize the warning signs of abuse earlier. This should certainly increase the number of referrals to social services from general practice of children in need, including those in need of protection. The likelihood remains, however, that a significant proportion of child protection concerns will be brought to the GP's attention if not by the child or adult carer, then by other agencies. In the final part of this chapter, I will consider the reactive role of the general practitioner in responding to enquiries about children from other agencies. It should be noted that exact procedures, referral and assessment forms, etc., are likely to vary from authority to authority. Practitioners are urged to refer to local guidelines where appropriate.

Section 47(1) of the Children Act 1989 places a clear obligation on local authority social services departments when they are informed or have reasonable cause to suspect that a child is suffering or is likely to suffer significant harm: 'the Authority shall make or cause to be made such enquiries as it considers necessary to enable it to decide whether it should take any action to safeguard or promote the child's welfare'. Medical advice from the child's usual medical carers must be included at all critical decision-making points and important views from health professionals must be included in discussions.

Under Section 27 of the same Act, there is a general duty of other agencies, including health authorities and NHS trusts, to assist social services department enquiries by providing relevant information and advice unless it would be unreasonable to do so.

PHCT members who are trust employees will generally have procedures laid down which they must follow if they have concerns about a family or they are asked to contribute to a social services enquiry, and contractor GPs are responsible for ensuring that their employees, too, are aware of local child protection procedures (para. 3.31).[8]

But what about the GP themselves? The expectations are clear (see Chapter 6c), although for independent contractors at least, these do not have the force of legal or terms of service obligations. Thus, *Working Together* paragraph 3.30 states that GPs have an important role in all stages of the child protection process, including 'sharing information with social services when enquiries are being made about a child'. The addendum to the 1991 edition of *Working Together, Child Protection: Medical Responsibilities*[10] is more emphatic and can be seen as an injunction both to doctors and social services departments: 'When a doctor has involvement with the statutory agencies it is *essential* that he or she is able to contribute to all stages of the decision making process, *including the decision whether to undertake an investigation* [my emphases], as doctors retain a continuing responsibility for their patients' (para. 2.17).[10] Again, in paragraph 5.2, we read, '. . . doctors are *required* [my emphasis] to participate at different stages of the child protection process . . .'.

General practitioners vary considerably in their interpretation of this guidance and Hallett[1] found GPs uniquely unwilling to collaborate at the enquiry stage. Social workers' expectations of GPs were allegedly so low that, in all but one of the 48 cases she studied, they had not even bothered to contact the GP in the first place, despite their apparent duty to do so. The stumbling block is generally the issue of confidentiality. There is a general discussion on confidentiality and its limits in Chapter 3, but certain key points with regard to child protection bear repetition:

> Doctors have a legal and ethical duty to maintain confidentiality and should not disclose information without consent unless disclosure can be justified in the public interest (e.g. in the best interest of the child) or is required by Court Order or Statute (para. 6.1).[10]
>
> There is no dispute that the child's interests are paramount, but the wish to maintain confidentiality may be strong. A doctor may be faced with this dilemma at any stage of the child protection process . . . At all stages, therefore, a doctor needs to make a balanced judgement between the justification for breaching confidence and the distress it might cause, and the withholding of information obtained within the doctor–patient relationship (para. 4.2).[10]
>
> If you believe a patient to be a victim of neglect or physical, sexual or emotional abuse and that the patient cannot give or withhold consent to disclosure, you should give information promptly to an appropriate responsible person or statutory agency, where you believe that the disclosure is in the patient's best interests. You should usually inform the patient that you intend to disclose the information before doing so. Such circumstances may arise in relation to children, where concerns about possible abuse need to be shared with other agencies such as social services. Where appropriate you should inform those with parental responsibility about the disclosure. If, for any reason, you believe that disclosure of information is not in the best interests of an abused or neglected patient, you must still be prepared to justify your decision.[11]

GPs might be contacted for information at the *initial assessment* stage (see Figure 6.1, p. 165 and Chapter 5d) where a child in need referral has been made by someone, particularly where there is a concern of significant harm. This might be a telephone contact or, in cases of lesser urgency, in writing. If a *core assessment* is deemed necessary, the GP and perhaps the health visitor will be asked to complete, or contribute to the completion of, an assessment form based on the framework parameters (see above), within the agreed timescale (the core assessment should be completed within a maximum of 35 working days from the completion of the initial assessment, or from when a strategy discussion decides to initiate S47 enquiries). Practitioners should be aware that their assessment contribution will generally be shared with family members, and with the child if appropriate. As mentioned, there are likely to be local variations in the details of this process. Some authorities, for example, may convene a planning meeting (similar to a strategy discussion) of involved agencies, when a core assessment of a child with complex needs is envisaged.

Where an initial assessment indicates the possibility of significant harm, a *strategy meeting or discussion* is likely to be convened. This is the multidisciplinary consideration of whether the information is sufficient and serious enough to warrant an investigation and, if so, how to conduct it (see Chapter 6a). In some cases the GP, even if not the referrer, may be asked to participate in this. Some GPs may get themselves invited to a strategy discussion if they know a family well and feel they have an important contribution to make on behalf of the child and/or the family. The GP's perspective and knowledge may prevent overprecipitate action by the statutory agencies, or conversely, convince those present of the urgency and seriousness of a situation. Strategy discussions do not generally include family members.

In extremely urgent situations, strategy discussions, as with initial assessments, may be held over the telephone. Although they may seem to be unofficial and informal parts of the process when conducted in this way, the same considerations with regard to safeguarding confidentiality apply:

- The GP should be satisfied as to the *identity* and position of the caller, as well as their *reason* for requesting the information. If necessary the GP may telephone the caller back, or request a fax on headed notepaper. This should not be used as a delaying tactic, however: *the GP should always act within a timeframe that is not detrimental to the interests of the child.* It is to be hoped that the joint working between health and social services envisaged in the 'new NHS' will make this kind of communication less fraught, whilst maintaining the confidentiality of the doctor–patient relationship within safe limits.

- The GP should ascertain from the enquirer whether members of the subject family are already aware of the enquiry. If so, the GP should obtain parents' (and/or a competent child's) *permission* before information is disclosed.

- If the family is unaware that information about them is being requested, the GP should consider disclosing information without consent *only if permission seeking may itself place a child at risk of significant harm* (para. 5.11).[8] The reasons why social services have not informed the family should thus be carefully ascertained before a GP inadvertently puts a child at risk by alerting them: conversely, often no overwhelming reason can be given and the GP can safely seek consent.

- The recipient of the information should be asked for a clear undertaking that they will use the information only for the purposes for which it has been disclosed.

- If the GP chooses to provide *written* information (a preferable course of action, except in urgent situations), the report should be sent only to a secured fax number, with the addressee alerted to receive it, or posted in an envelope marked 'Strictly confidential: for addressee only'.

- The GP may be in possession of information about a *third party* that is directly related to child protection issues, but does not relate directly to a child patient. The disclosure of such information, e.g. that a man is known to be sexually aroused to children, or has a known history of violence towards children from another relationship, is generally considered justifiable and, indeed, desirable if a continuing risk to children is thought likely.

- As with a written report to a case conference (see Chapter 6c) the GP who gives information over the telephone should be careful to distinguish between fact, observation, allegation and opinion. The *relevance* of the information given should also be considered: the GP should not withhold significant information concerning suspicious incidents or associated risk factors for abuse, but nor on the other hand should personal details superfluous to the enquiry be revealed without the informed consent of the person involved.

- The details of any telephone discussion should be noted as soon as possible: 'Those involved in discussions at any stage of the child protection process are advised to make *a written note of all contacts* with, and requests for information by, the statutory agencies...' A note of the contact should become part of the child or family's medical record held by the doctor (para. 2.10).[10]

- In making such notes, the GP should be mindful of the patient's *legal rights* under the Data Protection and Access to Health Records Acts to access medical records and reports. This consideration should also be borne in mind if details of a discussion are copied to the notes of other immediate family members, or if third parties' identities are recorded.

The issue of disclosure of information to a statutory agency, whether verbally or in writing, may seem something of a minefield, and the GP needs to proceed with care. But if the above considerations are borne in mind, I believe that the GP can respect both the rights and the limits to confidentiality, and thereby make a positive contribution to safeguarding the welfare of that child. Whilst the overriding aim of securing the best outcome for the child must be kept firmly in view, this can be done without necessarily jeopardizing the GPs relationship with the family, especially if those rights and limits are made clear at the earliest opportunity.

The information and judgements that the GP and the rest of the PHCT give may be enough in the early stages following a referral to reassure the statutory agency that no further action is necessary; alternatively, it may focus attention on a child's needs that can then be addressed in the context of supporting the family; or finally, it may provide the essential information necessary for the statutory agency to act in the best interests of the child by initiating a formal investigation.

References

1 Hallett C. *Inter-Agency Co-ordination in Child Protection.* London: HMSO, l995.

2 Meadow R. *ABC of Child Abuse.* London: BMJ Publishing Group, 1997.

3 Bridge Child Care Consultancy Service. *Paul: Death through Neglect.* London: Bridge Child Care Consultancy Service, 1995.

4 Waterhouse R. *Lost in Care.* London: Stationery Office, 2000.

5 Department of Health. *Diagnosis of Child Sexual Abuse: Guidance for Doctors.* London: Stationery Office, 1988.

6 Royal College of Physicians of London. *Physical Signs of Sexual Abuse in Children.* London: RCP Publications, 1991.

7 Department of Health. *Framework for the Assessment of Children in Need and their Families.* London: Stationery Office, 1999.

8 Department of Health, Home Office, Department of Education and Employment and the National Assembly for Wales. *Working Together to Safeguard Children: a Guide for Interagency Working to Safeguard and Promote the Welfare of Children.* London: Department of Health, 1999.

9 Dodgson C (Lewis Carroll). *Through the Looking-Glass.* 1872.

10 Department of Health, British Medical Association, Conference of Medical Royal Colleges. *Child Protection: Medical Responsibilities.* London: HMSO, 1994.

11 General Medical Council. *Confidentiality: Protecting and Providing Information.* London: GMC, 2000.

Chapter 5d

Child abuse and general practice 2: action

Stephen Amiel

1. The child's interests come first.

2. Relevant information should be shared with other authorized childcare professionals.

3. Concerns about possible abuse must be acted on: no action is not an option.

These points are part of the mantra of child protection. They inform all current child protection legislation and policy and thus appear in some guise or other in almost every chapter of this part of the book. *Partnership* is a fourth key principle: the need for *partnership between agencies and professionals*, which of course should go far beyond simply the sharing of relevant information, is emphasized throughout legislation and guidelines as being crucial for promoting children's well-being and safeguarding them from significant harm.

A good deal is made also of *partnership with parents and children*. Most general practitioners have little difficulty in seeing their relationships with all their patients as a form of partnership. The Family Rights Group[1] consider partnership to be marked by: mutual respect; rights to information; accountability; competence; and value accorded to any individual's contribution. Each partner is seen as having something to offer, power is shared, decisions are made jointly and roles are not only respected but backed by legal and moral rights. To a greater or lesser extent, GPs would have little quarrel with this formulation (although some patients would question the degree to which it applies in practice). When it comes to applying the same criteria to partnership with other agencies and professionals, things often seem more problematic.

For the primary health care team (PHCT), child protection puts partnership with both patients and other agencies to the ultimate test. It may seem that acting in accordance with the first three principles above cannot help but disrupt any sense of partnership with members of a child's family and often the child him or herself. In many instances, a social worker will start their relationship with a family with nowhere to go but up. For the GP, health visitor and other PHCT members, on the other hand, there are often grave concerns that initiating a child protection referral, or even responding to a child protection inquiry, will be disastrous for relationships that may have been built up over years.

This matters a great deal. When the GP or other PHCT member is faced with the possibility that a child may be suffering, or may be at risk of suffering, significant harm, the actions they take and the manner in which they take them may impact not only on the immediate safety of the child, but also—much more commonly—on the *quality of outcome* for the child and the family. Evidence in the Department of Health's *Child Protection: Messages from Research*[2] suggests that the quality of the relationship between a child's family and the professionals responsible is the most important condition for successful outcomes for children at all stages of the protection process. (The other precondition for success is, in most cases, the provision of services to enhance the child's general quality of life.) Positive outcome measures included improvements in health, living conditions, parenting skills, physical and mental development and rates of re-abuse.

The key message undoubtedly remains that the child's interests come first and foremost always, even if that occasionally means removing them from their parents: partnership with parents should never blind the professional to their duty to the child. In these extremes, alienating the parents may seem a small price to pay, although even here, co-operation needs to be attempted. In the vast majority of cases, however, children remain with their parents and, as will be discussed in Chapter 7c, the seeds that are sown at the onset of the child protection process will bear fruit—for better or for worse—later on.

According to *Messages from Research*, good relationships with families are more likely to be maintained and better outcomes thus achieved if:

- there is a conscious attempt to incorporate the family into the investigation and protection plan, by informing, involving and consulting them;

- there is an attempt to seek a measure of agreement about the nature and severity of the abuse;

- agreement is reached about the legitimacy of the enquiry and the solutions adopted;

- honesty, reliability and clarity are prioritized;

- family members feel that the child protection process is 'just', even if it seems to be working against their personal interests;

- parents and children are directed towards sources of support;

- delays and conflicts between agencies and professionals are minimized. (Arguably, many of these conflicts could be avoided if some of the above criteria were applied by professionals to each other as well as to families.)

In practice, it may be difficult for the GP and other PHCT members to achieve this comparatively harmonious approach with families, let alone with each other or with outside agencies, but these criteria are worth aspiring to wherever possible.

An important constraint on partnership with parents is apparent in the guidelines. *Working Together to Safeguard Children*,[3] which seeks to interpret the spirit and letter of child protection legislation says: 'All agencies and professionals should work co-operatively with parents *unless this is inconsistent with the need to ensure the child's safety*' (para. 1.13; my emphasis). This crucial proviso must be borne in mind at all times, although inevitably interpretations of what actions may compromise that safety differ between individuals and localities. Attention is drawn once again to the fact that local child protection guidelines and protocols should always be consulted.

In the remainder of this chapter, scenarios of varying severity, and the actions to be taken by the PHCT accordingly, will be considered with due regard to these introductory considerations. Confidentiality and its limits will also need to be considered at all levels of action. Whilst some reference to this will be made here, a more general discussion on confidentiality may be found in Chapter 3 (see also pp. 141–4).

What to do: low to moderate levels of concern

In Chapter 5c, I described various stages in the diagnosis of child abuse: listening to the patient; thinking the thought, 'Could this be abuse?'; asking supplementary questions; examination; preliminary investigations; reviewing the previous medical history; considering family and social circumstances; and considering the context of the presentation.

A single ambiguous indicator of abuse presenting to the GP will need to be interpreted in the light of what is gleaned during the above stages. If no similar indicators have been noted before, and other risk factors are not present, the GP should do the following:

- *Record all findings*, including important negative ones, and, where possible, a verbatim record of the explanation given by the child or carer for the symptom or injury.

- *Explain the findings* to the carer and, where appropriate, the child.

- Make a *follow-up appointment* with the GP and/or health visitor, with some mechanism for ensuring that a missed appointment is picked up.

- *Discuss the case* with practice colleagues—partners, health visitors (or possibly school nurses for older children) and practice nurses. Consent for professionals to share clinical information within a practice team on a need to know basis is generally thought to be implied, but it is good practice to tell the carer. It is in any case desirable to have a clear statement about the sharing of information in the practice leaflet.

- Check the *child protection register*. Practices should in theory have a record of all their patients who are on a child protection register, and it is considered desirable that their notes should be tagged in some way to alert the PHCT member (see Chapter 5c). With a newly registered family, or when the child is seen in an out of hours situation, checking the register may provide important information by which to judge the significance of a presentation. The following should be noted:

- if the child or sibling is already on the register, social services should certainly be informed at the earliest opportunity;

- the fact that a child is not on the register does not, of course, mean that abuse can be excluded;

- practices should be in possession of local Area Child Protection Committee guidelines that should give the telephone number for checking the register;

- checking the register does not constitute a referral to social services.

- If there remains some doubt about interpretation of the medical findings, consider *informal advice* from a more experienced colleague. This may be another GP with expertise in child protection, or a hospital or community paediatrician. Each health authority has a *designated doctor* (usually a senior local paediatrician) and *nurse*, amongst whose duties is the provision of medical advice and information on child protection, and their numbers too should be available in local guidelines. These posts are likely to be devolved to Primary Care Trust (PCT) level when the 2002 organizational changes to health authorites are fully in place.

There is an important point here. Child protection cases are rarely all or nothing situations where a practitioner either keeps everything to themselves or else has to trigger a formal full-blown investigation. Guidelines on medical responsibilities in child protection make this clear:

> Where uncertainty exists, doctors will often find it helpful to test out professional hypotheses before initial concerns about child abuse are shared with non-medical colleagues. Doctors should clarify their own thoughts about a particular case, and with advice as appropriate from a senior or more experienced colleagues, reach a critical threshold of professional concern. When a *critical threshold of professional concern is reached doctors must be prepared to share these concerns with the statutory agencies for further evaluation and discussion within a time frame which is not detrimental to the child's interests*[4] (my emphasis).

There is no set critical threshold of professional concern, of course. It has to be a matter of individual professional judgement, based on experience and training and will vary according to the individual and the situation. Reaching that threshold in a timely fashion is key to the practitioner's success in achieving a beneficial outcome for the child. Every GP must at the very least try to be aware of their limitations in assessing a situation of this potential gravity and feel able to seek professional advice accordingly.

- GPs should bear in mind their *duty of confidentiality*, whether preliminary consultation is verbal or in writing: this applies equally to medical and non-medical colleagues. Unless colleagues need to know the identity of an individual, e.g. to check their own records, information should be anonymized.

- *Statutory agencies* differ in their approach to informal enquiries from GPs, as they are bound under Section 47 of the Children Act to respond in an official capacity if they 'have reason to suspect' a child is suffering, or is likely to suffer, significant harm. Some GPs have been put off making such enquiries for this reason. In general, however, specialist social workers (child protection coordinators, child protection officers, etc.) are usually willing to discuss practitioners' concerns and provide advice on the understanding that a referral has yet to take place. The information should again be anonymized unless the identity of the individual needs to be known for the advice to be pertinent (e.g. so that circumstantial evidence can be shared confidentially and placed in what is perhaps a wider context of concern). Some social workers are happier to be asked 'hypothetical' questions about general issues rather than be faced with anonymized information about an individual.

- If a practice-employed *nurse, a GP registrar, locum or assistant* is presented with an isolated indicator of abuse, this should be discussed at the earliest opportunity with the responsible GP principal. Similarly, an out of hours GP working in a cooperative or deputizing service should ensure that attention is drawn in their report to any child protection implications of a patient contact. In general, details should be faxed to the responsible GP within 24 hours, rather than a note given to the patient or carer to pass on.

- Practice-attached or aligned *nurses and health visitors* will have their own trust procedures to follow in these situations. These procedures should always include informing the responsible GP.

- *Referral to a paediatrician* experienced in child abuse is a good option when the medical symptoms are not conclusive but are a cause for concern. A paediatric assessment may:[5]

  - *confirm the suspicion* of non-accidental injury;
  - reveal *associated* non-accidental injuries or evidence of *other forms of abuse* or neglect;
  - confirm a diagnosis of *accidental injury*;
  - identify a *medical problem* causing the symptoms or signs or explaining the concerns;
  - *provide the child* with an opportunity to be seen in his or her own right;
  - provide *information and support* for the family and child about the long-term impact of any injury—particularly in cases of child sexual abuse.

- At this point, the GP is genuinely uncertain as to the significance of the medical findings and a referral may be welcomed by the carer and/or child. The differential diagnosis, including abuse, should be *shared with the carer and/or child* if of sufficient understanding (unless it is felt that by doing so, the child might be put in immediate danger: see below).

- The referral to the paediatrician should be *unambiguous and comprehensive* in detailing the background as well as the questions being asked, bearing in mind the rights of the family to read what is written about them. Verbal referral should be followed up in writing. The written referral should also include:

  - clinical observations, including drawings if appropriate;

  - the child's explanation;

  - the parent's or escort's explanation;

  - details of other agency or professional involvement.

- A *full record* should be made in the child's notes of any verbal advice sought from a paediatrician and the advice received, with the date and time recorded.

- A *refusal* to attend a paediatric examination, or *failure to attend*, should be taken seriously, and should lead to consideration of a referral to a statutory agency.

What to do: allegation, disclosure or strong suspicion of abuse

I have said above that the point at which a critical threshold of professional concern is reached will vary according to the individual practitioner and situation. All forms of child abuse tend to be prolonged over time (indeed emotional abuse and neglect are rarely otherwise), and are often diagnosed only when an accumulation of evidence collected over perhaps a long period is examined after what may seem a minor incident or chance observation.

Thus, if *other incidents* of a similar nature have been recorded, or if there are *other risk factors* for abuse in the family, social circumstances or context of the presentation (see Chapters 5a–c), the practitioner has little option but to make a referral to a *statutory agency* (see below).

There are, however, other situations in which that threshold is crossed immediately and where a referral to a statutory agency is inevitable. These are:

- A clear *statement* from a child or accompanying adult that abuse has occurred.

- An *allegation* by one adult carer against another that a child has been abused.

- *Evidence of probable abuse or neglect* apparent from the history, examination or investigations.

- Evidence coming to light that an *adult poses a continuing threat* to other children (see p. 143).

Unless and until shown otherwise, the practitioner has in these situations to presume that the child or children unknown are suffering, or are at risk of suffering, significant harm (for a definition of significant harm, see Chapter 6a, p. 162), and act accordingly. What 'acting accordingly' entails will now briefly be discussed.

Which agency to refer to: statutory agencies

The statutory agencies that have powers to intervene in child protection matters are *social service departments*, the National Society for the Prevention of Cruelty to Children (*NSPCC*) and the *police*. In most situations, social services are the appropriate point of first contact, even when a criminal offence is suspected. In some areas, the NSPCC take a lead role, usually in close association with social service departments and both will work closely with police child protection teams. The police should be contacted first only in certain emergency situations, discussed further below.

What information to give to the statutory agency

The following information will need to be given at the time of a telephone referral and/or in the written referral that should follow.

- The *nature of the concerns*—whether they are thought to constitute abuse or neglect.
- *How and why* the concerns have arisen.
- *Corroborating evidence* for those concerns.
- *Family composition.*
- Relevant *background circumstances*, including any *disability* or sensory impairment the child may have.
- *Other perceived needs* of the family.
- *Other professionals* known to be involved with the family.
- Whether the child/ren may need *urgent action to make them safe* from harm.

Standard referral forms which follow the assessment framework parameters (see Chapter 5c) are available from social service departments: these will guide the practitioner further as to the information required.

Precautions to secure confidentiality over the telephone, fax or by letter should be as described on pp. 142–3 and 191. The identity or personal details of any third party informant should not be revealed without that person's permission.

What to expect from social services

Government guidelines,[6] giving clear timescales for a social services response to a referral of any child in need, are now clearly set out in the *Framework* document.[7] A referral is defined as a request for services to be provided by the social services department.

A decision as to *what response is required* has to be made within *1 working day*. Even if the response is one of no further action, this must be recorded as a decision and communicated to the referrer. In an emergency situation, decisions and preliminary feedback should obviously be even quicker.

If the decision is that more information needs to be gathered, an *initial assessment* is set in motion and must be completed within *7 working days* of the referral. This assessment must 'address the dimensions of the Assessment Framework, determining whether the child is in need, the nature of any services required, from where and within what timescales, and whether a further, more detailed core assessment should be undertaken' (para. 3.9).[7]

The initial assessment should include:

- Interviews with child and family members, as appropriate.

- Involvement of other agencies in gathering and providing information, as appropriate.

- Consultation with the supervisor/manager.

- A record of the initial analysis.

- Decisions on further action/no action.

- A record of decisions/rationale with family/agencies.

- Informing other agencies of the decisions.

- Statement to the family of decisions made, and, if a child is in need, the plan for providing support (para. 3.10).[7]

At the time of writing (2001), there has been no opportunity for the implementation of the assessment framework to be assessed. If the timescales prove to be workable (which many practitioners doubt), it should represent a huge advance for families in terms of reducing uncertainty and delay; and a great potential advance in terms of the child and family's needs beginning to be ascertained in a systematic, evidence-based and constructive manner. Whether those needs once ascertained can be adequately met is another matter.

More will be wanted more quickly from the GP by way of information, and early versions of the paperwork seem daunting. However, if more is expected of GPs, they in turn can expect more from social services by way of a speedy and comprehensive assessment, with action to follow.

The initial assessment will consider whether the concerns about a child's health and development, or actual/potential harm justify further enquiries, assessment and/or intervention. If further action is needed, it will also decide *when* enquiries and/or intervention will take place (see Chapter 6a).

If it is decided that a *further medical examination* is required, this will be arranged by social services, who will discuss the purpose of the examination and other relevant information with the paediatrician. A written report from the practitioner to the paediatrician should still be sent, with contents as detailed above (pp. 149–50). The *urgency* of an examination, who should conduct it, and where, and how the family will be involved, will also be discussed. Usually, a medical examination of *other children* in the family will also be arranged.

A decision *not* to conduct a medical examination should only be taken after the social worker and team manager have discussed the case with an appropriately experienced doctor.

If a child has a *disability* or sensory impairment, the local specialist child development paediatrician should be consulted to determine who should best perform the examination.

If it is deemed that a *criminal offence* against a child may have been committed, social services will coordinate their actions with the police. In less serious cases, they may after discussion decide that the best interests of the child will be served by a social services-led intervention, rather than a full police investigation.

The GP should also note the following:

- The information given by the GP should be used only for the purposes for which it was given.

- Information given by the GP should not be disclosed to a third party, including the family, if it contains personal information about a non-professional informant (e.g. a relative or neighbour), without the permission of that informant.

- The fact that the GP (or other professional) has made the referral will be made known to the family.

- Assessment framework forms completed by the GP or other professionals will be shared with the family.

- The information given by the GP or other PHCT member may be shared on a need to know basis with other members of the child protection team engaged in the investigation of possible abuse of the child concerned. The consent of the GP should be obtained before the information is provided to others who are not involved in the investigation, however.

What to say to the adult carer or competent child

'While professionals should seek, in general, to discuss any concerns with the family and, where possible, seek their agreement to making referrals to social services, *this should only be done where such discussion and agreement-seeking will not place a child at increased risk of significant harm*' (para. 5.6).[3]

Even in situations where the child or accompanying adult *discloses or alleges* abuse, fear and distress may be extreme and agreement to referral may not be easy to obtain. Fears are likely to centre around:

- The *implications of social services involvement.* Many parents and older children believe social services' only response to child abuse allegations is to remove the child from the family home. It is probably this fear more than any other that inhibits disclosure by children and non-abusing parents. GPs need to make it clear that they are obliged to make a referral, and are unable to give a promise of secrecy (see p. 120). On the other hand, they can be strongly reassuring that, provided the safety of the child is ensured, it is extremely unlikely that removal, even in the short term, will be necessary. Whilst no guarantee can be made either that there will be no police involvement or criminal charges, GPs should emphasize that referral to social services should generally result only in greater support being offered to the family. The likely sequence of events should be sketched out: initial assessment, which *may* lead to a more formal series of enquiries under Section 47 of the Children Act, which in turn *may* lead to a child protection case conference. The details of this process are set out in Chapter 6a. Some social service departments provide useful information leaflets explaining this process for families. These should be available to the PHCT to give out.

- *Retaliation* from the alleged abuser(s). These fears should be taken extremely seriously. If an older child or non-abusing carer expresses fears for their immediate safety should they return home, social services should be urgently consulted, or if they cannot be contacted, the police. This is discussed more fully below. Over and above the emergency situation, however, it unfortunately remains the case that the longer term protection of children and non-abusing parents may prove difficult to ensure, and the practitioner should acknowledge that this reality may inhibit cooperation, particularly if criminal proceedings are contemplated.

- The *severity and impact* of the injuries or abuse. The GP's role in examining the child is discussed in the Chapter 5c and may be critical in reassuring the child and carer, as well as identifying any immediate treatment that may be necessary. The practitioner should explain that a specialist paediatric examination will in all probability be required, what it will involve and what its benefits will be. The fact that other children in the household may also be checked as a precaution should also be mentioned.

When the *practitioner suspects* abuse or neglect, a professional judgement needs to be made as to whether sharing those concerns with the accompanying adult will place the child in immediate danger. There is no foolproof way to ascertain this and the practitioner who is in serious doubt should err on the side of caution, delaying confronting the accompanying adult with their concerns until social services have been contacted and a suitable plan worked out.

Some local authorities encourage GPs to contact social services without sharing their concerns or intentions, even with the non-abusing parent, in *all* cases of suspected child sexual abuse. The argument runs that in cases of child sexual abuse, in particular, a child may be intimidated into silence, or worse, if the abuser is given advance warning, and also that forensic evidence may be lost. On rare occasions this may be true, but more often this runs the risk of social services and the police arriving on the doorstep of the family unannounced, the family (including sometimes the child) feeling betrayed by the GP, and the relationship with that family suffering irreversible damage, especially if the abuse is not substantiated.

The GP, faced with a situation where they do not feel it is safe to confront the accompanying adult, or where local guidelines for child sexual abuse discourage them from doing so, may wish to consider two options that whilst not compromising the child's safety, allow at least a chance of retaining the family's trust:

1. *A high profile approach.* When informing social services, the GP can *ask to be involved in a joint visit* with them and the police. As with Mental Health Act assessments, a joint visit can be time-consuming, difficult to coordinate and distressing, but at least the GP can be open with the family at the earliest safe opportunity, rather than perhaps not seeing them again until they are confronted across the table at a case conference. The GP may also at the visit be able to provide information, reassurance and comfort to the child(ren) and non-abusing parent.

2. *A low profile approach.* The GP may express general concerns to the parent about the child, and say that they are unsure about the diagnosis, and that a *referral to a paediatrician* is called for. This can often be arranged by telephone to take place the same day: again it has to be a matter of professional judgement as to whether it can wait longer. There should also be an agreement for the GP and social services to be informed immediately if the child is not taken for the examination. The GP should, in addition to giving the paediatrician details as above (p. 150), clarify whose responsibility it will be to inform social services: the paediatrician should do it, but it is good practice for the GP to do so too. Most community paediatricians understand the importance of the GP's ongoing relationship with the whole family, and, given their own usually short-term relationship with (primarily) the child alone, are more than willing to act as the 'bad guys' in being seen to be responsible for informing social services. Telephone referrals to, and actions agreed by, a paediatrician should be noted, and followed up by letter, a copy of which should form part of the child's medical record.

In all cases, GPs should make a careful record of what is said to the child and accompanying adult(s), and their responses. Actions, their timing, reasons, responses and outcomes form a vital part of the medical record that the GP may need to call upon and answer for, especially if court proceedings follow.

Other considerations

- When a child is brought by an adult who does not have *parental responsibility*, or when an older child or adolescent *attends alone*, the GP should proceed on the basis of the principles discussed with regard to examination in the previous chapter.

- *Other members of the PHCT* will need to be informed of any referral to social services. The responsibility for informing other agencies or professionals involved with the family will usually fall to social services.

- If a practice-employed *nurse, a GP registrar, locum or assistant* is presented with an allegation or disclosure, or has strong suspicion that abuse has occurred, this should be discussed at the earliest opportunity with the responsible GP principal, provided that this can be done within a timeframe that is not detrimental to the child's safety. In the absence of the responsible GP principal, another partner should accept temporary overall responsibility for managing the case. A locum or assistant working alone may have to make a referral themselves if the urgency of the situation dictates it.

- An *out of hours* GP working in a cooperative or deputizing service should ensure that urgent attention is drawn to any child protection implications of a patient contact in their report to the responsible GP. Details should be faxed within 24 hours, rather than a note given to the patient or carer to pass on. This should be followed up by a telephone call to ensure the fax has been received. If the severity of the situation does not permit this, and/or the responsible GP principal or partner is unavailable, the coop or deputizing doctor should take emergency action, as below.

What to do: emergency action

For most children in most situations, action to promote or safeguard a child's welfare can be taken within the PHCT without recourse to statutory agencies. When a child is 'in need', social services have a statutory part to play in assessing and providing services to meet those needs, and the PHCT has an obligation to offer the family referral to them. Sometimes, when additionally a child is deemed to be suffering, or to be at risk of suffering, significant harm, a referral to social services will have to be made, and may lead to additional services being provided and/or action being taken to protect the child. In these situations, taking time to get things right, to reflect on the right course of action, to consult with colleagues, to make a careful and comprehensive assessment of need, and to work sensitively and cooperatively with parents, is not only permissible, but is positively desirable.

Very occasionally, that kind of time is not available. The *severity of a child's condition*, the *degree of continuing risk* of significant harm, or the *new risk following diagnosis or disclosure*, may necessitate immediate action on the part of the GP or PHCT member. In the final part of this chapter, the conditions and options for immediate action will be discussed.

Admission to hospital

Immediate admission to hospital may be necessary in cases of serious physical injury from non-accidental injury, serious neglect or sexual abuse. The practitioner's role is no different here than with any other seriously ill patient. A few additional points are, however, worth noting.

- Appropriate, immediate necessary medical care takes precedence over *evidential* considerations, and over issues of *consent* from an appropriate adult or competent child. 'In an emergency, you may provide medical treatment to anyone who needs it, provided the treatment is limited to what is immediately necessary to save life or avoid significant deterioration in the patient's health'.[8] Attempts should, however, be made to obtain such consent to treatment and admission if time and circumstances permit. For a discussion on consent, see Chapter 3 (p. 56) and Chapter 5c (p. 123).

- If a competent *child refuses* admission, an adult with parental responsibility may override the child's wishes (except in Scotland).

- If the *adult refuses* to allow the child's admission to hospital, the police and social services should be contacted as an emergency. The GP or PHCT member should have regard to their own safety as well as the child's and dial 999 if an adult tries to prevent a child's admission to hospital by removing them from the surgery premises.

- The accompanying *adult's response* when admission is recommended should be observed and noted, including where possible, a verbatim account of what is said.

- If time permits, the *referral letter* that accompanies the child to hospital should contain information as suggested on p. 149. Otherwise, further details may be sent later.

- Once the child has been stabilized and admission arranged, *social services* should be informed at the earliest opportunity. The admitting paediatrician and ideally the GP too should also inform the hospital social worker.

- Steps will need to be taken to ensure the well-being of *other children* in the household. This will usually be arranged by social services and/or the police.

- If the duty social worker cannot be contacted, the *police child protection* team should be contacted. Their office hours and out of hours contact numbers should be available in local guidelines.

- Hospital admission may serve several purposes, in addition to providing emergency treatment for the seriously injured or ill child. According to Speight,[9]

  - it permits the *assessment, documentation and investigation* of suspected child abuse;

  - it provides a temporary *place of safety*;

- in doubtful cases, it allows a *diagnosis* to be made;
- it can give valuable information by allowing *direct observation* of parent–child interaction and parental visiting patterns.

Emergency action by statutory agencies

'Where there is a risk to the life of a child or a likelihood of serious immediate harm, an agency with statutory child protection powers (local authority, police and the NSPCC) *should act quickly to secure the immediate safety of the child*' (para. 5.23).[3]

In general, an emergency referral should be made to social services (or the NSPCC in areas where they have a lead role in emergency work). The police should only be used as a first port of call where social services cannot be contacted or where there is an immediate threat of violence to the child, a non-abusing adult in the family or a member of the PHCT.

Planned emergency action should follow an immediate *strategy discussion* between social services, the police and other agencies, including the NSPCC where appropriate. The referring GP should have some input into this strategy discussion, which may take place over the telephone. Where immediate action is imperative, the strategy discussion may take place soon after.

Attempts will be made to secure the child's safety by securing the agreement of the alleged *perpetrator* to *leave the home,* or by taking action to ensure his removal (e.g. an Exclusion Order under the Family Act 1996).

At other times, if this is not possible, or if there is no other adult in the household able and willing to provide adequate care, the child may be *removed to a safe place,* either on a voluntary basis, or by obtaining an Emergency Protection Order (EPO). Social services departments will endeavour to place a child with a familiar adult (e.g. a grandparent) or failing that, an authorized foster parent. Similar arrangements will probably be made for other children in the household. (See also Chapters 6a and 6b.)

If necessary, the *police also have powers* under Section 46 of the Children Act to remove a child to suitable accommodation if necessary, but these powers are generally discouraged and in any case apply for a maximum of only 72 hours.

Occasionally, if it is felt that a *non-abusing adult's safety* cannot be ensured either, both she and the child(ren) may be temporarily accommodated elsewhere, e.g. in a women's refuge.

The GP, apart from their role in making the emergency referral and participating in the initial strategy discussion, will be approached for further information if, as is likely, further enquiries (under Section 47 of the Children Act) are made. They may also be required to provide to GP colleagues necessary medical information about those members of the family who may be temporarily accommodated elsewhere.

The GP should ensure that members of the PHCT have a clear *procedure* to follow in emergency situations, including making available the necessary *training opportunities.*

Emergency police and social services *telephone numbers* should be readily available and updated regularly.

Attempts should be made to keep in contact with the family wherever possible, including adults who may be suspected of abuse. The GP's role should not end with a referral and the immediate protection of the child. In many ways, this should be seen instead as the beginning of a new phase, working in conjunction with other PCHT members and outside agencies, but also working with family members, to secure the best possible outcome for the child. This is discussed further in Chapter 7c.

References

1 **Family Rights Group.** *The Children Act, 1989. Working in Partnership with Families.* London: HMSO, 1991.
2 **Department of Health.** *Child Protection: Messages From Research.* London: HMSO, 1995.
3 **Department of Health, Home Office, Department of Education and Employment and the National Assembly for Wales.** *Working Together to Safeguard Children: a Guide for Interagency Working to Safeguard and Promote the Welfare of Children.* London: Department of Health, 1999.
4 **Department of Health, British Medical Association, Conference of Medical Royal Colleges.** *Child Protection: Medical Responsibilities.* London: HMSO, 1994.
5 **Hodes D.** *ACPC Child Protection Procedures.* London: London Borough of City and Hackney, 1998: section 8.7.
6 **Department of Health.** *Quality Protects Circular.* Local Authority Circular (LAC). London: Department of Health, 1999.
7 **Department of Health.** *Framework for the Assessment of Children in Need and their Families.* London: DOH, 2000.
8 **General Medical Council.** *Seeking Patients' Consent: the Ethical Considerations.* London: GMC Publications, 1998.
9 **Speight N.** Non-accidental injury. In: Meadow R, ed. *ABC of Child Abuse.* London: BMJ Publishing Group, 1997: 5–8.

Chapter 6

What happens next?

Chapter 6a

The investigation of child abuse

Madeline Ismach

Introduction

Professionals interact with children and their families in different ways according to the nature of their contact and responsibilities. The key to making a positive and informed contribution to the safety of children is to have an understanding of the child protection system and be clear about your professional role. There are many reasons why GPs may give the identification of child abuse or neglect rather less attention than other medical responsibilities. Nevertheless guidance to GPs from the Department of Health indicates that GPs are a vital part of the professional childcare network and that there is a clear expectation of cooperation with child protection procedures. (See also Chapter 6c.)

The investigation of child abuse is a multidisciplinary affair. Each child abuse and child death inquiry has confirmed the crucial importance of multidisciplinary communication. The stark facts are that, when professionals fail to know and implement procedures and when information is not shared, a child may be placed at risk, sometimes with tragic consequences.

There are many complex tensions and pressures that may inhibit good communication. The web of legislation, guidance and structures which surround the provision of services for children both nationally and locally are in part a response to those. Primary among these is the *Children Act*, which was passed in 1989 and came into force in 1991. That year the Department of Health also published *Working Together*.[1] Updated in 1999,[2] this document interprets the Children Act and is intended to provide a guide to interagency cooperation.

The Children Act outlines the way courts and professionals should work with children and their families. The overriding purpose of the Act is to promote and safeguard the welfare of children within a framework which indicates that parents are responsible for their children and that these children are best looked after within their own families. Certain *basic concepts* are central to the legislation.

1. *The welfare of the child is paramount.* This issue is further defined by means of a welfare checklist which indicates relevant factors to consider in order to better identify what would be in a child's best interests. The checklist covers issues such as:

   - ascertaining the *wishes* and *feelings* of the child;
   - physical, emotional and educational *needs*;
   - the likely effect of a *change in circumstances*;
   - *age, sex* and *background characteristics* considered relevant;
   - any *harm* (s)he has suffered or is at risk of suffering;
   - the *capacity of the child's parents/carers* to meet his needs.

2. *Court orders* in relation to a child should only be made if it will be in the child's best interest and be better than not making an order, i.e. positive results will be achieved.

3. *Delay* in making decisions for children should be avoided.

4. Due consideration should be given to *race, religion, culture and language.*

5. *Children should participate* in and be kept informed of decisions in relation to their care.

6. Parents should be assisted where necessary in bringing up their children by the provision of services to support families. This should occur in *partnership with parents.* The issue of partnership is central to the Children Act and to current thinking about good practice for professionals. Partnership refers to cooperation, both between agencies and professionals and between professionals and families. (See also Chapters 5d and 6d.)

The concepts of *need* and *harm* and their implications for local authority action are further defined in the Act.

1. *Need.* Part III of the Children Act places on local authorities a general duty to safeguard and promote the welfare of children in their area who are deemed to be in need. Under the Act, a child is 'in need' if:

   - 'he is unlikely to achieve or maintain, or to have the opportunity of achieving or maintaining, a reasonable standard of health or development without the provision for him of services by a local authority';
   - 'his health and development is likely to be significantly impaired, or further impaired, without the provision of such services'; or
   - 'he is disabled' (Section 17(10)).

   (See also Chapter 5c.)

2. *Significant harm.* The impetus to investigate allegations of abuse comes from Section 47 of the Children Act. This section specifies that 'if a Local Authority is informed or has reasonable cause to suspect that a child is suffering or is likely to suffer significant harm, the Authority shall make or cause to be made such enquiries as it considers necessary to enable it to decide whether it should take any action to safeguard or promote the child's welfare'. It is the duty of other agencies to assist enquiries by providing relevant information and advice unless it would be unreasonable to do so.

   Significant harm is a concept introduced in the Children Act 1989 to help define more serious forms of ill-treatment. *Harm* is defined as '*the state of a child which is attributable to ill-treatment or failure to provide adequate care*'. It can encompass impairment of physical or mental *health* and/or impairment of physical, intellectual, social or behavioural *development*. From 2002, in recognition of the impact of domestic violence on children, the Children Act definition of 'harm' will also include 'impairment suffered from seeing or hearing the ill-treatment of another' (section 31(9)).

   Harm in relation to health and development is judged to be *significant* by comparing the health or development of the child in question with that which could reasonably be expected of a child with similar attributes and needs.

   To understand and establish significant harm, it is necessary to consider, as outlined in *Working Together*:[2]

   - the *family* context;
   - the child's *development* within the context of their family and wider social and cultural environment;
   - any *special needs*, such as a medical condition, communication difficulty or disability that may affect the child's development and care within the family;
   - the *nature of harm*, in terms of ill-treatment or failure to provide adequate care;
   - the *impact* of that harm on the child's health and development;
   - the *adequacy of parental care*.

   It is important always to *take account of the child*: their reactions and their perceptions, according to their age and understanding.

3. *Ill-treatment.* Four forms of ill-treatment are registerable according to the *Working Together* guidance:[2]

   - physical abuse;
   - neglect;
   - sexual abuse;
   - emotional abuse.

The nature and impact of these forms of abuse are discussed in Chapters 5a and 5b (see also Table 6.2, p. 183).

Failure to provide adequate care can apply not only to cases of obvious neglect but also when parents fail to make use of available services, to their child's detriment. An obvious example would be where parents do not ensure that their child receives appropriate and timely medical care essential to their child's well-being, to such an extent that the child is suffering, or likely to suffer, significant harm.

Investigating possible child abuse

The prime tasks of an investigation, according to *Working Together* 1991 are:[1]

- to establish the facts about the circumstances giving rise to the concern;
- to decide if there are grounds for concern;
- to identify sources and level of risk;
- to decide protective or other action in relation to the child and any others.

The Children Act and *Working Together* outline the issues that need to be dealt with when working effectively with children in a child protection framework. However, they have together added to the development of a formal procedurally driven system to investigate abuse. Inevitably the search for absolute certainty in professional practice has led to a sometimes unrefined 'catch all' system which can fail to distinguish levels of risk and to respond in an appropriately flexible way.

Increasing unease about the cost of such a system to both families and professionals has led to a range of responses. The Department of Health has issued a number of significant studies including guidance such as *The Challenge of Partnership in Child Protection: Practice Guide,*[3] which built on the policy laid out in *Working Together* 1991. This outlines in detail the way in which professionals, especially social workers, should undertake child protection practice, balancing the need to protect children with the recognition that the best way to do this is to involve and inform parents and children, while recognizing the parameters to partnership and where it may not be appropriate. The *Practice Guide* was followed in late 1995 by *Child Protection: Messages from Research,*[4] an account of 20 pieces of research which explore and report on outcomes of the current system. The findings included the fact that too many children and families are caught up in the child protection system and that far from protecting children, an investigation which highlights difficulties and which offers no solutions or support is likely to cause greater stress on the family. In a University of East Anglia study,[5] it was found that 44 per cent of investigations led to no further action at all and six out of seven children referred to the child protection system are filtered out and not placed on the register. These and other research findings have led to a swing of the pendulum towards a more positive *child in need approach.*

The general overview of *Messages from Research* indicated that children's safety following referral could be improved by:

- *sensitive and informed professional–client relationships* where honesty and reliability are valued;
- *an appropriate balance of power* where serious attempts are made at *partnership*;
- a wide perspective on child protection that is not simply concerned with investigating forensic evidence but also with notions of *welfare, prevention and treatment*;
- effective *supervision and training of social workers*;
- the general *enhancement of children's quality of life* by use of Section 17 and Part III of the Children Act to provide services to help children in need;
- the *making of enquiries into concerns* rather than the current investigative approach.

This has been taken up in different ways by agencies and individual professionals. Some local authorities have indicated that a lighter approach is needed, with all members of the professional network taking individual responsibility for establishing the level and nature of concern and referring more appropriately than previously to a range of community services. This may include coordinating multiprofessional meetings to set and monitor action plans. For other local authorities there has been little change in working practices. Inevitably it is likely to be the local authority social services department who sets the tone in a particular area as the principal agency in child protection.

In April 2001 the *Framework for the Assessment of Children in Need and their Families*[6] was introduced. This further refines the childcare system, building on the work coming out of *Messages from Research*. The framework is intended to provide 'a systematic way of analysing, understanding and recording what is happening to children ... within their families and in the context of the community in which they live'. The detailed parameters for the framework assessment are set out in Chapter 5c.

The framework provides a broader approach than that used previously and is initially focused on *establishing the needs* of the particular child referred (only one of which may be the need for protection from harm), then *aiming to meet those needs by providing services* to the child and their family.

This more holistic approach is intended to contribute to a more integrated inter- or multiagency approach as 'the safeguarding of children is not to be seen as a separate activity from promoting their welfare' (para 1.17).[6]

It is likely that GPs will need some knowledge of the assessment framework: they will be involved in making referrals and in contributing to aspects of the assessment process. Timescales are fairly rigorous and will be audited.

- *One working day* for a social services department to make a decision on a course of action or response to be made in relation to children in need referrals.

- *Seven working days* (maximum) for an *initial assessment* to be carried out and a decision to be made whether to initiate a child protection inquiry or a core assessment, whether to allocate resources, or whether to take no further action.

- A further *35 working days* (maximum) for a *core assessment* to have been completed, a child protection investigation completed, the needs of the child and family assessed, and appropriate intervention identified and implemented.

These timescales will undoubtedly impact on all professionals involved with the care of children in need.

Child protection is a difficult and imprecise area and for many professionals it is not their primary task. Indeed the very infrequency of its occurrence for some professionals may lead to the tensions and stress that occur between professionals as they struggle to fit into the currently prevailing system in their area. However, cooperation in child protection work is mandatory and all professionals should have training, knowledge of and access to locally specific procedures to enable them to make the best possible contribution to the process.

Although there will be local variations, the flow chart issued by Department of Health (Figure 6.1) is likely to be followed by most local authorities. Where the decision to refer has been made it is likely that the first port of call will be a duty social worker. In an emergency situation, referrals by phone or fax are appropriate. These should be followed up in writing: many social services departments will have standard referral forms, based on the framework parameters, for use by GPs or other professionals. From April 2001 local authorities are likely to have a permanent assessment team whose job it is to undertake enquiries into all allegations of child abuse and any short-term work involved with the task. They would usually carry the case to child protection conference when ongoing work is required. These teams are also responsible for the broader assessment of need, of which the need for protection is a part.

Studies in *Messages from Research*[4] indicate clearly that it is unlikely that a specific incident will in itself be a good indicator of the future welfare of a child. It is much more likely that a child's general environment and upbringing will give a far clearer understanding of the situation and more accurately predict the outcome for a particular child. It is precisely this perspective which may be lost in systems which focus too explicitly on a particular incident. Thus the provision of teams that are responsible for both safeguarding and promoting the welfare of children is intended to improve outcomes for children in need and their families.

Usually the duty social worker, as a way of ensuring that *network checks* are undertaken, will have specific forms to complete as part of an *initial assessment*, and will therefore want to elicit particular information. This involves all relevant professionals being asked for either general or specific information to enable the duty social worker to build up a detailed picture of the family in order that the level of risk to a particular child can be established and a suitable intervention planned.

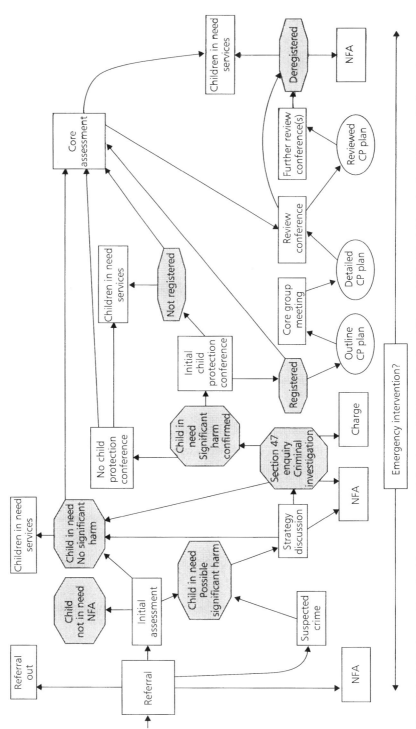

Fig. 6.1 Individual cases flowchart for assessment following a child in need referral (from ref [2]). CP, child protection; NFA, no further action.

It is important that GPs should have carefully thought through their own professional issues in advance in order to respond in a way which both meets their own professional needs and is in line with local procedures (see Chapters 5c and 5d).

Sadly, constraints in services mean that professionals sometimes feel obliged to designate referrals as child protection in order to obtain a service. This is generally unhelpful. It is critical that referrers are as accurate as possible and have, possibly through a process of consultation with colleagues or a designated doctor/nurse, a clear sense of their concerns. It is usually helpful to write down an exact record of the information or events which are the subject of concern.

There is however a place for *informal networking* in achieving this clarity. Each health authority has a designated doctor/nurse who should have current expert knowledge of child abuse. Usually the designated doctor is a paediatrician who can be consulted for advice. (These posts are likely to be devolved to Primary Care Trust (PCT) level when the 2002 organizational changes to health authorities are fully in place.)

Most social services departments have a lead officer in child protection often known as a child protection coordinator or child protection manager. This person usually has organizational responsibility for all child protection conferences in the area. Their staff or associates usually chair conferences independently. They are also available for consultation and training. It should be possible to hold an informal discussion of concerns with staff in these posts.

Some local authorities operate a 'patch' system: teams that are identified with, and have responsibility for, a particular locality or even a cluster of general practices. Making contact with the team manager or senior social worker in your locality prior to concerns arising and building a relationship with them will ensure that concerns can be properly considered as and when they arise. However, informal networking should not be used as a method of delaying a referral.

As implied above, there are local variations in these arrangements, and practitioners are advised to consult their local Area Child Protection Committee (ACPC) procedures which should detail the local variations.

The initial assessment will decide whether:

- *no further action* is required;

- there are *needs for services* that can readily be identified;

- there are complex needs requiring a *core assessment*;

- there is a possibility of significant harm and a *strategy meeting/ discussion* should be convened with a view to child protection enquiries being made.

In cases of extreme urgency, a strategy discussion can take place over the telephone, although the information shared, the decisions reached and the basis for those decisions, should be recorded by all parties to the discussion. Apart from social services and the police, a strategy meeting should include the referring agency and other agencies (e.g. education or health) as appropriate, unless the matter is so urgent that immediate action must be taken by police and social services to protect the child.

The strategy meeting or discussion should include consideration of:

- what *action* is needed to secure the child's *immediate and continuing safety;*
- the need for enquiries under Section 47 of the Children Act as part of a *core assessment:* what further information is needed about the family, and from whom;
- the need for a *police investigation;*
- how to best *gather information*—is there a need for the child's information to be given on video? (this would be done if allegations may constitute a crime leading to court proceedings and the video would then be evidence at a hearing);
- whether a *medical examination* is needed. This would entail referral to the designated local paediatrician. Other medical information from the GP/health visitor should be considered;
- the *involvement of the child* according to age and understanding;
- any issues of *race/language/gender/culture;*
- practical assistance to enable *family participation* and the sharing of information where this would not jeopardize the child or the investigation;
- identifying the *extended family* and any support they may offer;
- any *specific issues* which need to be considered, e.g. disability or the need for an interpreter;
- fitting the investigation into the *broader assessment framework.*

The issue of video disclosure interviews can be difficult. These are evidential interviews conducted in line with the *Memorandum of Good Practice* guidance[7] on the subject. They should be conducted by a trained police officer and social worker. The pressure not to miss evidence has led to the unnecessary use of video interviews. Very few have been used in court—the purpose for which they were designed. Some have been used in civil proceedings in an attempt to demonstrate that abuse did not occur as the child made no disclosure.

In general a video should only be made if the child is of an age and competence to give evidence and if there are indicators to suggest that an offence has been committed. Staff undertaking such interviews should have specialist training and be in a position to obtain regular practise.

In the majority of cases concerns will be either laid to rest or the need for services and support established. In a limited number of cases serious concern for the welfare of the child will be confirmed.

References

1 Home Office, Department of Health, Department of Education and Science, Welsh Office. *Working Together Under the Children Act 1989*. London: HMSO, 1991.

2 Department of Health, Home Office, Department for Education and Employment. *Working Together to Safeguard Children: a Guide to Inter-agency Working to Safeguard and Promote the Welfare of Children*. London: HMSO, 1999.

3 Department of Health Social Service Inspectorate. *The Challenge of Partnership in Child Protection: Practice Guide*. London: HMSO, 1995.

4 Department of Health. *Child Protection: Messages from Research*. London: HMSO, 1995.

5 Gibbons J, Conroy S, Ball C. *Operating the Child Protection System: a Study of Child Protection Practices in English Local Authorities*. London: HMSO, 1995.

6 Department of Health. *Framework for the Assessment of Children in Need and their Families*. London: Stationery Office, 2000.

7 Home Office, Department of Health. *Memorandum of Good Practice on Video Recorded Interviews with Child Witnesses for Criminal Proceedings*. London: HMSO, 1992.

Chapter 6b

Legislative framework for child protection

Alison Lowton and Gloria McFarlane

Introduction

Parts IV and V of the Children Act 1989 contain the statutory basis for child protection investigations. Within the philosophy of the Children Act, any action under Parts IV and V should (except in an emergency situation) follow from the preventative functions set out in Part III of the same Act. This contains the range of service provision that local authorities should provide for children in need and their families.

However, much of the familiar framework for child protection is not in the Children Act at all but is contained in *Working Together to Safeguard Children*.[1] *Working Together* provides the basis for the activities of the Area Child Protection Committee (ACPC), which is an 'inter-agency forum for agreeing how the different services and professional groups should co-operate to safeguard children in that area, and for making sure that arrangements work effectively to bring about good outcomes for children' (para. 4.1).[1] It also provides the statutory basis for child protection registers and child protection case conferences.

Working Together has the status of 'guidance', issued by the Department of Health, Home Office and Department for Education and Employment. Social services are required to act under the guidance of the Secretary of State for Health and as a consequence, guidance has virtually statutory force for local authorities. *Working Together* is, however, addressed to all agencies working with children.

The preventative role

Emphasis is increasingly being given to the preventative rather than the protective role of social services. Joint guidance has been issued instituting from April 2001 a new assessment framework[2] for children in need which will also have a multiagency approach.

It is important to recognize, however, that the provision of services to children in need and their families may also be the starting point for the local authority's role in child protection. There is a general duty on local authorities to take reasonable steps to identify children in need and to reduce the need for care proceedings. Local authorities either must or may make available a range of services to support children in need within their families. At some point, social services may come to the conclusion that the child may be more in need of protection than the other preventative services they may provide. To that extent, child protection has to be seen as part of the continuum of social services' more general responsibility towards children in need.

Investigation

There are two main duties to investigate imposed on social services by the Children Act, Sections 37 and 47. Section 37 is invoked as result of a court order and most often arises from private family proceedings where the court has concerns about the child's welfare or where social services have already had some involvement. Under the more commonly used Section 47, there is a duty to 'make such enquiries as [social services] consider necessary' where the authority has reasonable cause to suspect that a child is suffering or is likely to suffer significant harm or where the child is subject to an emergency protection order (EPO) or police protection. (A court must have the same belief in harm or likelihood of harm to the child to grant an EPO.)

The definition of 'harm' is very wide ranging. It includes not only ill-treatment but also the impairment of health or development. 'Significant' is not defined by the Act except that 'where the question of whether harm is significant turns on the child's health or development, his health or development shall be compared with that which could reasonably be expected of a similar child'. This means that comparisons are to be made with similar children—not children in similar circumstances (see Chapter 6a).

The purpose of the investigation is to establish whether or not the local authority should make an application for a care order or seek some other form of intervention through service provision and parental cooperation.

The authority must take reasonable steps to ensure they obtain access to the child. The authority does not have a right to enter premises where access is refused even with an EPO; however, if an EPO is granted an application can also be made to the court under Section 48 for a warrant to enter premises. Where access is refused or information on the child's whereabouts is denied, the authority is under a duty to apply for an EPO, care order, supervision order or child assessment order unless they are satisfied that the child's welfare can be safeguarded without so doing.

Part of the investigation will involve consultation with other agencies. Those agencies that are requested to assist by the local authority are under a duty to comply unless it would unreasonable to do so (Sections 47(9) and (10)). It is hard to see when it would be unreasonable to assist in a child protection investigation. The agencies listed are any local authority, housing authority, education authority and any health authority/NHS Trust. The list does not include grant-maintained or private schools, private or voluntary nurseries and other childcare organizations, private hospitals or clinics, police or the probation service.

GPs in England and Wales are now part of, and are increasingly accountable to, Primary Care Trusts (PCTs) (Health and Social Service Trusts, HSSTs, in Northern Ireland and Local Health Care Cooperatives, LHCCs, in Scotland, are broadly similar organizations) and the same duty to comply in a S 47 investigation may then reasonably be expected of them as of any other NHS Trust. Health authorites are enjoined (para. 3.26), through agreement with PCTs or equivalent, to 'ensure that the local health service contribution to inter-agency working is discharged'. In their role as commissioners of health services, PCTs are also expected to specify 'clear service standards for safeguarding children and promoting their welfare, consistent with ACPC guidelines' (para. 3.27). Paragraph 3.30 of *Working Together*[1] makes clear what is expected of the individual GP and the rest of the PHCT: their important role in all stages of the child protection process includes 'sharing information with social services when enquiries are being made about a child'.

Issues in the investigation

A child protection investigation may take a number of forms depending on the nature of the suspected abuse and the level, if any, of social services' prior involvement and knowledge. Broadly, it will involve information-gathering—either from written materials or interviews with professionals; interviews with family members; interviews with the child; and/or medical examinations. There are legal issues associated with all these approaches, which are briefly considered below. Not all child protection investigations will result in legal action. None the less, it is important to remember that they might and to avoid any obvious pitfalls.

By its very nature, a lot of the information collected by social services would in other proceedings be inadmissible in court—either because it is opinion and not fact or because it is hearsay (i.e. information given by one person but relayed to the court by another). However, any expert is able to give opinion evidence and the normal rule against hearsay does not apply in proceedings related to children. Social workers, teachers and doctors are all considered experts by the court.

Although one particular incident may trigger an investigation, there may be a long series of apparently unrelated, trivial incidents, reported to a number of different people. In assisting social services' investigations, this kind of information must also be provided so that patterns of behaviour can be identified. This is particularly important where there is apparent failure to thrive or other signs of neglect.

The standard of proof required in care proceedings is different to the standard required in criminal proceedings. For example, where a child is injured, a local authority does not have to prove who did it beyond reasonable doubt but that, on the balance of probabilities, it was non-accidental and attributable to lack of care by the parent.

Information from other professionals will predominantly be from teachers and health professionals. They may often regard their information as confidential or may have promised confidentiality to a disclosing child or adult. However, *Working Together* emphasizes that generally duties of confidentiality are overridden in respect of child protection (paras 7.32 and 7.33).[2] (See also Chapters 3 and 5c.)

Social workers may try to obtain information from other family members but cannot compel them to cooperate. Explanations from carers in cases of suspected non-accidental injury are vital to assess against the appearance of the injury. In cases of suspected sexual abuse, however, it is unlikely that social services will seek information from the carer until they can ensure that the child is not going to be silenced.

Information from the child is more problematic. Social services may interview a child without seeking parental consent, but this is unusual. If parents do not consent, social services would have to consider applying for an EPO. However, how much weight to give that evidence will depend on the individual child—how old they are; their ability to understand and to explain; their level of distress and so on.

Interviewing children (especially young children)—with or without a video—is difficult. If any part of the interview may be used in court proceedings (and especially if these are criminal) it is vital that it is the child that provides the information. In other words, the person conducting the interview must be careful not to make suggestions to the child or to appear to lead the child in any particular direction. This can be done verbally but can also be done in other ways and the use of anatomically correct dolls has caused particular problems. It can be argued, for example, that unless there is other evidence which strongly suggests sexual abuse, the introduction into an interview of such dolls is a way of leading the child, of suggesting to the child the sort of response the interviewer wants. The use of these and any similar props or tools should be done only in exceptional circumstances by someone with training. Generally speaking, great care must be taken in any discussion with a child about possible abuse, although there may clearly be situations where some attempt to direct the child is unavoidable.

There has been much emphasis, and controversy, on the use of video interviews. They are important in criminal proceedings to avoid the child having to give direct evidence but their usefulness as evidence in care proceedings is doubtful. They carry exactly the same difficulties as other forms of interview and again should only be conducted by someone with experience and training.

Other aspects of an investigation may include the need for a medical or psychiatric examination. If that is the case, parental consent is needed, unless examination is required as an emergency or the child is able to give informed consent. If consent is not forthcoming from a parent, social services may need to apply for an EPO and obtain leave of the court for the examination; this can only take place if the child agrees. Once an EPO or interim care order has been obtained, leave of the court for any examination or assessment will be required if any report is to be used as evidence. If any interview is to be videotaped, parental consent must be obtained. If the parent will not consent, social services will have to obtain a court order.

Following the investigation, the authority may decide that further action is required in order to protect a child. That is likely to be within the case conference framework.

Case conferences

A child protection conference should only be called after an S47 investigation. It is social services' (or the NSPCC's) responsibility to convene the conference although any concerned professional can ask for a conference to be held.

The only decision a child protection conference can take is whether to place or remove a child's name on the child protection register. It may make recommendations as to future action but the decision on that future action rests with social services as the agency with the statutory powers. There is a requirement to hold regular review conferences.

Membership of the conference in each case will vary depending on the particular circumstances. As a general rule, all agencies with specific responsibilities for the child should be invited. Because of this, it is often the first occasion when it is possible to build up a picture of that child's life. Those invited are entitled to the minutes which are otherwise confidential and only disclosable to non-participants with the consent of the chair.

Parents/carers are increasingly encouraged to attend. This poses difficulties, particularly for those professionals who will continue to have a relationship with the parents outside the child protection framework, particularly teachers and health professionals. There must be a clear procedure for parental attendance which deals with issues such as any grounds for refusing to allow parents to attend; confidentiality; and the role of any lawyer present (see also Chapters 6c and 6d).

As well as child protection conferences, social services may also hold strategy meetings. These are usually attended by the most immediately involved professionals but not by the parents. These meetings will consider more immediate actions to be taken to protect the child.

Immediate protection

There are two immediate ways in which children may be protected. The police have the power to remove a child to a safe place where they have reasonable cause to suspect that the child is suffering or will suffer significant harm if left, or if removed by a parent/carer from where they are (e.g. a hospital). This is not an order. It is a power which any police officer may exercise. A child may only be kept in police protection for 72 hours (usually in local authority provided accommodation).

Any person may apply to the court without notice for an EPO. The grounds are the same, although a local authority may also apply if access to a child is refused in the course of an investigation. An EPO lasts for 8 days (but can be extended on application to the court for a further 7 days). If the local authority thinks that the child requires looking after for longer, that either has to be with parental consent or by way of an interim care order. If a child has disappeared, the local authority may apply to court for a recovery order.

References

1 **Department of Health, Home Office, Department of Education and Employment and the National Assembly for Wales.** *Working Together to Safeguard Children: a Guide for Interagency Working to Safeguard and Promote the Welfare of Children.* London: Department of Health, 1999.
2 **Department of Health.** *Framework for the Assessment of Children in Need and their Families.* London: Stationery Office, 1999.

Chapter 6c

The child protection conference

Stephen Amiel

Introduction

Each year, in England alone, approximately 40 000 initial child protection conferences (CPCs) are held. For some, the CPC symbolizes the interagency nature of assessment, treatment and management of child protection. For many general practitioners, the conference epitomizes much of what they dislike, distrust and find frustrating about the child protection process. By and large, they appear to vote with their feet and stay away from them in droves.

As described in Chapter 6a, a great deal of work is done before, around and often instead of a CPC, some or all of which may involve the GP and the primary health care team. From the work of Gibbons and others,[1] it is estimated that in 1992, only a quarter of the 160 000 referrals to the child protection process in England reached the conference stage.

The filtering process that precedes a conference takes several forms. To recap briefly, following a referral to a statutory agency (social services, police or sometimes the National Society for the Prevention of Cruelty to Children (NSPCC)) immediate action will occasionally need to be taken if those agencies consider that a child's life is at risk, or there is a likelihood of immediate significant harm. In these cases, the child might be removed to a place of safety, either voluntarily, or as a result of an emergency protection order (EPO), or by being placed under police protection.

Usually, however, once an initial assessment has established that significant harm is a possibility, there is time for relevant records and child protection registers to be checked, relevant professionals to be consulted and a strategy meeting or discussion convened with a view to enquiries being made under Section 47 of the Children Act[2] as part of a core assessment. In roughly a quarter of cases, no further investigation will be considered necessary, although the need for further support and services may be identified. In the remainder (roughly 120 000 cases on Gibbons' figures[1]), sufficient concerns will remain to justify further enquiries.

In the investigation of suspected physical abuse, emotional abuse and neglect, those concerns will be put to parents as early as possible, usually on a joint family visit by social services and the police; consent to a medical examination and joint interview of the child will be sought; the circumstances of other children in the household will be considered, and plans usually made to investigate them too.

If sexual abuse has been disclosed or alleged, or is suspected on medical examination, the response following a strategy meeting may vary, according to whether the alleged perpetrator(s) is a member of the family. In this situation, contact may initially be with the non-abusing parent only, or, if both parents are alleged perpetrators, the child may need to be removed, at least temporarily, to a place of safety (see Chapter 6b). With lower levels of concern, or in the absence of a disclosure, the strategy meeting may decide to involve parents and child in a monitoring, assessment and, if necessary, a treatment process, reconvening the strategy meeting after a fixed period and leaving the option open at any time to proceed to interview, medical examination and conference if suspicions of sexual abuse reach a critical threshold.

By this point, the investigators should be able to decide, on the basis of the information gathered, the results of the initial interviews and the medical examination:

- if a significant degree of harm or risk of harm exists;
- if that harm is thought to be attributable to the child's parents/carers;
- what input or intervention is needed if that child is to stay safely with their parent/carer or, if that is not possible, what statutory action needs to be taken to safeguard the child;
- whether criminal charges are to be instigated (a police decision);
- whether a child protection conference needs to be convened.

In approximately 80 000 of the 120 000 cases investigated in 1992, no conference was felt to be necessary. At the other extreme, about 1500 children were separated from their parents even before a conference was held.

Functions and process of the initial child protection conference

In theory, according to government guidelines contained in *Working Together*,[3] an initial CPC should be convened within 15 working days of the strategy discussion. Gibbons and colleagues[1] found that in practice the interval was 34 days on average.

An initial CPC is not the place where a decision is made that a particular person has abused a child (a matter for the courts). Rather, its role is seen in *Working Together* thus:

> It brings together family members, the child where appropriate, and those professionals most involved with the child and family, following s. 47 enquiries. Its purpose is:
>
> - to bring together and analyse in an inter-agency setting the information which has been obtained about the child's health, development and functioning, and the parents' or carers' capacity to ensure the child's safety and promote the child's health and development;

Table 6.1 The tasks of the initial child protection conference.

- To *establish known facts* about the case
- To *share information* about the child and family
- To *evaluate the degree of risk* to all children in the family
- To make recommendations about what *immediate intervention* may be necessary to protect the child(ren)
- To make recommendations about what *services* should be provided on the basis of assessed needs, whether or not registration occurs
- To decide whether the child should be placed on the *child protection register*
- To appoint a *key worker* if the child is registered
- To make recommendations as to what areas a multidisciplinary, interagency *child protection plan* should address, and how and by whom they should be taken forward
- To appoint a *core group* of key professionals. This group will work with the family to obtain/complete a *comprehensive assessment*, which will inform the further detailed development and implementation of the child protection plan; the group will also agree how to monitor the child protection plan
- To set a date for the first *review conference*

- to make judgements about the likelihood of a child suffering significant harm in future; *and*

- to decide what future action is needed to safeguard the child and promote his or her welfare, how that action will be taken forward, and with what intended outcomes (para. 5.53).[3]

Table 6.1 sums up the tasks of the initial CPC.

The list of people invited to an initial CPC can be as daunting as the tasks they will face. It is recommended that, for the sake of both efficiency and confidentiality, only those with a need to know or a contribution to make should receive invitations. The guiding principles underpinning all child protection work, that the child's welfare is paramount, that professionals should work in partnership with family members and with each other, and that parental responsibility should be emphasized, also determine who is invited. Typically then, some or all of the following will be invited and/or expected to be present:

- *From social services:* the *chairperson* (occasionally from the NSPCC); *social worker* and their *team leader* responsible for the enquiries/investigation to date; *minute-taker.*

- *From health services: general practitioner; health visitor* and *nurse manager* (or child protection adviser); *school nurse.*

- *From education: teacher* and/or *head teacher; nursery worker; educational welfare officer.*

- *From law enforcement: police officer* (usually from the local child protection team); *probation officer.*

- *From the family: parent(s); child(ren); friend, relative* or *supporter.*

Depending on individual circumstances, the following may also be present: *hospital doctors* and/or *nurses* (where abuse was first diagnosed or suspected in hospital, or where the child is still an inpatient); *specialist paediatricians* and/or *psychiatrists* (where specialist medical examinations or assessments have already been carried out); an *adult mental health* services representative; a representative from the *housing department* (to deal with concerns about arrears, overcrowding or other housing inadequacy, harassment or homelessness); a *local authority lawyer* (where there may be legal considerations); *interpreters* or *community workers* (where there may be language difficulties or cultural considerations for minority ethnic families); *foster parents* (where, for example, emergency removal has already taken place); a representative of the *armed services*, in cases where there is a connection with the services.

In practice, an average of 10 professionals attend an initial CPC, representing about 80 per cent of those invited[4]. These averages conceal the fact that some conferences have almost double this number, which can inhibit decision-making and be particularly traumatic for participating parents. They also conceal wide differences in professionals' attendance records, notably general practitioners'.

The GP's role

Government guidelines, as Madeline Ismach has already pointed out (Chapter 6a), are unequivocal in stressing the importance of general practitioners' participation in the child protection process. *Working Together* states:

- The GP and other members of the primary health care team (PHCT) are well placed to recognise when a child is potentially in need of extra help or services to promote health and development, or is at risk of harm ... (para. 3.28).

- The GP and PHCT are also well placed to recognise when a parent or other adult has problems which may affect their capacity as a parent or carer, or which may mean that they pose a risk of harm to a child .... (para. 3.29).

- *Because of their knowledge of children and families, GPs (together with other PHCT members) have an important role in all stages of the child protection process, from sharing information with social services when enquiries are being made about a child, to involvement in a child protection plan to safeguard a child. GPs should make available to child protection conferences relevant information about a child and family, whether or not they—or a member of the PHCT—are able to attend* (para. 3.30; *my emphasis*).[3]

The addendum to *Working Together* 1991, *Child Protection: Medical Responsibilities*[5] reiterated this role in 1994. The Joint Working Party producing this addendum was made up of members of the Department of Health, the British Medical Association and the Conference of Medical Royal Colleges, and its guidelines acknowledged many of the dilemmas and difficulties facing doctors in child protection (see also Chapter 3). None the less, the GP, when involved by the statutory agencies in a child protection enquiry, whether or not as instigator of that enquiry, is seen to have little leeway:

> When a doctor has involvement with the statutory agencies it is essential that he or she is able to contribute to all stages of the decision making process, including the decision whether to undertake an investigation, as doctors retain a continuing responsibility for their patients (para. 2.17).[5]

Guidelines are no less unequivocal with regard to the GP's participation in the child protection conference. Thus:

- It is essential for doctors to contribute to this (part of the child protection) process and to recommendations on subsequent management (para. 3.3).

- Child protection conferences should be attended by those who have responsibility for the child and a definite contribution to make. The general practitioner with a continuing responsibility for the child and family has a major role (para. 3.5).[5]

The CPC may then benefit from the general practitioner's contribution in several ways, reflecting the GP's role as personal physician, as family physician, as primary physician, as custodian of the medical record, as a member of a primary health care team and as a patient advocate. (Chapter 3 deals in more detail with these attributes and their implications for family violence issues.)

Preparation of family members, including children where appropriate

- Prior briefing about what they can expect to happen.

- Encouraging them to meet the chair beforehand.

- Discussing and clarifying the contents of the GP record or written report, and its significance for the conference.

- Obtaining informed consent to the release of medical information where necessary.

- Explaining the limits of confidentiality.

Factual contribution

The GP can use the clinical record to inform the conference's assessment of the degree of risk to the child. This may include:

- details of the *incident(s)* which led up to the conference being held;

- the *index child's medical background*, with details of significant consultations/presentations, hospital attendances, failed appointments;

- background and similar details for *other children* in the family;

- relevant information on *parents/carers*;

- relevant information on *other significant adults and networks.*

Whether giving this information verbally or in a written report, the GP must clearly distinguish between what is *fact*, what is *observation*, what is *allegation* and what is *opinion*. Where there is positive information to give the conference, this should obviously be shared too.

Helping decide the degree of risk

The GP, having heard the contribution of other participants, can bring to the ensuing discussion a medical perspective based on their knowledge and previous experience in child protection matters generally, as well as their particular knowledge and experience of the family in question.

GPs are sometimes asked to interpret medical reports from other clinicians not present, for example paediatricians or accident and emergency doctors. As long as the GP is aware of the limits of their competence in doing this, and makes these limitations clear to the conference, this can provide a further useful contribution to the weighing up of risk to the child. (This should not be seen as a substitute for the relevant clinician attending themselves, however, particularly when complex and possibly contentious examinations for alleged sexual abuse are involved.)

Immediate intervention

Information shared at the initial CPC may sometimes reveal immediate child protection needs for the index child or for other children in the family that are not being met, or are being met inappropriately. Others should have the detailed knowledge of available legal options and local resources. However, the GP's knowledge and appraisal of, say, a non-abusing parent's ability to protect their child (and to cope generally) if the alleged abuser is removed from the home, may prevent an inappropriate and distressing removal of the child. Conversely it may correct an unwise and potentially dangerous assumption that the child will be safe at home. Where the child's temporary removal from the home is considered essential, the GP's knowledge of the wider family network may assist the conference in recommending a potentially far less traumatizing (both for the child and their parents) placement with a familiar relative.

Immediate support

The CPC is the interagency forum not only for assessing risk, but also for considering needs and what services and support should be provided to help meet those needs. When a child is *registered*, there is a formal commitment to a child protection plan involving a comprehensive assessment of the family's needs. This process may take many weeks, notwithstanding the apparently tight timescales dictated by the assessment framework, especially if assessment by child and family psychiatry services is required. The provision of therapeutic input may take much longer still. Some needs may be more pressing, or more readily identified at the conference stage and the GP can play an important part at the CPC in identifying them and helping to meet them. Specifically, they may agree to provide or arrange:

- *for the child:* developmental checks; immunizations; assessment for failure to thrive; referral for audiometry or optometry; referral to an enuresis clinic; sexual health check or contraception for older girls;

- *for the parents:* assessment/treatment/referral for physical health needs, mental health needs or substance abuse problems, any or all of which may be impairing their ability to care for their child.

More generally, the GP can add their weight, if necessary by agreeing to provide medical evidence in support of:

- rehousing/repairs;

- childcare support (nursery provision, family aides);

- benefits (certification, equipment grants, etc.);

- educational support (home tuition, 'statementing' of children for extra help at school, literacy or English language tuition for adults).

The GP's presence and opinions cannot, of course, guarantee that all of this will happen. Conversely, it should be noted that the CPC is not in a position to *require* a GP or any other agency to accept its recommendations for action.

More than one-third of initial CPCs will *not* end in registration, either because the alleged maltreatment does not justify it, or because there are no outstanding child protection concerns, or because further assessment is considered necessary before a decision can be made. The immediate needs of the family involved may be just as great: indeed, in some ways the role of the GP as the family's advocate in accessing services may be even more important here, as other agencies may be less willing to provide such services than if registration occurs.

The decision to register

In the minds of many professionals and most parents, the decision whether or not to place a child on the child protection register *is* what the CPC is about. Indeed Farmer and Owen[4] found that assessing risk and deciding on registration tended to monopolize CPCs, leaving an average of only 9 minutes for discussing the child protection plan. Undoubtedly, registration is an important consideration, which can have major repercussions whichever way the decision goes. The GP will, like other professionals at the conference, have to come down on one side or the other, justifying their decision to all those (often including the parents) who are present.

It is ultimately the chair's decision to place a child on the child protection register, but consensus will invariably be sought from all professionals at the CPC. The social worker responsible for the initial investigation and report will usually have made a recommendation about registration in that report to the conference, but this should not be considered binding, as new information and interpretations will invariably emerge at the conference.

Requirements for registration

Working Together (para. 5.64)[3] states that, in determining whether to register a child, the conference needs to consider the following question: '*Is the child at continuing risk of significant harm?*'

The test should be that either:

- the child can be shown to have suffered ill-treatment or impairment of health or development as a result of physical, emotional, or sexual abuse or neglect, and professional judgement is that further ill-treatment or impairment are likely; *or*

- professional judgement, substantiated by the findings of enquiries in this individual case or by research evidence, is that the child is likely to suffer ill-treatment or the impairment of health or development as a result of physical, emotional, or sexual abuse or neglect.

If the child is at continuing risk of significant harm, it will therefore be the case that safeguarding the child requires inter-agency help and intervention delivered through a formal child protection plan. It is also the role of the initial child protection conference to formulate the outline child protection plan, in as much detail as possible.

The conference should, if possible, establish a cause or causes of the harm or likelihood of harm. The decision to register siblings or other children living in the household may be justified if the cause could also be applied to them. (For a definition of significant harm, see p. 162.)

A written statement of the categories of abuse for registration should be available at the conference. Table 6.2 shows the four categories of abuse, which are discussed at length in Chapters 5a and 5b. It is recognized that in some cases more than one category may be appropriate.

Opinions about registration are sought from each professional in turn: dissent and the reasons for it should be recorded in the decision sheet and minutes circulated after the conference. If the chair overrules a majority opinion, the reasons for this should also be clearly recorded in the minutes.

If the GP or any other professional is unhappy with the way a conference has been conducted or the way in which a decision to register or not has been reached, they can,

Table 6.2 The categories of abuse for registration (from ref [3], paras 2.3–2.7).

Physical abuse

May involve hitting, shaking, throwing, poisoning, burning or scalding, drowning, suffocating or otherwise causing physical harm to a child. Physical harm may also be caused when a parent or carer feigns the symptoms of, or deliberately causes ill health, to a child whom they are looking after (factitious illness by proxy or Munchausen syndrome by proxy)

Emotional abuse

The persistent emotional ill-treatment of a child such as to cause severe and persistent adverse effects on the child's emotional development. It may involve conveying to children that they are worthless or unloved, inadequate or valued only insofar as they meet the needs of another person. It may feature age or developmentally inappropriate expectations being imposed on children. It may involve causing children frequently to feel frightened or in danger, or the exploitation or corruption of children. Some level of emotional abuse is involved in all types of ill-treatment, though it may occur alone

Sexual abuse

Involves forcing or enticing a child or young person to take part in sexual activities, whether or not the child is aware of what is happening. The activities may involve physical contact, including penetrative (e.g. rape or buggery) or non-penetrative acts. They may include non-contact activities, such as involving children in looking at, or in the production of, pornographic material or watching sexual activities, or encouraging children to behave in sexually inappropriate ways

Neglect

The persistent failure to meet a child's basic physical and/or psychological needs, likely to result in the serious impairment of the child's health or development. It may involve a parent or carer failing to provide adequate food, shelter and clothing, failing to protect a child from physical harm or danger, or the failure to ensure access to appropriate medical care or treatment. It may also include neglect of, or unresponsiveness to, a child's basic emotional needs

---

in addition to recording their dissent, make representations to the chair's line manager. Usually, the social services department Principal Officer for Children's Planning and Protection (designations may vary in different areas) is responsible for ensuring good and consistent child protection practice within the department. Representations can also be made to the Area Child Protection Committee (ACPC) directly or via the Local Medical Committee member representing GPs on the ACPC. Finally, it is open to the GP or any other professional to ask for a conference to be re-convened if concerns for a child's well-being continue or increase.

Parents or young persons may also appeal against the registration decision if they feel that registration criteria were not properly interpreted; if they believe the conference was not conducted properly; if they believe relevant information was not considered; or if they believe equal opportunities policies were not adhered to. These are complaints are, however, dealt with internally (see also p. 198). ACPCs should have written information on complaints and local mechanisms for progressing them.

Improving the CPC and the GP's contribution to it

As we've seen above, the *potential* contribution of the GP to the child protection conference is a significant one. Other professionals value the information the GP brings to the conference but, as indicated, the GP's input can be far more extensive and arguably more valuable than that. In many cases, the GP will be the only professional present with previous knowledge of and responsibility for the entire family. They can play an important part in ensuring that the focus of the conference stays not only on protecting the child from abuse or further abuse but also on the child as a member of a family often with multiple needs.

For parents or children attending the conference, the GP may be the most familiar and trusted professional present: the trauma, confusion and distress that so often accompanies the child protection process can be partially mitigated by the GP's presence, especially if some preparatory work is done with the family (see above) and if the GP is involved at the end of the conference in explaining decisions and next steps. This may not only help secure parental cooperation with child protection plans, but may also help the GP to maintain or improve their relationship with the family, even if the GP has supported registration.

Sadly, this rosy scenario is not that commonly seen in practice. Far too often, a self-fulfilling cycle of mutual suspicion (sometimes bordering on hostility), low expectations and minimal engagement seems to characterize the relationship of GPs and social service departments through most stages of the child protection process.

The GP, despite being well placed as a family doctor to notice indicators of abuse, apparently rarely does so, even with the enhanced role in child health surveillance and immunizations that many GPs now have. Hallett's study[4] of 48 registered cases of child abuse (albeit of school-age children) found that only four referrals were from GPs and in all of those, family members had presented reporting actual or suspected abuse. In this study, GPs accounted for only 1 per cent of enquiries to the child protection register. Birchall[6] found that fewer than half of GPs in her 1992 study had copies of local child protection guidelines or considered them useful.

At the enquiry/investigation stage, GPs were found by Hallett to be unique in their unwillingness to collaborate. One social worker described them as 'incredibly uncooperative because of their brief of confidentiality, so that's not a particularly good source [of information]'.[4] Significantly, social workers had stopped approaching GPs at all: in only one of the 48 cases was there a record of the GP even being contacted during the interagency check stage. GPs were rarely involved in medical examinations, even where suspected physical abuse was reported to them by parents.

In Hallett's study,[4] overall attendance by professionals at CPCs was good (77 per cent of those invited) 'with the predicted exception of general practitioners' who were present at less than 20 per cent of conferences. This was despite the fact that the majority of conferences were held in the early afternoon to facilitate attendance by single-handed

GPs. Most did not write or telephone information either. These figures actually compare favourably with GP attendance figures elsewhere, which in some areas dip well below the 10 per cent figure.

Unsurprisingly, GPs rarely figure in child protection plans either. They were only mentioned in two of the 48 cases in Hallett's study,[4] although 80 per cent of the children registered remained at home.

Hallett and Birchall[7] asked a wide range of professionals to rank each other's involvement and contribution to the child protection process. Social workers, teachers, educational welfare officers, lawyers, police, paediatricians, A and E consultants, health visitors, school nurses, psychologists and psychiatrists concluded about GPs:

- they have an essential/important role in child protection (stated by 90 per cent of respondents); this was a higher rating than police and paediatricians;

- they are the most difficult professionals to collaborate with; only lawyers figure higher than GPs as the group other professionals prefer not to collaborate with;

- their performance is rated 'poor' or 'very poor' by a higher percentage than any other group (48 per cent, compared with 34 per cent for teachers);

- they (together with teachers) approach child protection work with less urgency than other professions;

- they are able to agree with other professionals' concerns less often than other groups, with the exception of lawyers and psychiatrists.

Hallett concludes:

> It seems clear the mandate to work together is not widely accepted by GPs, who may have the status and independence to ignore it. It may be that despite the emphasis placed in official guidance on the importance of this role, they have, in fact, little to contribute and the system can and does function in the main without their active participation (p. 333).[4]

Hallett's bleak and contentious statement is worth examining further. Other professionals, as she herself acknowledges, have a different view, most of them seeing GPs as having an essential or important contribution to make in child protection. The extent of this potential contribution is set out and argued throughout much of this section. Her assertion that the system 'can and does function in the main' without GPs' active participation is arguable: the system's limitations in achieving satisfactory outcomes for children and families are clear and led to the extensive review in 1999 of *Working Together*.[3] It begs the question: 'how much better might child protection outcomes be if GPs were more actively involved?'

Plenty of reasons have been advanced, both by GPs themselves and by others, for the undeniable lack of GP involvement in the child protection process in general and the CPC in particular. Hallett's assertion that the profession, by virtue of its 'status and independence' has effectively chosen to reject the mandate to work together may have a point, but it ignores many other factors. Some of these are practical considerations, some relate to the nature of general practice, others to medical attitudes, education and training, and still others to the nature and conduct of the child protection process. Some lend themselves to relatively easy solutions or at least to better than nothing 'workarounds'; others are more intractable. In the rest of this chapter, some of these factors and solutions will be explored further. Chapter 3 offers a fuller discussion of factors relating to the nature of general practice, and Chapters 9c and 9d examine education and training issues.

Practical considerations

Timing, notice and venue of CPCs

Child Protection: Medical Responsibilities[5] states clearly that:

- whenever possible, child protection conferences should be convened at times when doctors can attend (para. 3.16);

- social service departments should be aware of GPs' 24-hour responsibility and the difficulties this may cause when calling CPCs at short notice (para. 3.9);

- conference venues other than social service departments should be considered, including doctors' own premises (para. 3.10);

- car parking needs, especially of those with on-call commitments, need consideration (para. 3.l0).

Many GPs say that implementing these seemingly small suggestions more widely would make a significant difference to their ability to attend. In general, however, the notice given even for initial CPCs should usually give GPs time to arrange cover, and review conference dates are usually set months in advance. The timing of conferences is particularly contentious in some areas: skilled chairs are in short supply and there are often too many CPCs for all to be held in the early afternoon. On the other hand, GPs are sometimes given no choice of times while other professionals (e.g. paediatricians) are considered more important to accommodate. Pressure of work for chairs and minute-takers is often cited as a reason for not holding CPCs nearer to the family and family GP: this problem is particularly acute in inner city areas and in isolated rural areas where social service departmental offices have been centralized. A 30-minute drive at either end of a 2-hour CPC with nowhere to park on arrival is a powerful disincentive for most GPs.

These problems are not insurmountable: representations by individual GPs to social service departments or by GP representatives to the ACPC can achieve considerable shifts towards a more GP-aware policy.

Length of CPCs

The standard pattern of care provided by GPs to their patients, consultations of 10 minutes or so repeated as necessary over a period of time, is far removed from the standard CPC format. The agenda is long, many professionals may have information to present as well as opinions to give, parents and sometimes older children must be heard, and difficult decisions may need teasing out; where there are several children in a family, each of these must be considered separately. For many GPs this may seem an excessive and wasteful use of time, a commodity which is often rightly regarded by them as their most precious and pressured one.

Undoubtedly, a poorly planned and poorly run CPC with uncertain objectives will become an overlong one, and when the outcomes are not seen to benefit the child or their family, the conference *will* be a waste of time, for all those present. There are, however, various administrative measures which can help. Again, these can be pressed for by GPs or their representatives, whilst recognizing that some have resource implications for social services departments that are unlikely to be overcome easily. They include:

- *prior circulation* of the social worker's and (with due regard to confidentiality) other professionals' written reports;
- the social worker's report to include a *genogram* and a tabular *chronology* in complex cases where there are multiple incidents or an emerging picture of neglect, with a separate chronology for each child;
- a clear *agenda*, with approximate time allocations to each part;
- specialist *chairs*, with the training and experience to work to a timed agenda, to encourage appropriate participation and to sum up effectively;
- for complex cases involving several children, consideration should be given to holding *separate, shorter* conferences;
- for *review conferences*: continuity of chairing to improve effectiveness; review and correction of *minutes* of the previous conference at the beginning of the meeting; prior circulation of an updated chronology.

Even if all these suggestions are implemented, CPCs will take time. I have argued above that the GP has a valuable part to play at different points of the conference, justifying their presence throughout. A lesser degree of involvement is, however, better than no involvement at all. In descending order of time involvement (although probably also in descending order of usefulness to the conference) this might be:

- *attending the first part* of the CPC, to present medical information, take questions and possibly express an opinion on risk, registration, etc.;
- preparation of a *written report* (see below);
- a *telephone* conversation with the conference chair or social worker, paying due regard to establishment of identity and issues of confidentiality. The name and

contact number for both the chair and social worker should be stated on the written invitation to the CPC;

- a discussion with the child's *health visitor* (if they have one) who can report to the conference on the GP's behalf.

Loss of income

Of all professionals present at a CPC, the GP is usually the only independent contractor, with a 24-hour responsibility for providing care to their patients. For the single-handed GP, attendance at a conference means finding and paying for a locum. For the GP in a group practice, cross-cover may be possible, but there is an equivalent opportunity cost.

Under current (1999) arrangements, attendance at social services case conferences is not part of the GP's General Medical Services obligations, and a fee is therefore payable. The amount varies according to the length of time away from the surgery. At the time of writing, the fee for more than 1 hour up to 3 hours out of surgery will pay the bulk of a locum's sessional fee, with a pro rata reduction for attendance of less than 1 hour. A mileage allowance is also payable.

Confusion surrounds whose responsibility it is to pay this fee: in different areas, it may be the local authority finance or social services department, the community health services trust or the health authority. Following the 1999 NHS reorganization, responsibility is likely to pass to Primary Care Trusts. The secretary of the Local Medical Committee, or its ACPC representative, should be able to provide up to date local information.

A standard claim form should be available from social services departments or the paying authority. This should be countersigned by the CPC chair.

A fee is also payable for the provision of a written report.

The written report

Child Protection: Medical Responsibilities[5] states (para. 3.22) that:

> Medical attendance is essential at some case conferences and desirable at most, but if attendance is not possible it is essential that medical views are represented at all child protection conferences. . . . the conference Chair should decide when medical attendance is essential or whether the submission of a report will suffice.

On current evidence of GP involvement, most chairs would be pleased even to receive a GP's report. For the GP, this is not necessarily a soft option, especially when a large family is involved. The following points should be noted:

- *Factual information* needs to cover the same ground as a verbal report to a CPC (see p. 179).
- As with a verbal report clear distinctions must be made between what is *fact*, what is *observation*, what is *allegation* and what is *opinion*.

- *Each member* of the family should be reported on *separately.*

- Whenever possible, the GP should *discuss the content* of the report with the parents and, where appropriate, with the child(ren), and *seek consent* to disclose personal and medical details.

- The GP's report, which will form part of the child's medical record, is subject to the 1990 Access to Health Records Act, and as such an adult with parental responsibility or a competent child (see Chapter 3) can apply for *access* to it. However, if disclosing the report is likely to result in serious physical or mental harm, or would disrupt the emotional well-being or development of the child, access may be refused. It may also be refused if the identity of an individual who has provided information would be revealed by disclosure.

- If the *post* is used to send the report, it should be clearly marked as 'strictly confidential: for addressee only' or equivalent and preferably sent by recorded delivery.

- If the report is *faxed,* it should be via a secure fax line, with the addressee ready to receive it.

- The GP should receive a clear undertaking that the recipient will use the report only for the purposes for which it has been compiled.

- The GP should be aware that the contents of the report will normally be made available to other participants in the CPC, including parents where present. Information that should not be shared with the parent or child for the reasons given above should be communicated to the chair separately.

- Social services have broadly similar access to records regulations as GPs and may limit information given to adults with parental responsibility or children on a similar basis.

- A GP's report to social services may be made available to professionals involved in a subsequent child protection plan. It should not be circulated with conference minutes, it should not be used without the *express permission* of the person providing the report, and may not be used for any other purpose without that person's permission.

- Different rules may apply when reports are to be used for care or other *court proceedings* (see Chapter 7a). GPs should note that social services have to disclose records in their possession if ordered to do so by the court, by guardians *ad litem,* the local government ombudsman or the Secretary of State.

- *If there is any doubt about the disclosure of information relevant to child protection in a report or other setting, the GP is urged to consult their medical defence organization.*

- Some social services departments will send the GP a *proforma* which details the information they require in a report: this may save time for all concerned.

- A claim form for completing the report may be sent with the report. This may forwarded to the paying authority or returned to the GP according to local circumstances.

Parental participation

Family rights groups (see Chapter 6d) argue for the fullest participation of parents in all stages of the child protection process, including the child protection conference. They do this with the full weight of research and government guidance. Many studies have found that where a conscious effort was made to incorporate the family into the investigation and protection plan, and an attempt made at some sort of alliance, outcomes for children were generally better.[8]

Whilst most professionals, including doctors, might consider parental participation in CPCs to be generally beneficial and their presence to have a positive effect on conference proceedings, there is no doubt that the presence of parents and children can sometimes present difficulties for professionals, particularly the GP.

Exclusion from a child protection conference is at the chair's discretion, subject to ACPC guidelines. Typically, grounds for exclusion might be:

- a parent/carer/child's presence is likely to be so disruptive or negative that the conference's work could not be conducted;

- it is felt that the presence of a particular adult would pose an unacceptable danger to the child or other parent/carer;

- a continuing police investigation or outstanding prosecution renders the police unable to be present at the same time as an individual;

- on previous experience, a person is thought likely to become violent;

- a person is incapable of participating because of substance abuse.

It should be noted that the need for professionals to disclose confidential information is not considered sufficient grounds to exclude parents or carers from an entire conference, although it is not unknown for a parent to be asked to withdraw temporarily. However, it is the chair's responsibility to provide professionals with ample opportunity to share their concerns about parent and child participation before the conference. Where confidential information that would be prejudicial to the child, one of the participating parents or a third party has to be shared with other professionals, this can be done by prior agreement with the chair.

In practice, many GPs have difficulties with parental participation because they feel it prejudices their relationship with them and there is anecdotal evidence that some absent themselves from CPCs for this reason. GPs, like health visitors and teachers, come to a conference because of a pre-existing relationship with the family and should in theory be key figures in helping the family after the conference. They can find themselves in a difficult situation when, in the presence of the family, they need to convey negative information or opinions and are then asked to 'vote' on registration. These difficulties are compounded when the GP initiated the referral, especially where, in cases of suspected sexual abuse, parents may not be forewarned that a referral to a statutory agency is to be made.

It is now recognized that some local authorities have taken partnership with parents too far. The Department of Health, in seeking to clarify and update *Working Together*, put it thus in its 1998 consultation paper:[9]

> Partnership with parents must be central to the child protection process. But it is also important that there is an opportunity for separate discussion to take place between professionals so that there is an opportunity for the sharing and analysis of key information about the child's safety and welfare. Evidence from the field indicates that partnership with parents has been interpreted to mean that professionals should never engage in analysis of a child's situation without the parents being present. This was never the intention (para. 6.8).[9]

It is hoped that this change of emphasis, together with the move towards focusing throughout the child protection process on needs and family support rather than on incidents and investigations, will make the process and outcomes more acceptable and productive for families and professionals alike. It may allow the CPC to become a forum where, notwithstanding difficult things being said and difficult decisions like registration being made, the relationship between the GP and family is preserved or even strengthened.

When a conference decides there is a need for a child protection plan, a *core group* of key agencies and family is usually established. Whether this group's role is primarily that of monitoring the implementation of the plan, or of producing it, the GP can be an influential member, although in practice they are rarely asked to join. Core group meetings are smaller, shorter and more informal than most CPCs and can more readily be arranged to take place at a convenient time and location for the GP, health visitor and family.

Conclusion

The 1999 rewriting of *Working Together*[3] acknowledges many of the flaws and shortcomings of the child protection process. Cooperation and joint working by all agencies is still seen as an 'essential prerequisite for the safeguarding of the welfare of children'. However, a significant shift in focus is envisaged, with the emphasis now on a wider, more proactive view of vulnerable families' needs; the better targeting of support, based on an assessment of those needs; and earlier intervention to deal with difficulties before they escalate into abuse.

The child protection process is, then, about more than investigating an incident, apportioning blame and separating the child from the abuser. Likewise, the child protection conference is no longer seen as being primarily about deciding on registration. Rather, the CPC needs to be seen as part of an ongoing process of assessing and meeting a family's needs, albeit from the perspective of the child who has suffered harm and with the overriding aim of protecting that child from further harm. Its key functions are now more clearly those of drawing up a child protection plan, using the key worker and core group to achieve desired outcomes for the child.

Registration has been seen by many professionals as the only way to obtain resources for these families and the CPC has not infrequently become an interprofessional battle-ground on this front. Similarly, conflicts over deregistration have sometimes dominated review conferences, with some professionals seeing deregistration as being driven by scarcity of resources and performance norms.

The changes to *Working Together* and the use of the assessment framework may go some way towards countering the culture of cynicism that I believe is at the heart of GPs' lack of involvement in the child protection process. There are undoubtedly practical obstacles, issues of knowledge and training, ethical conflicts, and interprofessional preconceptions and prejudices, all of which are amenable to at least partial resolution. Arguably, the organizational and financial amalgamation between health and social services in Primary Care Trusts and eventually into Care Trusts may do a good deal over time to remove these obstacles. GPs need in the meantime to be convinced that these changes in emphasis in the child protection process are not merely changes in rhetoric, but will be matched by the provision of more adequate resources, and that outcomes for their patients will be better as a result. If they can be so convinced, their participation in the child protection process should become proportional to its importance and be seen by them as a valid and effective investment of their time and expertise.

References

1 Gibbons J, Conroy S, Bell C. *Operating the Child Protection System: a Study of Child Protection Practices in English Local Authorities*. London: HMSO, 1995.

2 *Children Act 1989*. London: HMSO, 1989.

3 Department of Health, Home Office, Department of Education and Employment, the National Assembly for Wales. *Working Together to Safeguard Children: a Guide for Interagency Working to Safeguard and Promote the Welfare of Children*. London: Department of Health, 1999.

4 Hallett C. *Inter-Agency Co-ordination in Child Protection*. London: HMSO, 1995.

5 Department of Health, British Medical Association, Conference of Medical Royal Colleges. *Child Protection: Medical Responsibilities*. London: HMSO, 1994.

6 Birchall E. *Report to the Department of Health: Working Together in Child Protection*. Stirling; University of Stirling, 1992.

7 Hallett C, Birchall E. *Co-ordination and Child Protection, a Review of the Literature*. London: HMSO, 1992.

8 Department of Health. *Child Protection: Messages from Research*. London: HMSO, 1995.

9 Social Care Group, Department of Health. *Working Together to Safeguard Children: New Government Proposals for Inter-Agency Co-operation. Consultation Paper*. London: Department of Health, 1998.

Chapter 6d

Child protection: the family perspective

Bridget Lindley

Introduction

The families of children who are the subject of child protection investigations often experience personal crisis, as well as fear, anger and bewilderment at the procedures in which they find themselves involved. Some may have had experience of being involved with social services before; others may be involved for the first time. They may be panic-stricken at the way that the procedures seem to be taking over their family life, and may fear that any contact with professionals will result in their child being removed from them.

In these situations, family members often feel very isolated. This isolation is exacerbated when they lack information about the specific allegations being investigated, about the procedures and likely outcomes of the investigation, and about what they are expected to do to overcome the child protection concerns. They often lack legal advice at least at the initial stages of the investigation. They may also lack the ability to express their views about what has happened, and about ways in which they believe that their child can be protected in the future. Professionals need to be aware that, in their panic, these families may not be thinking clearly. They may need help to understand the nature of the child protection concern, why it presents a risk to their child, and to explore ways in which their child can be protected in the future. For example, in the case of domestic violence the woman may not have addressed the emotional impact on her child of witnessing violence, and may need a lot of support to help her decide how to protect her child from this in the future. Similarly, if the home situation is breaking down, relatives may need to be encouraged to come forward to offer support or care for the child for a period of time. If families are left to sort things out on their own, they may fail in their task, not just because they are likely to be experiencing some sort of personal crisis which led to the original investigation, but also because they may be very traumatized by the process itself.

The Department of Health's research in the 1990s on the effectiveness of the child protection system confirms that the most important condition for success in child protection work is the quality of the relationship between the child's family and the professionals responsible. It stresses that an alliance is needed:

> which involves parents and, if possible children, actively in the investigation, taking account of their views and incorporating their goals into plans. Failure to achieve this level of cooperation helps to explain why some children remain safe when others do not.[1]

The family's involvement is also essential from a practical and legal point of view: they are an important source of information about the child under investigation; they frequently care for the child during and after the investigation (an estimated 82 per cent of those registered on a child protection register remain at home[2]); and those with parental responsibility (usually the parents/carers) also have a legal right to be involved because they retain their parental responsibility throughout the child protection investigation. The local authority does not acquire it unless an emergency protection order or care order is made. Their agreement should therefore be sought for any plan that is to be implemented outside the court process.

That family members should be involved in the child protection processes is therefore indisputable. However, it is not an easy task. Parents may be too shocked, angry and bewildered to be receptive to social services. Professionals may also lack the time and skills to engage them in the process. Previous attempts to integrate partnership between local authorities and families into practice have been consolidated and developed in the government's guidance in *Working Together* 1999.[3] The rationale for, and the commitment to, this is discussed at length in its Chapter 7:

> Families have a unique role and importance in the lives of children, who attach great value to their family relationships. Family members know more about their family than any professional could possibly know, and well-founded decisions about a child should draw upon this knowledge and understanding. Family members should normally have the right to know what is being said about them, and to contribute to important decisions about their lives and those of their children. Research findings brought together in *Child Protection: Messages from Research* endorse the importance of good relationships between professionals and families in helping to bring about the best possible outcomes for children.... Where there is compulsory intervention in family life, parents should always be helped and encouraged to play as full a part as possibly in decisions about their child (paras 7.2–7.3).[3]

This guidance is quite directive about how this should be implemented in practice. It stipulates that there should be a presumption of openness, joint decision-making and being willing to listen to families and capitalize on their strengths, but always subject to an overarching principle to always act in the best interests of the child (para. 7.6). It states clearly that agencies and professionals are expected to be honest and explicit with the child and family about professional roles, responsibilities, powers and expectations, and about what is and what is not negotiable (para. 7.7). Specific mention is made of ways in which families may be enabled to participate actively in the decision-making process: through the use of family group conferences (FGCs);[4,5] through referral to advice and advocacy services, both locally and nationally; through the sharing of all the information they need to help them understand the child protection process; and through sensitivity to varying family patterns, lifestyles and childrearing across different racial, ethnic and cultural groups (paras 7.13–7.24).[3]

In addition to the general discussion about the principle of partnership, there are specific requirements about the support and involvement of families in individual cases at every stage of the process, as follows.

Stages in the child protection process

Initial assessment

When the local authority decides what action to take in response to a referral of any child in need, the guidance states that parents' permission should be sought before discussing a referral about them with other agencies, unless such 'permission seeking' may itself place the child at risk of significant harm. The process of initial assessment should also involve speaking to the family, and social services' decisions about the next course of action following the initial assessment should normally be discussed with the family unless such a discussion places the child at risk. The family should therefore be aware of what is happening during the initial assessment and following it (paras 5.11–5.17).

Children in need

If this further action involves a core assessment of the child's needs, the *Framework* document[6] is designed to ensure that families are fully involved in this process, their parenting capacity and family and environmental factors being central to the identification of needs and appropriate services. Detailed guidance is given on how to maximize the chances of fully engaging them in the assessment, with particular emphasis on the need to give them information, both verbally and in writing, about the process of assessment. Suggestions are also made about how to encourage their involvement where there is resistance to it.

Child protection enquiries

If further action involves S 47 enquiries being conducted (see p. 162), then subject to the proviso of protecting the child from further harm, the presumption of openness, honesty and joint decision-making raises similar expectations about information sharing, and the empowerment of parents.

One of the tasks of the strategy discussion is to decide what information about the strategy discussion will be shared with the family (unless such information sharing poses a risk to the child) (para. 5.28). It adds that the decision about who to interview, when and for what purpose, should be taken bearing in mind that the way that interviews are conducted may have a significant impact on the likelihood of maintaining a constructive working relationship with the family (para. 5.29).

Social services departments are expected to explain and give written information about the purpose, process and outcome of S 47 enquiries to the parents and child, and be prepared to answer questions openly unless to do so would affect the safety and welfare of the child. This information should include details of how advice, advocacy and support may be obtained from independent sources (para. 5.43). The aim, as far as possible, should be to conduct the enquiries in a way which allows for future constructive working relationships with families (para. 5.44). This includes an implicit acknowledgement of the parents' parental responsibility by stating that interviews with children should normally only be undertaken with the parents' knowledge, except in exceptional circumstances, for example if there was a possibility that a child might be coerced into silence (para. 5.37).

The outcome of S 47 enquiries should be recorded, and parents should be given a copy of the record, in particular in advance of any conference which is to be convened (para. 5.45). If the child is adjudged not to be at risk of continuing harm, but is still being monitored because there are lingering concerns, the purpose of this monitoring should be clear and parents should always be informed about the nature of any ongoing concerns (para. 5.47). Similarly, if the agencies involved with the child agree that the child's future safety and welfare can be guaranteed without the need for a formal child protection conference and plan, for example because the parent is being cooperative, the guidance suggests that family members should be invited to meet with professionals to agree on what future actions should be undertaken and by whom, and with what intended outcomes. It mentions the potential usefulness of FGCs in this context (para. 5.50).

Child protection conferences

There is a clear expectation that parents and wider family members will normally attend *child protection conferences*. However, it is acknowledged that, exceptionally, the chair may decide to exclude a family member, in whole or in part, following criteria set out in a protocol drawn up by the Area Child Protection Committee (ACPC). Where a family member is excluded they should be helped to communicate their views by another means.

Working Together[3] adds that parents should be 'helped fully to participate' and that their involvement should be planned carefully. The chair is given the specific task of meeting family members in advance to ensure that they understand the purpose of the conference and what will happen (paras 5.57–5.59).

There is a new expectation that parents will be given a copy of the social worker's report in advance of the conference, although there is no mention of a minimum time for advance disclosure. There is a similar expectation in relation to the reports of other professionals (paras 5.61–5.62). However, there are no sanctions or penalties for those failing to give advance disclosure, the absence of which can be disempowering for parents attending conferences.

Parents should be helped in advance to think about what they want to convey to the conference and how best to get their points across on the day, which might include providing their own written report (para. 5.62). Social services should also give them information about local advice and advocacy agencies, and should explain that they may bring an advocate friend or supporter to the conference (para. 5.57). The role of such an advocate for parents is not discussed in any detail but there is an expectation that this will be outlined in a local protocol drawn up by the ACPC, to include provision where parents may, for example, have learning difficulties or where English is not their first language.

Child protection register

If a child's name is placed on the register, the conference should make recommendations about how 'parents (including all those with PR) and wider family members should be involved in the planning and implementation process, and the support, advice and advocacy available to them'. The outline child protection plan should also be clear about who has responsibility for what actions, including actions by family members (para. 5.68–5.69). Family members should therefore have an understanding of what is expected of them and what they can expect of others.

The core group

It is acknowledged that parents and family members may find it difficult to agree to a child protection plan in a formal conference. The *core group* is therefore regarded as an important forum for working with them and they are expected to be members of it (para. 5.77). The key worker, who has the task of ensuring that the core group draws up and implements a full child protection plan, must 'make every effort to ensure that the parents have a clear understanding of the plan, that they accept it and are willing to work to it'. It should take their views into consideration, in so far as they are consistent with the child's welfare. They should be given a copy of the plan in their first language (para. 5.83). There is considerable emphasis placed on the importance of parents having full information about the concerns and how they are expected to overcome them. It is considered good practice for a written agreement to be drawn up with parents, setting out as part of, or in addition to, the original plan, the respective roles and responsibilities of family members and different agencies in implementing the plan (para. 5.88).

Appeals and complaints

There is still no provision for appeal against registration. In rare cases, parents may be able to challenge a decision to register if they can establish grounds for judicial review, but this is exceptional rather than routine.

Complaints about the work of individual agencies will continue to be addressed and dealt with by the agency concerned, but there is a new expectation that there should be a formal procedure to deal with complaints about the management of a conference. These will be addressed initially to the chair of the conference, but will be passed on to the social services department, who must process them in accordance with a complaints protocol drawn up by the ACPC (para. 4.18). There is, however, no requirement that an independent person or body should consider the complaint, nor that the family member may make oral representations at a panel hearing.

Conclusion

Working Together is issued under Section 7 of the Local Authority Social Services Act 1970, which *requires* local authorities to act in accordance with guidance issued by the Secretary of State unless there are exceptional circumstances to justify variation. As we have seen, it is prescriptive about how family members should be supported and enabled to participate throughout the child protection process.

When the appropriate services or support for families are not forthcoming, the detailed expectations of the guidance may need to be cited to challenge the lack of provision. Although the direct involvement of GPs in the process may be limited, family members may consult them at any stage of the child protection process. Whilst the limits of their confidentiality (determined by their reporting duty to social services about any evidence of risk to a child) need to be clearly explained to family members, GPs are in a good position to support them, and indeed advocate for them to obtain the services and information to which they are entitled under the new framework. The practical intervention of GPs on their behalf may therefore be a crucial factor in achieving a positive working relationship with the local authority which, as we have seen, is the key to the successful protection of children at risk.

References

1 Department of Health. *Child Protection: Messages from Research.* London: HMSO, 1995.
2 Department of Health. *Children on Child Protection Registers for the Year Ending March 1997.* London: DOH, l997.
3 Department of Health. *Working Together to Safeguard Children.* London: Stationery Office, 1999.
4 Morris K, Marsh P, Wiffin J. *Family Group Conferences—a Training Pack.* London: Family Rights Group, 1998.
5 Marsh P, Crow G. *Family Group Conferences in Child Welfare.* Oxford: Blackwell Science, 1998.
6 Department of Health. *Framework for the Assessment of Children in Need and their Families.* London: HMSO, 2000.

Chapter 7

The aftermath

Chapter 7a

Legal options

Vera Mayer

Introduction

Having concluded a child protection investigation pursuant to Section 37 of the Children Act, or after obtaining an emergency protection order (see Chapter 6b), the local authority will have to decide whether they need to intervene in the life of a family by way of applying for a (further) statutory order. This is a drastic step, in as much as it takes any proceedings concerning children out of the realm of private law (which deals, in the main, with disputes between a child's relations about residence and contact, and protection of a parent and a child from violence of another parent) and into the realm of public law—i.e. the state intervening in family life. Whereas members of a family can make decisions about where a child will live and who he/she will see without involving the courts, the state can not intervene in decisions about children without resorting to the courts.

As soon as a local authority brings proceedings in respect of a child the court (always the family proceedings court, the equivalent of a magistrates court, where all public law proceedings start) appoints a *children's guardian* (commonly still known as a guardian ad litem or GAL)—normally an experienced former social worker belonging to the Children and Family Court Advisory and Support Services (CAFCASS)—to represent the interests of the child. The children's guardian is represented in court, as is the local authority and the parents, by a solicitor or counsel (a barrister).

In making public law orders (i.e. a supervision order or a care order, or interim, orders for these), the court has to be satisfied that the 'threshold criteria' have been crossed. Threshold criteria is a term of art, always used in public law proceedings. The threshold is that beyond which a child has been found to have suffered significant harm, or has been found to be likely to suffer significant harm (this is often used for newborn babies whose siblings have suffered significant harm). Saying that the 'threshold criteria' have been satisfied means that the above findings have been made and that the court now turns to consider whether an order should be made.

Prior to a decision as to which order the court should make, consideration must be given to a decision as to whether *any* order is necessary. The court will only make an order if the welfare of the child dictates that making an order is better than not making an order at all (Section 1(5)).

Having decided on the information before it (see below) to make an order, the court will have to review the full range of orders available to it and go from the lesser to the greater; in other words, if a lesser order suffices, a greater (more draconian order) should not be made.

In this chapter I shall discuss the following legal concepts:

- parental responsibility;
- interim orders;
- split hearings;
- assessment under an interim order;
- care plans;
- supervision orders;
- care orders.

Parental responsibility

This is a concept that has been introduced by the Children Act, although it had a precursor in previous legislation. It is defined by Section 3(1) of the Act as 'all the rights, duties, powers, responsibilities and authority which by law a parent has in relation to the child and his property'. In reality, it gives a person the right to make all major decisions in respect of the child—from changing the child's surname to where he/she is educated, where they live, access to their medical records and school records, and indeed all decisions about their upbringing.

Parental responsibility is acquired in the following manner:

1. All *mothers* have it as of right.
2. All *fathers* who were either married at the time of the child's birth or married the mother after the child was born have it as of right.

3. *Unmarried fathers* can acquire it either with written proforma consent of the mother or by order of the court. Whether they get it from the court or not depends primarily on their attachment and commitment to the child and their motives in applying for the order.

4. Any person other than the parent acquires parental responsibility if the child lives with them under a *residence order*. This, of course, makes sense; say grandparents acquire a residence order in respect of their grandchild, they should be in a position to dictate major decisions for him/her, so long as he/she lives with them. Parental responsibility which is acquired through a residence order terminates with the termination of the residence order.

A court will always enquire who has parental responsibility for a child. For the general practitioner (and other health professionals) too, establishing who has parental responsibility may be very important. For example, an estranged father with parental responsibility, who has no communication with the mother, can gain access to the child's medical records without the mother's consent.

The notion of parental responsibility is also important in public law, because under an interim care order or a full care order the *local authority* shares parental responsibility with the mother, and with the father if he has it. By sharing parental responsibility, the local authority can make decisions (authorized by the court under an interim care order and without the authority of the court under the full care order) that completely override the parents' decisions.

Interim orders

Under Section 38 of the Children Act, if the court is satisfied that there are *reasonable grounds* for believing that a child is suffering or is likely to suffer significant harm, and that such harm is attributable to the care (or lack of it) of the child's parents or those who are in *loco parentis*, it can make an interim care order (ICO) or an interim supervision order (ISO).

A court would make an interim rather than a final order when more time is needed for the gathering of further information, for carrying out further assessments and for appropriate planning for the future. It is vital to remember that once a final order is made, particularly a final care order, the courts no longer have any part in the monitoring of the care of the child unless fresh proceedings are brought.

More often than not, when a local authority decides to intervene, it applies for an ICO. This gives the local authority the right to share parental responsibility with the child's parents (or carers) and control all decisions about the child in the interim period. Under an ICO a child may stay at home or be removed to an alternative placement; it can also be removed from home to an alternative placement without further application to the court. Under an ISO, the local authority does not share parental responsibility with the parents or carers.

Although the threshold criteria are the same for an ICO and an ISO—i.e. are there *reasonable grounds* for finding that a child has suffered or is likely to suffer significant harm—the orders differ, and the difference is significant. An ISO is often applied to 'scare' the carer into action and into cooperation with the local authority without removing the child. An ICO is applied when the draconian power of removing a child is considered absolutely necessary.

The court can exclude a violent or otherwise abusive carer from a home under the provisions of an ICO (Section 38A). Rather than removing a child, a court, in certain circumstances, will prefer to remove the alleged abuser, so as to minimize the trauma to the child by removing it to an alternative home.

All interim orders can be made initially for a period of 8 weeks and then have to be renewed at court at 4-weekly intervals. This ensures minimization of slacking in planning for the child and the court retains control over the timetabling of the legal proceedings.

Split hearings

The split hearing is a fairly recent phenomenon, the result of decisions by judges who forever strive to reduce delays and minimize costs (not always possible simultaneously) in public law proceedings. It applies to cases where there are suspicions of physical abuse rather than emotional harm. So, for example, if a child is alleged to have suffered a shaking injury, a non-accidental fracture or sexual abuse the court will look in the first stage into the circumstances of the injuries/abuse only, without looking into the family circumstances or psychological profiles of the alleged perpetrators of the abuse.

The evidence for the first part of a split hearing of this nature often involves medical evidence, since the first question always is, 'Is there an injury?' and if so, 'Is it non-accidental?' The other question in the first part of a split hearing is, 'Who is the perpetrator?' This is determined on a factual basis: who had the opportunity?, who had the motive? and so on. Only when these questions are answered would the court go to the second part of a split hearing and decide where the child should live and under what court order.

One of the main reasons for split hearings is the fact that abuse is often committed by one member of the family, unbeknown to other members. If findings are made (for example about a mother's boyfriend sexually abusing her daughter or a mother fracturing her baby's leg unbeknown to the father), the non-abusing member may well need time and professional support to come to terms with the findings and with the fact that his/her family unit is likely to be split up. Thus, there is usually a gap of some weeks between the two parts of a split hearing.

Assessment under an interim order

At the end of the first part of a split hearing, or at the end of a hearing which does not necessarily start as a split hearing, the court often finds itself short of information for the final disposal of the case. For example, although abuse, physical and/or emotional, has been found to have been perpetrated, the court is in no position to say whether it is likely to be perpetrated again. Again, it may have been found that child A, who no longer lives with the family, has been abused, but there is now a new child, child B, and questions as to his/her protection are unanswered. Is a mother who failed to protect child A now (say with the passage of time or change of partner) able to protect?

In these circumstances, the court has power (Section 38(6)), to order the local authority to carry out a further assessment, including an assessment at a residential institution. The conditions for ordering such an assessment are that, firstly, it is an assessment involving the child, secondly that it is only for the purpose of gathering further evidence for the court and thirdly, that it is primarily an assessment and not an exercise in therapy. The funding is by the local authority.

Care plans

Before dealing with final orders, I should mention another term of art—the '*care plan*'. This is a detailed document that the local authority must put before the court on an application for a final order. The care plan must give information about the intention of the local authority in respect of the child's:

- *residence*;
- *legal status* (e.g. if he/she is to be adopted or remain in long-term foster care);
- *when* is he/she likely to be placed;
- how likely are they to be placed with carers of *similar ethnic origin*;
- how often is he/she to have *contact* with members of the natural family.

The care plan is a vital document, as once the court makes a final care or supervision order, the proceedings have come to an end. In cases of a final care order a child may remain in the care of a local authority for years without their cases being referred to the court for review; the care plan is then the only guideline as to what should happen to this child.

Final supervision order

This does not allow the local authority to share parental responsibility with the child's mother or others who hold it. It does, however, give the local authority various powers to see the child and order the child to attend certain places, live at certain places and to participate in certain activities. (This is not a comprehensive list—see Schedule 3 to the Children Act.) A supervision order can be made initially for a period of 1 year and can then be extended for 2 further years; thus it is not an efficient method to monitor long-term concerns.

Final care orders

A final care order gives the local authority full powers to pursue their care plan. The legal proceedings come to an end, the children's guardian is no longer involved, and the courts have no say in what happens to the child. The powers of the local authority are virtually unfettered when it has a final care order. The local authority still has statutory reviews (twice a year) to monitor the progress of the care plan; no outsiders however are there to criticize and move matters on. Most readers have no doubt heard horror stories of children being forgotten in the care system. Although it is less frequent now than say 25 years ago, it is, sadly, not a rare occurrence.

Significantly, parental responsibility is vested in the local authority on the making of a final care order. In theory parental responsibility is to be shared with the parents. It remains the right of the parents to decide major decisions such as the child's religion, change of surname or emigration, for example. However, the reference to 'shared' parental responsibility is somewhat deceptive. While the parental responsibility of the parents subsists for the duration of the order, the local authority have the power to determine the extent to which the parents exercise their responsibilities. Where the care plan is for adoption the local authority will usually seek parental agreement. However, where withheld, the local authority may apply to the court for an order dispensing with parental agreement. Legitimate grounds for such an order include: where the parent cannot be found or is incapable of agreeing; where agreement is withheld unreasonably; where the parent has persistently failed without reasonable cause to discharge parental responsibility; and where the child has been abandoned, neglected or ill-treated and rehabilitation of the child to the home is unlikely. In reality once a final care order has been granted the local authority determines the scope for parental involvement.

It ought to be remembered, however, that any person with parental responsibility (including the local authority), and the child, can apply to the court for the *discharge of a care order*. An application for discharge of a care order is the only mechanism to review the situation of a child in care, albeit not necessarily a legitimate one. To illustrate, a parent struggling with alcoholism or drug abuse would be unlikely to have any prospect of succeeding on such an application, yet he or she could make the application to ensure that any failure of duty to the child by the local authority is addressed. Incidentally (and importantly), legal aid is available to parents of a child who is subject to an application for a care order regardless of the merit and regardless of the parents' means.

Legal options available against the abuser

On first analysis *criminal proceedings* may appear to be the most appropriate option in dealing with an abuser. However, in reality there are significant difficulties in pursuing prosecution. The primary obstacle is satisfying the criminal burden of proof. It is for the prosecution to prove the case 'beyond reasonable doubt'. To do so would require the child to give evidence in the vast majority of cases. The ordeal of recounting the abuse (even where the evidence is taken in an ostensibly 'user-friendly' room and conveyed to the jury by a television link) only heightens the trauma already suffered. Bearing in mind the high standard of proof required, acquittal can have a devastating effect on a child whose greatest fear (other than anticipation of repeated abuse) is to be disbelieved. Also, on a practical and by no means lesser note, the pursuance of criminal proceedings will delay the commencement of essential therapy and counselling, as such work could be seen as contaminating the evidence of the child (see Chapter 7b).

Instead abuse may be proved in the family courts on a lesser civil standard, i.e. 'on the balance of probabilities'. The burden is satisfied providing the judge considers it more likely than not that that the person accused perpetrated the abuse.

The outcome of public law proceedings brought by the local authority will impact on the options available to the non-abusing parent. Where the abuser is, for example, a non-resident father, a positive finding of abuse will greatly assist the resident parent in opposing an application by the abuser for contact with the child. Similarly, the same principle applies to an application by the resident parent to vary an existing order for contact. Additionally, the finding would support an application by the non-abusing parent for a residence order.

The merits of pursuing civil proceedings such as personal injury claims are limited. However, victims of violent crimes may obtain compensation via the Criminal Injuries Compensation Board. Clearly physical and sexual abuse are within the definition. The application should be made on behalf of child victims by the non-abusing parent (with parental responsibility) or a representative of social services. It is advantageous that a successful claim is not dependent on conviction. Generally a complaint made to the police will suffice. However, such a complaint may not always have been made, if for example the abuser is within the same household and reconciliation is being attempted. In such circumstances a comprehensive account must be given of the injury and events culminating in infliction. On the premises that an award is in the best interest of the child and the resident abuser will not benefit financially, a decision will be reached on whether an award should be made. This option is a useful method of compensating the child directly.

Where does the GP come in?

Over and above their role in the prevention and early detection of abuse, the GP has an important part to play if, and when, legal proceedings are considered or undertaken.

Firstly, *knowledge and understanding* of the presentation, symptoms and signs of the various forms of abuse will enable the GP to ask appropriate questions, seek out corroborating evidence, and elicit other signs. Serious suspicion should be conveyed to the local authority forthwith. The GP may in this way not only uncover a need for further action to protect the child, but also, should the need arise, provide important evidence for the courts to consider later.

Secondly, the *accurate recording* of all information, particularly in cases where sexual abuse is suspected (but also in cases of other physical harm and injury, or domestic violence), is of great importance in the event of legal proceedings. The early disclosures and statements in abuse cases are particularly vital; later, they are likely to be contaminated by questioning of an anxious parent and their evidential value will reduce substantially.

Thirdly, the GP may play an important role in *advising and supporting* anxious and distressed parents and children faced by local authority powers and the powers of the courts.

The role of the medical practitioner in the court process cannot be overestimated. The specialist knowledge of lawyers and the judiciary is limited to the law. For this reason the observations and knowledge of a medical expert will often be relied upon and may be crucial to the ultimate outcome. As a general guide, expert evidence tends to comprise:

- admissible evidence of *facts observed* (e.g. the physical injury);
- *interpretation* of the fact (explanation of possible causes);
- *opinion* evidence (e.g. opinion as to the actual cause).

The doctor writing his notes or report, or indeed giving oral evidence, may refer to statements made to him by the child or other person not called as a witness. If the reference is made with the intention of proving that the statement by the other person is in fact true, it is *hearsay*. Alternatively if the reference is made only to show that the statement was actually made, it will not be hearsay.

It is a rule of law that hearsay evidence is generally inadmissible. While this rule is effective in criminal proceedings, it does not apply equally to civil proceedings. Furthermore, evidence relating to the upbringing, maintenance or welfare of a child is admissible in family proceedings. Notably such evidence extends beyond what the child may have said, to include previous statements of any person and need not necessarily be first hand hearsay. Consequently, the medical practitioner is at liberty (subject to confidentiality guidelines—see Chapters 3 and 5c) to state any admissions or disclosures made to him or her by any person associated with the child in question. However, it is worth remembering that the more remote the statement, the less weight will be attached to it as evidence. In any event I would suggest that the medical practitioner include any statements, particularly in original medical records, as the judge will consider any questions as to the weight of the evidence.

I shall now consider *record keeping, report writing* and the giving of *oral evidence* in turn, with a view to providing (by no means exhaustive) guidance on what information will be useful in a legal context.

Record keeping

Comprehensive medical records provide an invaluable catalogue of facts and observations that may suggest or indeed rebut a history of abuse. It is important to remember that seemingly trivial concerns noted on one occasion, if recurring may take on a very different complexion, pointing to either physical or emotional abuse, or as is often the case, a combination of the two. Good medical notes alone are relevant to proceedings but are also useful documents for any expert asked to write a report for the purpose of proceedings.

- Notes should be made *contemporaneously* or as soon as possible after the child presents at the surgery.

- The *date and time* of attendance should be stated along with details of the *person accompanying* the child.

- The *purpose for the attendance* should be logged along with any account given for the injury/illness in question.

- A *verbatim record of statements* made is always preferable.

- It will be highly relevant if a *child* gives an explanation in his or her *own words* as opposed to the account given by an accompanying mother or father.

- *Explanations or prompts given by an accompanying adult* should also be noted.

- It is assumed that doctors will note any *examination* undertaken, *diagnosis* and medication or *treatment* prescribed, with appropriate *diagrams*.

- It will also be extremely helpful to attempt to *date any injury* observed.

Such information is vital but additional, seemingly less relevant, observations can be rather telling. For example, observations of the appearance and/or behaviour of the child and the accompanying adult may place the injury or illness in context, particularly when considered in conjunction with any past complaints. There are no fixed rules on writing good medical notes. I would simply suggest that all observations, however small, are comprehensively, contemporaneously (and legibly!) recorded.

Providing reports

The report writer must bear in mind two things:

- that his or her *primary duty is to the court* rather than the person instructing;

- that *any opinion given must be honestly held*. It is vital that the doctor providing a report, whether as the child's GP or as an expert witness does not mislead, even by omission, as *objectivity is an essential element of a good report*.

The opinion expressed should not resemble an argument, and where based on insufficient material, this should be stated along with the fact that the opinion is merely provisional. Much guidance can be drawn from the letter of instruction sent by the instructing solicitor. The letter ought to clearly identify the purpose for which the report is required, setting out specific questions and issues of fact to be addressed.

An expert may give an opinion on any relevant matter on which he or she is qualified to give evidence. It is permissible for an expert to give evidence as to the truthfulness or accuracy of the child or accompanying adult. However, the judge will decide on the issue of precisely who caused the harm to the child. For example, a doctor may observe a certain injury and indicate a number of potential causes. He may even, and where possible should, state which of those causes he believes is the relevant one. In general, the GP will be appearing as a professional witness rather than as an expert witness, and opinions of this nature will not be expected to the same degree, and should not be offered unless the GP feels they can readily support them. However, it would be beyond any doctor's expertise and remit to go on to identify the person whom he believes inflicted the injury.

Evidence in court

Preparation is unquestionably vital for the GP appearing in court, whether as a professional witness or as an expert. Part of that preparation necessarily entails updating oneself on any developments in the case that could alter an opinion previously held. The doctor appearing as an expert witness should be aware that it is entirely plausible that different experts may rely on different information and therefore reach differing conclusions. With this in mind the individual expert should be prepared to comment on the opinions of other witnesses, both lay and expert. Where multiple experts are called it may be beneficial for all to confer in advance of the hearing to establish the prominent issues and areas of agreement. Further, there is no shame in stating that a particular issue is beyond the witness's expertise. Indeed it is far more constructive to make such an admission as an opinion of the expert could affect the final placement of the child, with disastrous consequences if ill-founded.

Conclusion

Public law proceedings underpin child protection and prevention of abuse. GPs are optimally placed to identify the symptoms of abuse at an early stage, and for this reason have an invaluable contribution to make to subsequent legal proceedings. While recognizing the potential impact of care proceedings on the child and the family as a whole, medical practitioners can assist in a legal context by compiling detailed evidence of abuse from the initial stage of identification through to report writing and oral evidence at the final hearing. From a legal perspective, the most helpful approach for the medical practitioner to adopt is one of objective yet thorough observation of the spectrum of abuse indictors.

Chapter 7b

Therapeutic options

Danya Glaser

Introduction

The aims of the therapeutic response to child abuse and neglect are to address both retrospective and prospective issues. The experience of being abused or neglected leaves a more or less well-healed wound, whose nature is psychological and more rarely also physical. The more raw the feelings, the more urgent is the therapeutic need. Past abuse or neglect may well have an effect on the child's future development as well as affecting their vulnerability to further abuse. Beyond physical injuries, the effects of abuse and neglect are psychological, emotional or behavioural. As well as healing, therapeutic responses are, therefore, also regarded as (tertiary) prevention, by promoting the child's coping and reducing future vulnerability. Given the child's inherent dependency on adult carers, and their likely membership of a family, therapeutic endeavours need to attend not only to the child's individual needs but must include, with equal importance, the needs of the adult carers and the family.

In terms of therapy, most attention has been accorded to the aftermath of *sexual* abuse although there is increasing evidence of the long-term psychological harm associated with physical abuse, neglect[1] and emotional abuse.[2] Moreover, many children have experienced more than one form of abuse[3] even if initially only one form is evident. Thus, whilst well-documented therapeutic approaches for certain forms of abuse have been developed, in practice the children not infrequently require additional help.

There are two dimensions which need to be considered—the *developmental* dimension and the systemic or *relational* one. A child's age and developmental stage, both at the time of the abuse and at the point at which therapy is offered will determine and inform the nature of help offered.

In thinking about child abuse and neglect, it is useful to consider the abuse relationships within a triangle consisting of the child, the abuser and the primary carer(s) (Figure 7.1). This triangle is naturally embedded within several other contexts, including the family, social network and cultural group.

Some forms of abuse constitute discrete (even if repeated) events. Others form an integral aspect of the relationship between the abuser and the child to the extent that the abuse or neglect comes to characterize the relationship. In 'event abuse', typically sexual

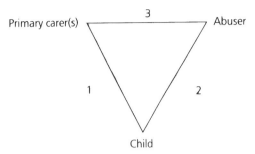

Fig. 7.1 The abuse triangle.

abuse and non-accidental injury, the abuser and the primary carer are not usually the same person although they may be closely related or, at least, well known to each other. Emotional abuse, neglect and those forms of physical abuse which are a habitual part of harsh discipline, are more properly considered as 'relationship abuse'. Here, the abuser and primary carer are more likely to be the same person, which has serious implications for protection of the child.

Protection from abuse can, in theory, be achieved in one of three ways:

1. The abuser, or his/her circumstances change so that the abusive interaction or behaviour is lessened or ceases.

2. All interactions between the abuser and the child are supervised.

3. The child is separated from the abuser, by one or the other leaving home.

The first way is difficult to achieve, and is certainly not possible in the short term. Supervision is only a realistic option when there is limited contact between the child and the abuser. The third option may be the only way of protecting a child. In sexual abuse this will often allow the child to remain with the non-abusive parent. This is relevant to the axiom, often and appropriately applied to some forms of abuse, that protection must *precede* therapy. However, if the abuser and the primary carer are one and the same person, then initial protection may well require a separation of the child from the primary carer/abuser, which would add to the child's loss and likely trauma. In emotional abuse and neglect, therefore, the initial therapeutic involvement is working *towards* protection, rather than following protection, with the recognition that for the foreseeable future, the child will probably continue to be abused or neglected.

The principles, practice and evaluation of treatment (or therapy) for *sexual* abuse have been the most clearly developed. The reasons for this are not entirely clear. Neglect and physical abuse are more common and do undoubtedly lead to sequelae requiring therapy. It may be that, with the former having been in the province of social workers and the latter often in the hands of paediatricians, psychological approaches and therapies have been less developed. The following section will therefore describe in more detail considerations relating to therapy following sexual abuse. Contrasts relating to other forms of abuse and neglect will then be addressed.

Sexual abuse

A comprehensive therapeutic approach to the aftermath of sexual abuse needs to address the following:

- pre-abuse circumstances;
- peri-abuse factors;
- post-abuse circumstances.

Pre-abuse circumstances include the nature of the child's attachments and the care given to the child, as well as family relationships. It could be said to apply particularly to side 1 of the abuse triangle (Figure 7.1). *Peri-abuse* factors refer to the abuse itself and include the nature and severity of the abuse, its duration and its frequency. In interactional terms, peri-abuse circumstances describe the nature of the relationship between the abuser and the child, during the period of the abuse, and the relative power, dependency, trust and fear between the child and the abuser. It applies particularly to side 2 of the abuse triangle. *Post-abuse* circumstances describe the response of the abuser and, crucially, of the non-abusing parent or carer, to the discovery or recognition of the abuse. The relationship, if any, between the non-abusing carer or parent and the abuser is very likely to affect their responses to the child and the abuse (side 3 of the abuse triangle). Following the discovery of abuse, it is possible to predict that the closer the relationship between the primary carer and the abuser, the worse is the outcome for the child.[4] Closeness here does not connote only love or affection, and includes also dependency and fear.

Therapy for sexual abuse

Child sexual abuse has three important elements: the secrecy and usual absence of independent witnesses during the abuse; the denial of the abuse by the alleged abuser when it is discovered; and the consequent, not infrequent, disbelief in the child's account. As there is no postsexual abuse syndrome,[5] therapy for sexual abuse is no straightforward matter, nor is a standard, programmatic approach useful. There are issues concerning purpose, recipients, content, treatment modality and process, including duration.[6]

Purpose

The aims of therapy are based on fulfilling the needs of the child. Following the discovery of, and protection from, sexual abuse, the child's immediate needs are:

- to be *believed*;
- *not to be blamed* for the abuse, for not disclosing earlier or for disclosing now;

- to be *protected* from further abuse;
- to be *informed* about developments in the post-disclosure process, including any legal proceedings;
- to be enabled to *talk* about the abuse.

In the longer term, the child's needs are to live in a permanent setting, either in the original or an alternative family.

Treatment is essentially psychological, apart from rare occasions where serious injury occurs as part of the abuse or when a child contracts a sexually transmitted disease or falls pregnant. Psychological treatment is orientated both retrospectively, dealing with the aftermath and effects of the abuse, and prospectively with the aim of ensuring the best possible future adjustment for the child. There is empirical evidence indicating that mothers who were seriously abused in childhood, and who received therapy that helped them to be able to talk coherently about their own abusive childhood experiences, do not go on to abuse their own children.[7]

Recipients

Children who have been abused by strangers or non-family members are more likely to be protected by their family, and are therefore not liable to child protective measures by social services. Despite their frequent need for support and therapy,[8] they and their family therefore tend to miss out on this process. Apart from the child, there are other important members of the abuse and family network who need to be considered in planning a systemic treatment approach or programme. They include, next to the child, the *mother, non-abusing parents* or *primary caregiver(s)*. These persons are inevitably disturbed by the discovery of the abuse. There is now ample evidence indicating that the prognosis for the child is significantly determined by the mother's support for the child.[9,10] Conversely, the mother's emotional distress adversely affects outcome for the child.[11] The child's *siblings*, who may have been silent witnesses, unknown victims or merely 'forgotten', have their own needs. Finally, the *abuser* will require treatment if he is able to admit to the abuse and particularly if he wishes to continue to maintain a meaningful relationship with the child. At different times in the process, these members of the child's family may be seen together, singly or in different combinations, depending on need.

Content

The minimum requirement of post-abuse help to a child is to offer opportunities for the child to talk about the abuse and the *feelings* associated with the experience, including the inevitable *guilt* and *confusion, shame* and *isolation*. There is also always a need to address issues of *sexuality*, about which children who have been sexually abused hold many misconceptions. For instance, boys who have been abused by a man often fear that they had been 'recognized' as homosexual by the abuser, or that the abuse has changed them into homosexuals.

There are many reasons for children feeling that they are to blame, despite the fact that the children are, by definition, not guilty. Reasons include the children's erroneous belief that they should have been able to stop the abuse or to report it earlier. Other children feel guilty for disclosing the abuse, particularly if the consequences are distressing for the mother or are perceived to have caused a subsequent family break-up. Some children come to feel guilty for the subsequent imprisonment of the abuser.

Many children have additional therapeutic needs which may only be found if specifically looked for. A significant proportion (approximately 35 per cent)[12] of children who have been sexually abused suffer from post-traumatic phenomena or actual *post-traumatic stress disorder.*[13] In this condition:

- unwanted vivid recollections of the traumatic event(s) intrude into the child's present, either during the waking state by way of flashbacks or triggering reminders, or during sleep as nightmares;

- the child fearfully avoids possible reminders of the abuse and its circumstances;

- the child may be generally more anxious and aroused.

Inappropriate sexualized behaviour is the commonest sequel of sexual abuse, particularly in younger children. It includes talk about genitalia and sexual activity, and behaviour rarely seen otherwise, such as inserting fingers, objects or a penis into the vagina or anus, and oral–genital contact.[14] This behaviour may be exhibited towards another child, a doll or sometimes an adult. It also includes more commonly seen genitally-orientated behaviours such as looking at, touching or drawing genitalia or simulating sexual intercourse fully clothed. In the sexually abused child, these behaviours are more likely to be repeated, to become a preoccupation for the child, or to be accompanied by coercion of another child in the activity. These sexualized behaviours are particularly difficult to manage and treat.

Other issues include *circumstances in the child's life* before the abuse, such as a poor relationship with the primary caregiver or *neglect*, which will have rendered the child more vulnerable to abuse. Until the child is permanently and safely settled after the abuse is discovered, the child may be more preoccupied with the question of *where they are going to live* and the *nature of their future contact* with their family and with the abuser. Indeed, while the child is 'in transit', these latter concerns may stand in the way of the child feeling able to become fully involved in therapy concerned with the actual abuse.

Children, and particularly adolescents, suffer from *depression* following a history of sexual abuse; others move on to *drug abuse* and deliberate *self-harm*. Childhood *prostitution* is another outcome. There are reported associations between a history of sexual abuse and *eating disorders*, especially bulimia nervosa. Specific therapeutic work will be required here.

Treatment modality and process

The child

Some issues concern the abused child's feelings, thoughts and experiences and are more appropriately addressed with the abused child, either individually or in a group. On present evidence, there is not a clear-cut advantage to group or individual therapy for sexually abused girls, in terms of overall outcome. Children report preferring group therapy over other modes such as individual or family therapy.[15]

Groups   The actual group *environment* is an important component of the treatment process. Belonging to a therapy group reduces the children's sense of isolation, shame and stigma. It offers the opportunity to share one's experiences in a safe setting. It is reassuring to hear about the guilt and self-blame that other group members have also experienced, even if these feelings are not thereby alleviated fully. Children often find the peer group an enabling environment in which to talk about difficult issues. This includes finding an appropriate language with which to talk about the abuse. Learning about sexuality, in a peer group, reduces the embarrassment.[16]

The group setting is also useful in helping to identify those children who will require further, individual therapy.

Over the age of 6 years, groups are best offered to boys and girls separately and the work is most appropriately carried out with four to six children of a similar age and developmental stage, within 2–3-year age bands. They require structure, a pre-planned programme of content and activities,[17] and two cotherapists of whom at least one should be female. Groups for boys are reported to require particularly firm structure and containment. Some older adolescents benefit from longer term and less structured groups in which there is more opportunity to reflect on experiences.[18] Although several children are treated simultaneously, group work offers little actual saving in therapist time, requiring careful planning, actual preparation and regular supervision. There is also a need for parallel work with the children's carers.

Parallel work with carers   It is extremely useful to offer parallel group or individual work for the children's carers. This helps to ensure that the children will actually attend. The children's group process is affected adversely by irregular membership, particularly so when the group is time-limited and based on a programme. It is also important for the carers to know about aspects of the content of the child's therapy, for instance sex education, which the child may wish to continue to discuss. Parents or carers of children who have been sexually abused have many concerns and unanswered questions which can begin to be addressed in a carers' group.[19]

Individual therapy   Some children who are extremely troubled and whose difficulties include a deep sense of guilt, low self-esteem or difficulties with attachment, resulting from poor experiences of being parented may, in addition, require individual therapy. As with group therapy for children, it is important that the child's caregiver is seen alongside the child. *Cognitive behavioural therapy* (CBT) has been shown to be especially useful for the treatment of post-traumatic stress disorder and for sexualized behaviours of younger children.[20]

Therapy and the law   If a child is to give evidence in a criminal trial of an alleged abuser, there are certain cautions regarding the child receiving therapy before the trial.[21] Group treatment pretrial is probably best avoided in order to avoid the subsequent complaint that the child's evidence has been 'contaminated' by the accounts of other children. While it is now accepted that the child's treatment take precedence, prior consultation with the Crown Prosecution Service is advisable, via the police child protection team. Careful notes need to be kept by the therapist.

The non-abusive parent

There are many troubling issues which arise for the mother, or other non-abusive parent, following discovery of sexual abuse.

- There are feelings of guilt at not having been aware of the abuse or for not having acted earlier on suspicions of abuse.

- For various reasons which include guilt, possible memories of her previous own sexual abuse, and the consequences of believing the child, the mother may have serious difficulties in believing the child's account.

- If the abuser has been known to the non-abusing parent, was or is in any form of emotional or biological relationship with the non-abusing parent, and especially if the alleged abuser is denying the allegation of abuse, there is a serious dilemma for the mother or non-abusing carer(s) in deciding whose side to take or whom to choose.

- If the mother believes and supports the child, this may be at a considerable cost to her, involving, as it may, losses of relationship and income, and fear of, and even threats or attack from, the abuser.

There is therefore a need to provide therapy for the non-abusing carer who is often, at the crisis time of disclosure, more needy than the child. Groups for mothers are often particularly helpful in enabling the participants to share their dilemmas and co-construct solutions. These groups are more than self-help groups and require the leadership of therapists.

The mother needs to actively support the child, not only by believing but also by protecting the child. The latter is measured by the mother's capacity to separate from the abuser, at least until the abuser takes responsibility and receives treatment.[22]

The abuser

For the protection of other children, and particularly if there is an intention for the abuser to return to an unsupervised or meaningful relationship with the child, there is a need for therapy. Given the addictive nature of sexually abusive activity, the best which therapy can be expected to achieve is a full recognition by the abuser that he has the potential to abuse children, and that he needs to guard indefinitely against this danger, by a number of means.

Much therapy for abusers is carried out in groups, one of whose advantages is that group members are in a good position to discourage minimization and denial by other members, while retaining a degree of mutual compassion and support. For therapy to commence, there is a prior requirement for the abuser to begin to admit to the abuse. Therapy deals with various aspects of *denial* which include denial of:

- the extent of the abuse, the number of victims and the frequency of the abuse;
- the abusive nature of the sexual contact;
- the discomfort, distress and harm which the abuse has caused the victim;
- responsibility for the abuse.

Therapy explores *antecedents* to the abuse in the abuser's own past childhood history. This is likely to include one or more harmful experiences including emotional, physical or sexual abuse, exposure to parental/domestic violence, neglect or disruption of primary attachments. Therapy for abusers needs to balance compassion for their own past victimization with an insistence on the *taking of full responsibility* by the abuser for the abuse. Other specific issues in addressed in therapy are:

- victim awareness;
- to explore in detail the abusers' distorted thinking about abuse that includes reframing it as an expression of love or as instruction for the child;
- exploring the cycle of precipitating stimuli which lead to abuse, as well as the grooming behaviour which the abusers develop in relation to their child victims;[23]
- helping the abuser to develop alternative ways of responding to the temptation to sexually abuse children.

Convicted abusers may receive treatment as part of a custodial sentence or following discharge from prison. It is possible, in some cases, for treatment to form part of a probation non-custodial order. This is clearly preferable for the majority of adolescent abusers.

Adolescent abusers   It is now increasingly recognized that a significant proportion of sexual abusers are adolescents, mainly boys, who are older brothers, cousins, uncles or baby-sitters of the children whom they abuse.[24] The hope that this could be regarded as a benign, transient phase of adolescent development is mistaken. Many adult abusers describe their activity commencing in adolescence. Without treatment, adolescents who have sexually abused younger children must be considered to continue to pose a serious risk. The dilemma for those who are parents of both the abuser and the abused is a particularly difficult one. The success of treatment for adolescent abusers is especially dependent on the capacity of the parents or carers of the young person to challenge the adolescent's denial and support treatment for him. The treatment of young abusers is discussed in more detail by Eileen Vizard in Chapter 9b.

Therapy for relationships

As well as dealing with individual issues, either in individual work or in separate groups of children, mothers or abusers, there is also a need to facilitate therapeutic communication about many painful and unresolved issues between the various members of the family network surrounding the abuse. This includes the mother and child, where the child might question why the mother had not protected the child; the non-abusing parent and abuser; and, if the abuser is able to acknowledge responsibility for the abuse and the child is willing to meet him, therapeutic conversations between the child and the abuser.

Whole family meetings are also important. The purpose here is to facilitate more free communication between family members who are living together, all of whom know about aspects of the abuse but often find difficulty in talking about it. There are also other aspects of *family functioning*, which, if relevant, benefit from therapy.[25] They include inappropriate intergenerational *boundaries, disorganization,* parental *neglect and unavailability,* and styles of *problem-solving.* Family work can only usefully include the abuser if he has taken responsibility for the abuse.

It is particularly important that the various modalities of treatment, which may overlap or be offered consecutively, are coordinated and that the various therapists continue to communicate with each other as well as with the general practitioner, statutory agencies including social services, the police and lawyers, if any of these are still involved.

Following abuse, there is often a need for different therapeutic inputs for some considerable time, although this might well be intermittent. Different needs arise at different stages in the child's development, such as the onset of puberty. It is often not possible to rely on one comprehensive and definitive treatment programme which will encompass and successfully anticipate all future therapeutic needs.

Treatment for other forms of abuse and neglect

There are no specific treatment approaches for children who have been physically abused and neglected. The direct psychological consequences of *physical abuse* and neglect include low self-esteem with a sense of worthlessness, bad self view in which the child believes they are bad and often behave according to this belief, or a sense of shame and humiliation. Following serious injury, some children may also experience post-traumatic phenomena. These need to be acknowledged and addressed therapeutically and specifically related to the child's experiences. In practice, this does not happen as systematically as following sexual abuse.

Emotional abuse and emotional neglect

Emotional abuse and emotional neglect are found independent of, or in conjunction with, physical abuse and neglect. Here, there is a variety of non-physically mediated, harmful parent–child interactions which pervade and characterize the relationship and whose severity calls for intervention.

Physical abuse and neglect are particularly associated with two variants of emotional abuse:

- *emotional neglect* and *poor parenting.* This latter includes age-inappropriate expectations and impositions on the child, setting of inconsistent or no boundaries, and punitive discipline.

Other variants of emotional abuse include:

- the specific *negative targeting*, scapegoating and rejection of a child who is believed by the parent to deserve this;

- *failure to recognize and respect the child's own feelings*, perceptions and psychological boundaries;

- *impeding the child's socialization* or *mis-socialization* of the child.[26]

Three *parental risk factors* are particularly associated with emotional abuse and neglect of their children, namely *mental ill-health, substance abuse* and *domestic violence.*[27]

Children who have been emotionally abused and neglected show a variety of difficulties in all domains of their development and functioning including emotional, behavioural, cognitive/educational, social/peer relationships and physical development. The pattern of associations between the various forms of emotional abuse and specific forms of childhood disorders and difficulties is still being explored.

Treatment of emotional abuse and emotional neglect therefore needs to address three aspects:

- *Parental risk factors* which may be known to adult services but which are sometimes not known to those initially dealing with the children's presenting difficulties.

- The various aspects of emotional abuse characterizing the *parent–child relationships.*

- The *children's own difficulties,* for which children are often referred to child and adolescent mental health services.

With body and life-endangering physical abuse, as with sexual abuse, treatment follows protection. With emotional abuse and neglect, which may or may not be associated with chronic physical neglect and abuse, treatment cannot await protection since the latter is itself dependent on successful treatment. Only in those cases where therapeutic intervention does not bring about sufficient change within the child's time limits, is protection by statutory measures and separation from the parents considered.[27]

Conclusion

Psychological and psychiatric treatment following various forms of child abuse and neglect is a complex and long-term process. A programmatic treatment approach or 'packages of care' are not appropriate since there are no clear-cut post-abuse syndromes. Research and clinical experience have, however, pointed to patterns of difficulties and disorders associated with a history of abuse that are recognized sufficiently frequently to indicate a systematic search for these difficulties in abused children. Specific forms of treatment are continuing to be developed. Treatment needs to address the child's own difficulties as well as carefully considering the child's family and wider contexts. Abuse and neglect are often so pervasive in the child's development that effective treatment may need to continue to be available and offered at several points in the child's subsequent life. It calls for a multi-professional approach and cooperation between the many agencies involved.

References

1 **Kaplan S, Pelcovitz D, Laruna V.** Child and adolescent abuse and neglect research: a review of the past 10 years. Part I: Physical and emotional abuse and neglect. *Journal of the American Academy of Child and Adolescent Psychiatry* 1999; **38**: 1214–22.

2 **Bifulco A, Brown G, Adler Z.** Early sexual abuse and clinical depression in adult life. *British Journal of Psychiatry* 1991; **159**: 115–22.

3 **Ney P, Fung T, Wickett A.** The worst combinations of child abuse and neglect. *Child Abuse and Neglect* 1994; **18**: 705–14.

4 **Berliner L, Elliott D.** Sexual abuse of children. In: Briere J, Berliner L, Bulkley J, Jenney C, Reid T, eds. *The APSAC Handbook on Child Maltreatment*. London: Sage, 51–71.

5 **Kendall-Tackett K, Williams L, Finkelhor D.** Impact of sexual abuse on children: a review and synthesis of recent empirical studies. *Psychological Bulletin* 1993; **113**: 164–80.

6 **Glaser D.** Treatment issues in child sexual abuse. *British Journal of Psychiatry* 1991; **159**: 769–82.

7 **Egeland B, Jacobvitz D, Papatola K.** Intergenerational continuity of abuse. In: Gelles R, Lancaster J, eds. *Child Abuse and Neglect: Biosocial Dimensions*. New york: Aldine de Gruyter, 255–77.

8 **Grosz C, Kempe R, Kelly M.** Extrafamilial sexual abuse: treatment for child victims and their families. *Child Abuse and Neglect* 2000; **24**: 9–23.

9 **Everson M, Hunter W, Runyan D, Edelsohn G, Coulter M.** Maternal support following disclosure of incest. *American Journal of Orthopsychiatry* 1989; **59**: 198–207.

10 **Runyan D, Hunter W, Everson M.** Maternal Support for Child Victims of Sexual Abuse: Determinants and Implications. Washington, DC: National Center on Child Abuse and Neglect, 1992.

11 **Cohen J, Mannarino A.** Factors that mediate treatment outcome of sexually abused preschool children: six and 12 month follow-up. *Journal of the American Academy of Child and Adolescent Psychiatry* 1998; **37**: 44–51.

12 McLeer S, Dixon J, Henry D, *et al.* Psychopathology in non-clinically referred sexually abused children. *Journal of the American Academy of Child and Adolescent Psychiatry* 1998; 37: 1326–33.

13 Trowell J, Ugarte B, Kolvin I, *et al.* Behavioural psychopathology of child sexual abuse in schoolgirls referred to a tertiary centre: a North London study. *European Journal of Child and Adolescent Psychiatry* 1999; 8: 107–16.

14 Lloyd Davies S, Glaser D, Kossoff R. Children' sexual play and behaviour in pre-school settings: staff's perceptions, reports and responses. *Child Abuse and Neglect* 2000; 24: 1329–43.

15 Prior V, Lynch MA, Glaser D. *Messages from Children: Children's Evaluations of the Professional Response to Child Sexual Abuse.* London: NCH Action For Children, 1994.

16 Glaser D, Frosh S. *Child Sexual Abuse.* London: Macmillan, 1993.

17 Nelki J, Watters J. A group for sexually abused young children: unravelling the web. *Child Abuse and Neglect* 1989; 13: 369–77.

18 Furniss T, Bingley-Miller I, Van Elburg A. Goal-oriented group treatment for sexually abused adolescent girls. *British Journal of Psychiatry* 1988; 152: 97–106.

19 Rushton A, Miles G. A study of a support service for the current carers of sexually abused girls. *Clinical Child Psychology and Psychiatry* 2000; 5: 411–26.

20 Jones DPH, Ramchandani P. *Child Sexual Abuse: Informing Practice from Research.* Abingdon: Radcliffe Medical Press, 1999.

21 Home Office, Crown Prosecution Service, Department of Health. *Provision of Therapy for Child Witness Prior to a Criminal Trial: Practice Guidance.* London: Crown Copyright, 2001.

22 Heriot J. Maternal protectiveness following the disclosure of intrafamilial child sexual abuse. *Journal of Interpersonal Violence* 1996; 11: 181–94.

23 Hawkes C. Linking thoughts to actions: using the integrated abuse cycle. In: Kemshall H, Pritchard J, eds. *Good Practice in Working with Violence.* London: Jessica Kingsley, 1999: 149–67.

24 Vizard E, Monck E, Misch P. Child and adolescent sex abuse perpetrators: a review of the research literature. *Journal of Child Psychology and Psychiatry* 1995; 36: 731–56.

25 Elton A. Working with substitute carers. In: Bentovim A, Elton A, Hildebrand J, Tranter M & Vizard E, eds. *Child Sexual Abuse within the Family: Assessment and Treatment* London: John Wright, 238–51.

26 Glaser D. Emotionally abusive experiences. In: Reder P, Lucey C, eds. *Assessment of Parenting: Psychiatric and Psychological Contributions.* London: Routledge, 1995: 73–86.

27 Glaser D, Prior V. Is the term child protection applicable to emotional abuse? *Child Abuse Review* 1997; 6; 315–29.

Chapter 7c

Picking up the pieces

Stephen Amiel

Introduction

This chapter looks at the tasks and issues facing the GP and other members of the primary health care team (PHCT) in the aftermath of a child protection referral. As such, its title is misleading and outdated, or at least I hope it is. Or at least I hope it soon will be. Implicit in it is the notion that the buck stops with us, and that much of what the GP and the rest of the PHCT have to do after a child protection referral has run its initial course is about damage limitation.

This notion, which may owe a little to self-pity and prejudice, but which owes more to collective past experience, goes something like this. If abuse is not proven, if the child is not placed on the child protection register, we are left with the task of cleaning up the mess once the multiagency circus has left town. We have to meet as best we can the needs of the child and family that have been identified along the way. We have to try to minimize the harm done by the child protection process itself, particularly the harm done to relationships: within the family; between the family and ourselves (especially if we made the referral to social services in the first place); and with other professionals and agencies. We have to cope with feeling ignored, with not being believed, or with being wrong.

If abuse is proven (the notion goes), the child may at best be protected from further harm. Some needs may be identified and, providing the child is put on the child protection register, some support and services promised, but these rarely materialize within an acceptable timeframe, or at all. The child protection process further traumatizes the child and their family, already in crisis as evidenced by the abuse. The family may be split up altogether: the child may be accommodated, facing the further perils of the care system; the non-abusing parent may be left destitute and unsupported; and the abuser may be left untreated and probably at large to abuse again. The family, or part of it, disappears from our list, or else we are left trying to retrieve irreparably damaged relationships. Relationships within the PHCT may be strained by conflicting loyalties towards family members or recriminations over what went wrong. Already difficult relationships with other agencies may deteriorate further as review conference dates are changed arbitrarily, referrals do not happen, and so on. We are left feeling guilty for missing the abuse or for letting things get that far, or sometimes doubting that we did the right thing by finding it.

The core of this notion is borne out by a good deal of research evidence on the outcomes of the child protection process,[1,2] some of which is discussed elsewhere in this book. This evidence also suggests that other agencies, especially social services, feel just as let down and unsupported by GPs as the other way round.

Research evidence like this was instrumental in stimulating the theoretical and attitudinal shift in child protection thinking over the past decade that has been highlighted in other chapters of this book. With the introduction of the assessment framework,[3] the reworking of official guidelines[4] and the move towards social services integration with health and/or education services, the organizational underpinning for this shift ought to be in place. Inevitably though, there will be a lag between what ought to be, and what is. This lag has a great deal to do with the inadequacy of resources (in social services departments as well as for the service needs identified). Undoubtedly, however, it also has something to do with a lag in shifting the attitudes and perceptions of all of us at ground level, professionals and public alike.

In time, families we care for, and we ourselves, may see firsthand the benefits of early referrals to social service departments of children thought to be in need, rather than waiting for those children to become children in need of protection. We may all become convinced that referrals of children in need are neither stigmatizing nor threatening, but are received sympathetically, in a spirit of constructive partnership between all concerned; that the needs of the child are rapidly ascertained and then met swiftly and appropriately, wherever possible by supporting and strengthening the family; and that much child abuse and many child removals are thereby prevented. There will, in short, be no pieces for us to pick up.

Until that time arrives, I suggest that the role of the GP (and the rest of the PHCT) in the aftermath of a referral will remain a challenging one, even if that referral is made with the enthusiastic consent of family members, with no child protection concerns on the agenda. When a referral is made because child abuse is suspected, alleged or apparent, the GP's work should only just have begun. Early referral of children in need is hugely important and can—using a familiar disease model—play a part in the primary prevention of child abuse. Equally though, the GP and other PHCT members can make a major contribution to secondary prevention (controlling disease in an early form) and tertiary prevention (preventing complications and/or mitigating the disabling consequences of a disease).

Notwithstanding the changes we are now seeing in the child protection landscape, tertiary prevention with regard to child abuse—proven, unproven or unfounded—may still involve the GP in attempting to prevent the complications and mitigate the consequences of the child protection process itself, as well as of the abuse. Those consequences may affect the child, other family members, the team and the GP.

In the remainder of this chapter, I will briefly recap on the contribution the GP can make to meeting the needs identified in the assessment process. I will address the GP's involvement around any continuing child protection concerns. Finally, I shall look at some of the issues facing the practice team in the aftermath of a child protection referral.

Meeting needs

In contributing to a core assessment, the GP and others will have an opportunity to identify what they see as a child's *needs*. They may be asked to comment on the severity of those needs; the capacity of the parents to meet those needs without support or services; the likely effects on the child's health and development were the needs not to be met; the urgency with which they should be met; and how best they feel those needs might be met.

Some of the needs identified may be specifically *health-related* (see also Chapter 6c) and may be met directly by the GP and the rest of the PHCT:

- *for the child:* developmental checks; immunizations; assessment for failure to thrive; referral for audiometry or optometry; referral to an enuresis clinic; sexual health check or contraception for older girls.

- *for the parents:* assessment/treatment/referral for physical or sexual health needs, mental health needs or substance abuse problems, any or all of which may be impairing their ability to care for their child.

Often though, needs identified will centre around concerns for a child's emotional or psychological well-being, relationships within the family, or general parenting capacity: such concerns will often have led to a referral being made in the first place. If an initial assessment confirms or increases those concerns, a core assessment may include a reasonably in-depth study of the family by specialist workers, often a multidisciplinary team of social workers, clinical psychologists, family therapists, etc: this study will help inform decisions about further action that may need to be taken (see Figure 6.1, p. 165). Under the new assessment framework guidelines, this work will have to be completed to a strict timescale (within 35 working days of an initial assessment).

However, resources to meet the *therapeutic* needs that may thereby be identified are rarely so forthcoming. Whilst some family assessment centres may undertake limited ongoing work, usually family members will have to be referred elsewhere. The GP may well in these circumstances feel the need to initiate this process, although the timing and exact nature of the referral may be dictated by further stages of the child protection process. Prior discussion with social service and/or family centre colleagues who are already involved with the family is, of course, desirable in these situations. It should be considered obligatory when there are ongoing formal child protection enquiries or proceedings, and when a child has been registered.

If, following a referral, continued social services involvement is considered unnecessary, the GP or health visitor may still consider there to be a need for, and will therefore need to initiate, some therapeutic input for family members. Even where such involvement continues, however, for example after registration, the GP's and health visitor's contribution in deciding on an appropriate referral, providing background information for the referral, chasing up appointments, and sometimes helping to ensure that appointments are kept, can be a vital one. As I have suggested in Chapter 6c, GP and/or health visitor membership of the core group of key agencies and family members can be effective and an efficient use of time in this regard.

There are a huge and sometimes bewildering variety of therapeutic resources that may be appropriate to children and families, either as individuals or as a family. There is also, however, huge *variation* across the country in the availability of these resources. Any of the following services may be considered:

- *child and adolescent* psychiatry, psychology, psychotherapy and counselling;
- *adult* psychiatry, psychology, psychotherapy and counselling (including specialist services for substance abuse, anger management etc.);
- *relationship* counselling;
- *family* psychiatry, family therapy.

Increasingly, Community Trusts, Mental Health Trusts and Primary Care Trusts (PCTs) provide directories of mental health services available locally: these often provide referral guidelines and pathways to assist practitioners.

Therapeutic options for children, adult survivors of abuse, and abusers are discussed in detail in other chapters of this book (see Chapters 5b, 7b, 8a and 9b).

The assessment process will often highlight (and may add to) a family's need for *support* and *information*, either in addition to, or instead of, therapy as such. Here too, the range of options is wide and variable.

Support may come from the *statutory* sector (health, education and social services), the *voluntary* sector and from *self-help* organizations. It may come in the form of financial assistance, drop-in groups, home visitors, language classes, toy libraries, survivors' groups, telephone or internet-based support services, support workers to assist with hospital visits, baby-sitting circles, and even peripatetic workers who come to live with a struggling family for a period.

At the time of writing, various government initiatives in support of children and families are being piloted in areas of high social deprivation, with a view to national roll-out, as part of an overall strategy to reduce child poverty, health inequalities, social exclusion and teenage pregnancies. As well as attracting significant new central funding, they are designed to draw together health, education and social services, and voluntary and self-help provision, providing information, support (both from professionals and peers) and services in an accessible, non-stigmatizing and seamless way.

The GP and other members of the PHCT may be already becoming familiar with some of these initiatives, for example:

- *Sure Start:* local programmes for parents-to-be and parents of 0–3 year olds, providing better access to family support, advice on nurturing, health services and early learning. Specific objectives include: reduction by 20 percent in Sure Start areas of the proportion of children re-registered within the space of 12 months on child protection registers; care and support programmes for mothers with postnatal depression; guidance on breastfeeding; and a reduction in hospital admissions for gastroenteritis, respiratory illness and severe injury.

- *The Children's Fund:* support for 5–13 year olds and their families, with the aim of preventing drug abuse, truancy, exclusion from school, crime and future unemployment. Services will combine *improved identification* of children with difficulties, through integrated assessment approaches, improved data sharing or common referral systems; and *increased support* through mentoring, counselling and advice services, parenting education, support for children of single parents, and work with individual children through multidisciplinary teams in schools and health centres.

- *Connexions:* careers advice and youth support services for 13–19 year olds. By 2003, a network will be in place of personal advisers as well as on-line and telephone services providing help and guidance on 'anything stopping you getting on in life'.

These may well become significant resources that practitioners' patients will access for themselves, or that team members may direct them towards. A full evaluation is pending: whilst their aims and objectives can hardly be faulted, and whilst the new money promised may even be real, there are already some concerns that resources are, or will be, diverted from more basic but less glamorous areas, like health visitor establishments in PHCTs, and social worker establishments in local authority social services departments. For Sure Start at least, core services include outreach and home visiting; advice about family health, child health and development; and help for children and parents with special needs in getting access to specialized services. This runs the potential risk of duplication and unnecessary overlap, confusion as to responsibilities, doubts over accountability, and mixed messages being given by different agencies, if liaison and cooperation between Sure Start programmes and existing agencies, including PHCTs, are not given a high priority.

Social services departments and health visitors are more likely than GPs to have up to date knowledge of the resources available locally and the GP's role in accessing them on behalf of families may be peripheral. Two points are none the less worth making.

First, the practical help and emotional support that can be brought to bear in this way may be of inestimable value in protecting children within a vulnerable family. In my view, some knowledge of what is out there and how to access it is as appropriate and valuable as anything else in the GP's armamentarium. More specifically, the GP may also be of help in providing medical evidence in support of:

- rehousing/repairs;
- childcare support (nursery provision, family aides);
- benefits (certification, equipment grants, etc.);
- educational support (home tuition, 'statementing' of children for extra help at school).

Second, and conversely, the GP and health visitor, when faced with an apparently limitless choice of helping agencies, services and resources, may be tempted to *over-prescribe* these for families, both because they genuinely believe in their value and because of an understandable desire to lighten their own load. As with any prescription, however, the patient needs to be convinced that it is appropriate to their particular needs, and that it will benefit rather than harm them. For this to happen, they need to be part of the decision-making process, rather than the passive recipient of a list of what is good for them.

Also, as Balint observed,[5] the GP (or the health visitor) is often the prescription themselves: the emotional as well as practical support a vulnerable family can gain from a familiar and trusted professional, by virtue of that familiarity and trust, can also be of inestimable value.

As has been discussed elsewhere in this book, the relationship of a family doctor with a family that is failing, whether violence is a symptom of that failure or not, is rarely straightforward or easy. We have argued for our relationship with all patients to be based on: clarity; honesty; respect for their autonomy; positive regard for them, for what they have achieved or have tried to achieve; understanding of the difficulties in the way of their achieving more; their right to confidentiality as well as their need to understand its limits. We have discussed the early indicators of abuse and how to organize the practice to assist in the prevention and early detection of abuse. We have highlighted the positive contribution the GP can make to supporting the family through the investigative process, without compromising the protection of its more vulnerable members or distancing ourselves from professional colleagues.

With these prerequisites in mind, and hopefully in place, members of the PHCT will have positioned themselves as best they can to preserve meaningful and constructive relationships with family members, even those who we might have been instrumental in exposing as failing, or abusing.

Continuing child protection concerns

Our usefulness as *advocates*, both for the family and its individual members, has already been highlighted above in the discussion of needs: such concrete demonstration of support may itself help to re-establish or strengthen relationships. This advocacy role continues to be of crucial importance *when a child is registered.*

The core group and the child protection plan

Registration, it will be remembered (see p. 182) signifies that a child is at continuing risk of significant harm, and that the child requires interagency help and intervention delivered through a formal child protection plan. Within 10 working days of the initial child protection conference (CPC), the *core group*, coordinated by the social worker appointed as *key worker*, should be convened. The core group should comprise representatives of the key agencies who have continuing involvement with the family, as well as family members, and should meet sufficiently often thereafter to discharge its key functions. These functions are as follows:

- to *provide a forum* for working with parents, wider family members and children of sufficient age and understanding;

- to *develop* the *child protection plan* as a detailed working tool, and to *implement* it, within the outline plan agreed at the initial CPC;

- to determine what steps need to be taken, and by whom, to complete the *core assessment* on time;

- to *refine* the plan as needed;

- to *monitor progress* against the agreed objectives of the plan;

- to produce *reports for child protection review*, providing an overview of work undertaken by family members and professionals, and to evaluate the impact on the child's welfare against the objectives set out in the child protection plan. (See paras 5.77–5.79, 5.92.)[4]

It is recognized that a formal conference is intimidating for most families, and securing agreement to the details of a child protection plan may be much easier within the smaller, more informal core group. Indeed, key professionals too may find this setting more conducive to forging important partnerships, both with family members and each other. It is also easier in the core group setting to avoid the misunderstandings and splitting that can also be generated (sometimes deliberately) between the various parties.

Whilst membership of the core group should not be seen as an alternative to one-to-one consultations with family members, I have argued that it can be a valuable use of a GP's time. In any case, it is unusual for a core group to meet more than once or twice in the standard 3-month interval between an initial and a review case conference. Social workers are, in my experience, usually more than happy to convene a core group meeting at a time and location convenient to the GP: the surgery is often a closer and less intimidating location for family members, health visitors and teachers too.

The core group provides a good opportunity for the GP:

- to help *formulate and refine* the core assessment and child protection plan;

- to bring his/her *knowledge of the family* and local resources to bear in order to help ensure that the plan; (i) adequately reflects the needs identified, and (ii) has realistic, specific and achievable objectives;

- to *clarify roles and responsibilities* (including their own) for completing the core *assessment*;
- to clarify roles and responsibilities (including their own) for implementing the *child protection plan.*

And, at subsequent meetings:

- to *update* other professionals on developments with the family since the last meeting or conference, including positive steps taken by family members or possible further concerns that may have emerged;
- to *be updated* by other professionals in turn;
- to *progress* chase referrals, provision of services.

And, in general:

- to *support* family members, within a multiagency forum;
- to *facilitate working together* with other professionals;
- to contribute to the core group's *report to the review conference.*

There will be situations where the GP is unable or unwilling to be part of the core group: this does not, of course, preclude liaison with other professionals on behalf of family members. At the very least, details of important health-related developments concerning family members, referrals made or reports received, should always be passed on to the key worker, who has the lead in coordinating interagency work with the child and family.

The child protection review conference

Within 3 months of the initial case conference, and at no more than 6-monthly intervals thereafter, every child on the child protection register should be subject to a review conference.

The purpose of the child protection review conference is to

- 'review the safety, health and development of the child against intended outcomes set out in the child protection plan;
- to ensure that the child continues adequately to be safeguarded;
- to consider whether the child protection plan should continue in place or should be changed' (para. 5.91).[4]

In deciding whether the child is at continuing risk of significant harm, the responsibility to that child of those who are involved is as onerous as it is in the initial case conference. For the GP, the same considerations apply too: the reader should refer to Chapter 6c for a discussion of the ways in which the GP can contribute before, during and after a conference.

The GP may be faced with considerable pressure from various quarters to support *de-registration*. Most parents are desperately keen for their child to be de-registered, for obvious reasons, although some fear the withdrawal of support and services that they suspect will follow; key professionals involved with families see de-registration as formal validation of their work with them; some social work managers may be keen to reduce the child protection caseload their social workers are carrying, and may also fear being seen as an outlier relative to other local authorities' registration figures; and the pressure from government expectations such as those attached to initiatives like Sure Start (see above). As was pointed out in *Messages from Research*,[2] the emphasis can too often be, 'What must be done to get them off?' to the detriment of 'What are their needs?'

The potential dangers to the child if these pressures are succumbed to are clear. At an individual family level, the completion of a core assessment following initial registration may not yet have been followed by adequate measures to reduce the risk of significant harm; some parents may be anxious to remove their child and themselves from professional scrutiny because of continuing abuse; or a social worker, keen to close as many cases as possible before they leave their post, may wishfully think that a family is coping better than it actually is. More generally, there may be very good reasons why some areas have higher than average registration figures: minor demographic differences, small pockets of particularly high deprivation, the rehousing of 'problem' families in certain estates, even the registration of one or two large families, may distort figures, leading to a wholly inappropriate drive to de-register. Moreover, it is a matter of concern to many professionals in the field that registration figures should be used as an outcome measure of success in Sure Start areas, at least in its first few years of operation. The likelihood is that registrations will actually *increase* at first, as families in need come forward.

As well as inappropriate pressures to de-register from different quarters, there may also be pressure to *maintain* a child on the register for the wrong reasons, principally to ensure the continued provision of services and support. In theory though (and increasingly in practice), de-registration should *not* lead to the automatic withdrawal of help. It should also be pointed out that sometimes de-registration *increases* the help that families actually get. By removing a major source of friction between families and social services, de-registration can lift the barrier to effective working with families.

At a review conference, a decision may be made to *continue* registration under the same category/categories; to *change* the category/categories; or to *de-register*. De-registration should only occur:

- If *a review conference judges that a child is no longer at continuing risk of significant harm requiring safeguarding by means of a child protection plan*, for example:
  - the risk of harm has been reduced by action taken through the child protection plan;

- the child and family's circumstances have changed; or

- reassessment of the child and family indicates that a child protection plan is not necessary.

- If the child and family have moved permanently to another local authority area (in which case the receiving local authority must hold a CPC within 15 working days of being notified of the move).

- If the child has reached the age of 18, has died or has permanently left the UK.

Dates for review conferences are usually set well in advance, but if a GP is unable to attend in person, a *written report* (see pp. 178, 188–90) should be sent to the conference chair. The GP may be asked to give in this report their opinion on de-registration. Given that this would obviously have to be offered before a conference discussion takes place, I would advise caution in offering this opinion too readily.

A fee is payable for attendance at a review conference or core group meeting, or for a written report (see p. 188).

As with the initial decision to register, *dissent* on a decision to de-register may be voiced by any professional present and should be recorded in the minutes (see p. 184). These minutes should be distributed to all those invited to the review, not just those who were present. Parents and young persons may also appeal in certain limited circumstances against the conference's decision (see p. 183, 198).

Finally, whether de-registration is agreed to or not, the GP and other PHCT members need to keep in mind the possibility of *re-abuse* occurring. Between *a quarter and a third of children are known to have been re-abused* after they came to the notice of child protection agencies;[2] for sexual abuse, the figures may be even higher.[6] This staggeringly high proportion certainly called into question the effectiveness of the existing child protection system, and the evidence confirming it[7–10] was one of the important triggers for the reforms to the child protection process that are now in train.

The figures for re-abuse also highlight the importance for the GP and the rest of the PHCT of organizing their thinking and their practice so as to optimize the prevention and early detection of re-abuse, as well as initial abuse. In the final part of this chapter, I will summarize some of the organizational and housekeeping issues for the practice in the aftermath of a child protection referral.

Part 8 reviews

If a child dies and abuse or neglect is known or suspected to be a factor, or a child is permanently and seriously harmed through abuse or neglect, and concerns arise about the way local professionals and services worked together, there is likely to be a review (usually called a '*Part 8 review*') conducted by the Area Child Protection Committee (ACPC). A review can be requested by any professional if it is felt that there are important lessons for interagency working to be learned from a case, or an inquiry can be ordered by the Secretary of State for Health.

Professionals including GPs may have their records relating to the case sequestered to guard against loss or interference; and independent practitioners such as GPs will be expected to provide reports of their involvement. Each relevant service is required to undertake a separate management review of its involvement, and designated professionals will review the practice of all involved health professionals and providers within their PCT or equivalent area. An overview report commissioned by the ACPC will bring together all the reports and other information, and make recommendations for future action, which, like the individual management reviews, should be fed back to the individuals and agencies involved. Although case reviews are not in themselves part of a disciplinary process, they may indicate that disciplinary action should be taken.

Part 8 reviews are not supposed to be like, or feel like, a trial or an ordeal, notwithstanding the above: rather, they are intended as a learning exercise, where good practice is shared as well as areas for change identified. The recommendations in *Working Together* for 'day to day good practice to ensure that [Part 8] reviews are conducted successfully' apply equally for GPs and others who wish to avoid them (for the child's sake, of course, but also for their own):

- 'establish a culture of audit and review. Make sure that tragedies are not the only reason inter-agency work is reviewed;

- have in place clear systematic case recording and record-keeping systems;

- develop good communication and mutual understanding between disciplines ... ' (para. 8.32).[4]

Issues for the practice team

Medical records

In Chapter 5c I discussed ways in which the practice might organize itself to facilitate the prevention and early detection of child abuse. I dwelt at some length on the importance of comprehensive, accurate and accessible records, and how useful they can then be, particularly when tagging and cross-referencing is used (see pp. 129–32).

Good records can help in:

- identifying vulnerable children and families;

- making a diagnosis of child abuse or re-abuse;

- focusing the response of the practice team appropriately when family members present.

They are particularly important when:

- family members may see different doctors in the practice;

- other team members use the same record to access or record information;

- referrals to specialists or other agencies are made;

- information is sought by other agencies;

- a family moves to another GP's list;

- court proceedings require the GP to write a report or appear as a witness.

They may, of course, be vital to the GP themselves in the event of a complaint or an inquiry.

Following the initial resolution of a child protection referral, by whatever route (see Figure 6.1, p. 166), several issues with regard to the medical record may need to be considered.

- The records of *all* household members should be *reviewed and updated:* information presented at a conference or emerging in the course of an assessment may be relevant to the health, well-being and/or safety of any or all family members. Existing information in the record may need to be re-interpreted and shared with social services if not already done so. In certain circumstances, the records of extended family members or close family associates may need to be looked at too.

- If a child is *registered*, this should be recorded, together with the category/categories for registration. If following a review conference, the category/categories are *amended*, this should be recorded (with computerized records, it is recommended that an additional new entry is made, rather than the former entry altered).

- Similarly, in the event of *de-registration*, it is recommended that the original entry concerning registration is not deleted, as it forms an important part of the historical record, although of course the fact of de-registration needs to be noted too.

- The name and contact details of the child's *key worker* should be recorded accessibly.

- If a child is the subject of child protection enquiries, but is *not registered*, or if the siblings of a registered child are not themselves registered, this should be recorded in the notes. In the latter case, some indication that there is another child in the household on the child protection register should be available to members of the team on a need to know basis: this may take the form of an explicit note, including the reason for registration, or may simply signpost the clinician to the relevant details in the registered child's notes.

- If a child is accommodated elsewhere, or some members of the family are moved for their own safety, or choose to move, *transfer of the medical records* should be viewed as priority (see p. 128).

- Issues of *confidentiality* have to be balanced against issues of the child's and other family members' *safety* and impact on the detailed implementation of all the above. General principles of confidentiality and its limits with regard to child protection have been discussed elsewhere in this book (see Chapter 3).

Case conference minutes

Working Together regards the written record of the child protection case conference as 'a crucial working document for all relevant professionals and the family'. Minutes should include:

- the essential facts of the case;
- a summary of the discussion at the conference, which accurately reflects the contributions made;
- all decisions reached, with information outlining the reasons for decisions;
- an outline or revised child protection plan enabling everyone to be clear about their tasks (para. 5.74).[4]

GPs should note the following:

- Minutes should be circulated as soon as possible to all those invited to the conference, *including family members* (although the latter will not receive notes of those parts of the conference from which they might have been excluded). They provide an important source of information to the GP unable to attend, particularly as family members may wish to discuss their contents.

- GPs who did attend the conference should *check the minutes* carefully for accuracy and inform the chair immediately of any inaccuracies they are aware of. These will in general be corrected at a review conference, or by letter to all participants if no review is planned. It should be emphasized that conference minutes, in addition to being a working document, also constitute a quasi-legal record which may form the basis for court proceedings or inquiries. Despite the professionalism of minute takers and the chairs who are supposed to check them, errors of omission or commission are not uncommon.

- *Minutes are confidential* and should not be passed by the GP to any third party without the consent of the chair or the key worker. Occasionally, a solicitor acting for a parent in court proceedings may request copies of the medical record from the GP and case conference minutes will form part of that record. Having said that, some social service lawyers argue that, technically, under the Access to Health Records Act 1990, minutes do not qualify as a health record (as they were not prepared by, or on behalf of, a health professional as defined in the Act) and therefore do not need to be, and should not be, disclosed. Most parents will have seen the minutes anyway, but if they have not, the GP should take advice from their defence organization before disclosing them to parents' legal representatives. They should in any case bear in mind before disclosing any of the record, the proviso in the Act that permits the withholding of information that might cause serious harm to the physical or mental health of the patient or any other individual. British Medical Association guidance[11] also points out that if the medical record identifies a third party who is not a health professional, that individual's consent must be sought before that information is released, although the seeking of that consent is not a requirement under the Act. This may be particularly important when the safety as well as the confidentiality of family members, neighbours, etc. who have provided information may be at stake.

- *Copies of the minutes* should be made and put in the records of all the children in the household who were discussed at the conference, whether registered or not. Copies should also be placed in the records of the parents, subject to them being party to the minutes in the first place, and subject to the removal of notes relating to any part of the conference from which they might have been excluded. There are delicate issues around third party confidentiality involved here. It might, for example, be considered good practice to remove clinical or other information about a sibling or parent from the copy of the minutes going into another sibling's notes: on the other hand, that information might be considered essential to protect that sibling from the risk of significant harm themselves. While the Access to Health Records Act can be used to prevent lay access to this information about third parties, is it proper even for other health professionals to have access to this? At the time of writing, there seem to be no clear-cut guidelines on this, and the GP should refer to general discussions both in this book and elsewhere, using these to help inform their decision on a case by case basis.

- When family members change doctors, conference minutes should be sent on with the rest of the medical record.

Communication and learning within the PHCT

For over 20 years I have worked as part of a first-rate primary health care team comprising GPs and GP registrars, employed practice nurses, practice-attached health visitors and district nurses, practice counsellor, and adult care social worker. We have had in the past and, at the time of writing, are about to have again, a social worker with responsibility for children and families attached to the practice. We all work from the same purpose-built premises and can if needs be access the same, now fully computerized, medical record.

While this may in many ways be an ideal configuration to help prevent and detect child abuse, it is not an option for many colleagues, and is not wanted by some even if it were. But nor is it in my experience a guarantee that the child protection process will be smooth, effective and painless, for anyone.

It is thankfully rare for child protection cases to go so very badly wrong that a Part 8 review is necessary (see above). In my experience, though, it is equally rare in a case of child abuse for everything to go right. More often, while there is not a disaster, there is a feeling either between or within agencies that things could have been done better.

Within the practice team, mechanisms need to be in place which, if they cannot always prevent that feeling, can at least help the team to deal with it, and just as important, learn from it.

- *Communication* needs to be worked at constantly. Full and accurate records are essential, and tagged/cross-referenced records can be very valuable, but significant developments need to be communicated personally to those who need to know, within the practice team as much as outside it. A telephone call, an internal e-mail, a note in a tray, a word over coffee, can all be vital supplements to the written record.

- It cannot be assumed that all *documentation* (accident and emergency department reports, reports from child guidance clinics, adult services, etc.) will be copied to other members of the team involved in the care of the child. This too should be checked and team members should be shown or copied relevant documents that they need to see.

- Chapters 9c and 9d discuss in some detail ways in which *child protection training* can be improved for general practitioners and practice teams. Hodes and Weir in Chapter 9c describe their success in implementing practice-based workshops where awareness of child protection is raised, and experiences and uncertainties are shared. To a degree, this kind of learning can be woven into the everyday work of most practices. Regular *practice team meetings*, involving reception staff as well as clinical staff, are a good forum for discussing and improving practice procedures, for sharing information about local resources, or alerting team members to particular concerns about children and families. They also help to facilitate *team-building*: understanding each other's job better, its constraints and pressures as well as what it can bring to the task, can be an important part of increasing the effectiveness of, and trust between, team members. Detailed clinical information about families should not be discussed in front of non-clinical members of the team.

- Discussion within the practice team of what went wrong in the aftermath of a child protection case has tended to be a private affair between the protagonists, or has not happened at all. Doctors are typically poor at giving constructive criticism to each other, possibly because they are typically even worse at taking it; and there are probably even fewer examples of harmonious interdisciplinary exchanges of this kind, particularly when the doctor is on the receiving end. In the new NHS this is, we are told, all changing, as practices, in common with all other health service organizations, become obliged to engage in and demonstrate the various components of *clinical governance*.

- Obligation or not, the principles of clinical governance can certainly be of help in setting up and implementing practice systems for dealing with the aftermath of child abuse, as well as for preventing it. 'The creation of a *blame-free culture* of lifelong learning based on reflective practice' may sound like educationalist jargon to many, but its essence is an important prerequisite for helping team members to deal with and learn from difficult child protection cases.

- Other components of *clinical risk management* have been discussed elsewhere in this book: developing effective *communication* systems; liaising with other practitioners; managing and making *registers of vulnerable patients*; and suitable *training* for staff. A difficult child protection case will often be suitable for analysis by the practice team as a '*significant event*', whether it constitutes a 'near miss' or indeed where there are successful aspects that provide learning opportunities for the rest of the team.

- Critical *self-examination* is supposed to be part of the blame-free culture. The emotions that a child abuse case may leave a practitioner with can make this self-examination a difficult business, notwithstanding the presence of a supportive practice team. Neighbour talks of *housekeeping*,[12] a process where the practitioner acknowledges what he is feeling, tries to work out where those feeling originate, and asks himself what needs to be done about them. Housekeeping, with its connotation of cleansing, involves the practitioner in trying to dissipate the stress from the left-over feelings of previous consultations to prevent contamination of subsequent ones.

- With child abuse, these feelings can be overwhelming, especially, but not exclusively, when things go wrong. The difficulty in coming to terms with getting things wrong can be compounded by feelings of revulsion, anger and fear, which can spill over into overprotectiveness of one's own children, difficulties in one's own personal relationships, or a sense that abuse is everywhere. Some practitioners will have suffered abuse or neglect in their own childhoods: for them, the resonances of a child abuse case can be particularly painful. Acknowledging these feelings, being able to share them with a colleague or other professional, or with a family member, and being reassured that they are normal, sounds easy enough. It also has to be acknowledged, however, that many practitioners find this very difficult. Some may find support outside their practice or family from young principals' groups or Balint groups.

- When a practitioner feels that their emotional equilibrium or even their psychological health has been affected significantly, help may need to be sought elsewhere: occasionally a colleague may need to initiate this on their behalf. Even those practitioners who set aside their traditional reticence when it comes to asking for help for themselves, may, however, find it difficult to access occupational health services: these, certainly for GPs and their staff, are fairly embryonic. Putting this right is now correctly considered a government priority,[13] attracting modest new resources: a telephone advice service should already be available and a full range of services should be in place by 2002 (arrangements may vary in different parts of the UK).

References

1 Hallett C. *Inter-Agency Co-ordination in Child Protection.* London: HMSO, 1995.

2 **Department of Health.** *Child Protection: Messages from Research.* London: HMSO, 1995.

3 **Department of Health.** *Framework for the Assessment of Children in Need and their Families.* London: Stationery Office, 1999.

4 **Department of Health, Home Office, Department of Education and Employment, the National Assembly for Wales.** *Working Together to Safeguard Children: a Guide for Interagency Working to Safeguard and Promote the Welfare of Children.* London: Department of Health, 1999.

5 **Balint M.** *The Doctor, His Patient and the Illness,* 2nd edn. London: Pitman Medical, 1964.

6 **Sharland E, Jones D, Aldgate J, Seal H, Croucher M.** *Professional Intervention in Child Sexual Abuse.* London: HMSO, 1995.

7 **Cleaver H, Freeman P.** *Parental Perspectives in Cases of Suspected Child Abuse.* London: HMSO, 1995.

8 **Farmer E, Owen M.** *Child Protection Practice: Private Risks and Public Remedies—Decision Making, Intervention and Outcome in Child Protection Work.* London: HMSO, 1995.

9 **Thoburn J, Lewis A, Shemmings D.** *Paternalism or Partnership? Family Involvement in the Child Protection Process.* London: HMSO, 1995.

10 **Gibbons J, Conroy S, Bell C, Gordon D.** *Development after Physical Abuse in Early Childhood: a Follow-Up Study of Children on Protection Registers.* London: HMSO, 1995.

11 **British Medical Association.** *Access to Health Records Act 1990—Guidelines for Doctors.* London: BMA, 1991 (revised 1995).

12 **Neighbour R.** *The Inner Consultation.* London: Kluwer, 1987.

13 **Department of Health.** *The Provision of Occupational Health and Safety Services for General Medical Practitioners and their Staff.* Leeds: Department of Health, 2001.

Chapter 8

The late sequence of child abuse

Chapter 8a

Survivors of childhood abuse: why should primary care be involved?

Gill Wakley

Introduction

'I can't see what it's got to do with me,' said one general practitioner as he sat unwillingly in a small group on an up-dating course, 'I am perfectly well aware of the places I can refer people to'. The experiences of some of the other doctors in the group changed his attitudes to identifying prior sexual abuse. He heard about some patients who had large numbers of investigations for somatic complaints. They had often not attended for these investigations, only later to insist they were done urgently. They were difficult patients, alternately demanding or compliant. They made the doctors feel that they must help, but often alienated them. Eventually the doctors had been able to hear about early experiences of abuse. Then the difficulties began to make sense.

Patients may be extremely reticent about their history of childhood abuse. Seven case histories of patients who had large numbers of somatic symptoms appeared in a paper in the *British Medical Journal* in 1990.[1] Staff obtained the history of childhood sexual abuse unexpectedly at a late stage after the patients had investigations and interventions in many specialities. Causality is always difficult without objective and clear evidence but it was noticeable that the case notes originally contained almost no psychosocial details. Other papers have concentrated on:

- psychological disturbances;[2]
- chronic pain;[3]
- abdominal or pelvic pain.[4]

It is often difficult to separate the effect of childhood abuse from generalized family dysfunction. Salmon and Calderbank[5] reported on the relationship of childhood physical and sexual abuse to adult illness behaviour in 275 undergraduates. Abuse was associated with increased somatic complaints and hypochondriasis. Other samples, selected because of their contact with health professionals for psychiatric help, eating disorders or chronic pelvic pain, have found more marked associations with previous abuse.

What is sexual abuse?

Definitions affect the quoted prevalence rates. Some observers include any type of sexual behaviour that occurred in childhood, even that between children of similar ages. A useful definition occurs in a report of prevalence in Great Britain in 1985 from Baker and Duncan.[6] The study used a Mori poll to obtain a prevalence of 12 per cent for girls and 8 per cent for boys. The definition used was

> A child is sexually abused when another person who is sexually mature, involves the child in any activity which the other person expects to lead to their own sexual arousal. This might include intercourse, touching, exposure of sexual organs, showing pornographic material or talking about sexual things in an erotic way.

Many of the prevalence studies suffer from bias. The numbers are likely to be exaggerated if estimates are obtained from replies to questionnaires in magazines, or from patients attending psychiatric specialists. Rates of 25–40 per cent are quoted, which seem very high. However, when childhood physical abuse was first described, it was thought to be very rare. It takes time for people to lose their reluctance to divulge previous abuse, and for professionals to consider it possible. A paper from Geneva reported on the experiences of 13–17 year olds from 17 schools.[7] The information was obtained from 1193 self-administered questionnaires that included factual descriptions of sexual activities and specific forms of child sexual abuse; 33.8 per cent of the girls and 10.9 per cent of the boys reported at least one sexually abusive event.

Until recently, the picture of sexual abuse that most professionals held was of a relationship between a young teenage girl and an older man. The man was thought likely to be a stranger or a relative such as a step-father. It is now clear that abuse usually occurs at a much younger age. The abuser is usually well known to the victim, and is, most often, the father. In the paper from Geneva, 46.5 per cent had experienced the first event before the age of 12 years and one-third reported more than one abusive episode.[7] Vaginal or anal penetration of very young children is a distressing image. The effects of genital touching, fellatio or signs of sexual arousal in the adult, may be just as agonizing and long-lasting to the survivors. The abuse of boys is not as common as in girls but has been poorly reported in the past. Investigations have shown it to be more frequent than we thought previously.[8]

Presentation

It has become easier to talk about abuse, but it is always difficult. Media attention has helped to make the subject more visible. After reading an article, or watching a programme about abuse, those involved feel less isolated. They are less likely to feel that they are the only ones with this dreadful secret.

Health professionals need to be ready to listen when patients make the first tentative steps towards revealing their secret. The doctor or nurse hearing the account may have difficulty in accepting firstly, that such terrible things could happen, and secondly, that the events could happen to ordinary people. The listener may feel too distressed to be able to help the patient, or may deny that it could have happened.

Survivors attending for counselling later in life are often bitter about the way in which their revelations were received. Remarks made at the time (such as 'She said that it was normal for little girls to want to be their dad's wife') are frequently remembered many years later with anger.

Judgemental statements or comparisons with other histories of abuse are counterproductive. The listener cannot know what it is like to feel distressed about such events. Patients are the experts on how they feel. The events revealed may vary enormously and it is the *patient's feelings* about the occurrences that matter, not what actually happened.

Finding out

Most doctors and nurses have had little professional training in sexual medicine. Their knowledge and attitudes have been acquired along the way and are shaped mainly by their own personal experience.[9] Most health professionals think that they are able to discuss sexuality openly with patients. However, when training is carried out, it becomes apparent that they are only comfortable when the sexual activities being discussed fall within the boundaries of their own experience. Discomfort will discourage them from even beginning to take a sexual history, let alone delve into past history.[10]

Asking direct questions is rarely of use and can be counterproductive. It is more difficult for the patient to raise the subject later after initial denial of childhood abuse. The first step is to be aware of the possibility. Some of the clues have been suggested already and include:

- psychiatric disturbance;
- eating problems;
- somatization;
- chronic pain.

Other indicators include:

- current sexual problems;
- frequent changes of contraceptive methods;

- complaints of vaginal or anal discharge or soreness without abnormality;
- parenting difficulties;
- low self-esteem.

Jehu[11] in his book describing therapy with women who were victims of childhood abuse, concluded that low self-esteem, feelings of guilt and depressive episodes were common in women who had survived childhood abuse. Patients also frequently described dysfunctional sexual and interpersonal relationships. He used a questionnaire to assess these patients and establish their psychological distress. The questionnaire is several pages long and is clearly not of use in a primary care setting. Jehu suggests that all patients should be asked about sexual abuse. This *might* signal to patients that the doctor or nurse was comfortable discussing the issue. However, patients may not be ready to reveal such information, or may feel that the problem has been diminished by being asked about routinely.

Having identified someone as having features suggestive of prior abuse, how can the subject be introduced? Using open-ended questions such as 'How is your sex life?' or 'Is this affecting your relationship?' shows that the doctor or nurse is willing to hear intimate problems. The book *Sexual Health Promotion in General Practice*[12] gives some general guidance on starting to take a sexual history in different situations.

A more specific enquiry such as 'Did anything happen to you when you were young that might have affected how you feel now?' may provoke a response that can be defensive ('I don't know what you mean') or revealing ('Well, I suppose it might have done').

If disclosure is made, it is important that the listener acknowledges the difficulty that the patient has had in talking about it. The story should be heard without exclamation, judgemental attitudes or excessive emotion. If the doctor or nurse cannot bear to hear the story, how can the patient bear to tell it?

Barriers to disclosure

Part of the difficulty in telling anyone about abuse is the sense of personal responsibility for what has happened. Although the patients were children when it happened, somehow they feel that *they* should have been able to stop it. They feel that it was something about themselves that made the abuse occur. The excitement that accompanies sexual stimulation or secret activity is suppressed but makes them feel more responsible for the events. If they were very young, or had dealt with it by withdrawing emotionally, they may be unsure about what happened exactly.

The events were part of a special relationship with the abuser and not open to public inspection. They find it difficult to trust. The abuse betrayed that confidence that children should have in adults, and the following case illustrates how difficult it may be to feel that *any* relationships are trustworthy.

Case

T. originally disclosed his history of abuse to his wife when, at the end of her tether, she threatened to leave him. His wife persuaded him to see his doctor. He was hesitant and reluctant to talk. During several appointments, he was able to give a factual account of what he could remember. He had been brought up mainly by an aunt and returned to his parental home as a young teenager, only to get into trouble. He was put into care, where he was abused. Despite the distressing nature of his account, very little emotion escaped him. He could not let the doctor close enough to share in how hurt he had been. He was eventually able to express his anger towards his mother who had not only failed to protect him, but had rejected him twice. He continues to have difficulties communicating with his wife, in case she rejects him. He is still afraid of showing affection towards his teenage daughter, although he tries to take more interest in her activities. He has made a better relationship with his younger daughter, and has made great efforts to become a responsible adult. He remains distant from the doctor who, like other women, might let him down, and prefers to consult other partners with physical complaints when essential.

Often the difficulties with relationships are apparent in how the health professional is treated. Appointments are made and not kept, inappropriate demands are made, or patients appear superficially compliant, only to sabotage treatment at every turn. They may behave as though consultations are social or sexual encounters. They fail to ask for appropriate help because they feel too worthless. In particular, they may either avoid physical examinations that expose that part of their body involved in the abuse or want it constantly examined. It is a diagnosis to consider in any patient with an unexplained 'fat file' of voluminous medical records.

Help for the patient

Some patients will have already dealt with the impact of prior abuse. It may be mentioned in passing, and appears not to affect present functioning. However fascinating, it is inappropriate to fasten onto the remark if the patient does not see it as relevant to the present complaint.

Others will not be ready to tackle it. For some patients, just telling the story, being heard and acknowledged, is often enough for the present. To insist that these patients must 'go for therapy' may be quite harmful. It implies that the listener cannot bear the distress that the patient has. Often patients behave in a child-like manner making health professionals react in a parental or authoritarian way. Taking control reinforces the patients' sense of lack of control and their low self-esteem. It is important that the types of help are offered without pressure to take any of them up at that time. Hooper[13] sent a questionnaire about sexual abuse to all his general practice patients between 20 and 60 years of age. Four hundred and eighteen (65 per cent) replied with 14 per cent admitting childhood sexual abuse had happened to them. Only one patient took up the offer of counselling.

The doctor or nurse may offer help within the primary care setting.[14] The work can be difficult and demanding and should not be undertaken without extra training and support. The case reported below illustrates some of the difficulties both patient and doctor may face. The patient is unusual in that transference has required long-term treatment in the original primary care setting. Most patients can be treated briefly, or referred for more specialist help.

Case

S. attended for a cervical smear. In response to an open-ended enquiry whether there were any problems, she told the doctor that she felt sex was dirty and that she should not be doing it. The doctor offered to see her for a longer talk. Although otherwise happily married with two children, she felt unattractive, fat and disgusting. The doctor looked at her rather thin body, and worried about anorexia. The more the doctor heard about the need for absolute control, how no-one came up to her exacting standards at work, and felt the neediness within the patient, the more worried she became. This was a disturbed patient, surely beyond her competence to manage in a primary care setting, despite her extra training. The doctor discussed referral with the patient—but this was totally unacceptable, and to S., felt like rejection. The doctor went on seeing the patient, who became clearly anorexic and dangerously thin. S. lost her job and became more disturbed. The doctor discussed the transference difficulties with a psychoanalyst, and took the case to group discussion. At times the situation became almost unbearable for both patient and doctor. The patient became profoundly depressed, curling up in a fetal position on the floor, and attempted suicide several times. Admitted to hospital, the patient's defences against external control were so effective that the staff initially labelled her manipulative, not recognizing her deep distress. Eventually the doctor managed to persuade a psychiatrist of the patient's illness, and gradually the patient learnt to trust enough to show her torment. On neuroleptic drugs the distress was muted, the weight increased. The emotional deprivation of her upbringing was explored with the doctor. A sexually abusive episode between the patient when a teenager and an older married man was often discussed but never seemed to make sense. Eventually after 4 years of struggling to understand the conflicts and emotions, sexual abuse at an early age by the father was revealed.

After 5 years of intermittent consultations, this doctor was often seen as the alternative mother figure. The patient was searching for the mother who would be good enough, with whom she could have a loving relationship, who would protect her and care for her. The 'mother' also holds the secrets of adult sexuality, which the patient saw as frightening and unobtainable. Whenever S. contacted her biological mother, she was disappointed again and became distressed. Her need for contact with her general practitioner increased, and she also feared rejection and abandonment whenever the doctor was going to be unavailable. Eventually the patient resolved many of her difficulties, and as her own children grew into young adults became much less reliant on the alternative 'mother' figure.

Brief therapy

Brief therapy or interactions can help many people. Few general practitioners or practice nurses in primary care have the time or inclination to give up long periods of working (or leisure) time to the needs of just one patient among many. Health workers dealing with other aspects of the care of a patient, such as secondary care specialists in sexual or reproductive medicine, also have other priorities. So skills in brief therapy are important. Spending a few extra minutes—about as much as would be needed for a physical examination—can be very effective.

Traditional medical training produces doctors who think they should be knowledgeable and in control. Helping people with a history of sexual abuse requires humility (you do not know how she/he feels) and ignorance (you do not know what happened). Each patient encounter is unique and listening needs to be done in an atmosphere of trust and acceptance. Do not listen uncritically but in a spirit of enquiry. What does this part of the story mean to that person? How does it feel to be with him/her while it is being told? Does the feeling during the consultation shed any light on how that person relates to other significant people in his/her life? If you feel impatient and dismissive, overburdened or angry, this may be how other people feel with this individual. Do the particular words chosen reveal clues about the functioning of that person? Feeling 'sore' or 'numb' or having a 'burning' pain can help to move the enquiry into a more psychological direction. Does the examination give clues about how the patient behaves with a partner—perhaps making the doctor or nurse feel abusive or protective in turn?

The response to explanations or suggestions helps the doctor or nurse understand the functioning of the patient and the ability to move forward. We have all come across patients for whom nothing is ever right, and who counters every suggestion with reasons why it will not work. Sometimes all that can be offered is a listening ear and tolerance of the damage that has occurred after the abuse.

Health workers are familiar with the concept that illness is a complex interplay of physical, emotional and social factors. They weigh the impact of each in every consultation. People choosing a doctor or nurse are asking for all of these factors to be considered, not just the psychological (when they might choose a psychologist or counsellor) or the social (when they might choose marital therapy).

Skills in brief interactional psychosexual therapy are outlined in the introductory chapter by Ruth Skrine in 'Psychosexual Medicine' edited by Rosemarie Lincoln.[15] They are derived from the Balint[16] studies of 'using the doctor as treatment' and have been developed by the Institute of Psychosexual Medicine.[17] Information about training can be obtained from the Institute.[18] The British Association of Sexual and Relationship Therapy[19] and some postgraduate departments[20] offer training for specialist management of sexual problems.

One of the advantages of help being offered in a primary care setting is the continuing availability of the therapist when the work needs to be done in stages. People can do a little work, resolve some of the problems, and return for further help at a later date. After disclosure, the patient can work at her/his own pace through the resolution of the issues of guilt, shame, anger and excitement. Life events that precipitate a request for further help can be:

- new relationships;
- pregnancy or childbirth;

- children reaching the age at which they themselves were abused;

- children going to school or leaving home;

- the death of a parent;

- personal illness;

- a hysterectomy;

- bleeding from piles or other significant sign of dysfunction of the abused part of the body.

Each time the patient presents, the knowledge of previous work done is there, ready to be resumed when appropriate. Sometimes, just a remark such as 'this must be difficult for you in particular' is all that is needed for the patient to gain insight into why problems are newly apparent. Beware of putting too much emphasis on sexual abuse as a cause of all her/his problems! It is just as likely to be a new cause, so start again in ignorance of the aetiology of the problem. Just because someone has been abused in the past, does not mean that she/he is not having 'mother-in-law problems', financial difficulties or pelvic inflammatory disease, in the present.

False memory syndrome

One of the advantages of using an open-ended questioning approach is that you do not impose your views or biases on patients. Allowing patients to give a history in their own words and concentrating on the interaction between the patient and health professional is the best protection against obtaining an erroneous account of any condition. Leading questions such as 'Were you ever abused sexually?' are best replaced by 'Did anyone ever do anything to you that might have led to you feeling like this?' Not only does this allow patients to explain in their own words what happened, but also avoids the difficulty of defining what sexual abuse means for any individual. A well adjusted and secure individual might dismiss a single episode of witnessing 'indecent exposure' as 'just one of those things'. Another individual might be more sensitive and regard it as shameful, abusive and inhibiting to subsequent sexual intimacy. There are many instances of where the bias of interviewers has resulted in false accounts of events and we have all come across patients who give totally different histories when they are seen by another health worker.

Sometimes a victim can use 'false memory syndrome' to withdraw an account previously given because they need a defence against too much distress. The defence needs to be examined for what it is—and respected if the pain cannot be tolerated.

More frequently, those accused of being abusers use it as a defence. Actual confrontations between victim and abuser are not a useful way of resolving feelings, especially when the abuse continues to be denied. Imaginary confrontations (where the victim pretends the abuser is present and tells him what he/she feels) *may* reduce guilt and shame. Denial of the accusations is likely to lead to deeper feelings of responsibility by the victim, confusion about what actually happened, or an increase in the anger. Unless legal proceedings or the protection of others is at stake, the actual truth of what happened is not relevant within a medical or nursing consultation. It is important to examine what the events, real or not, mean for the functioning of the patient in the present.

Some patients are histrionic and produce stories that are not truthful in order to gain attention. Doctors and nurses can usually identify this—but not usually on the first few encounters! The difficulties of diagnosing Munchausen syndrome in the early stages are well known, and false stories about prior sexual abuse can fall into this category. The lack of consistency in the account can give clues that the story may be fabricated. Inappropriate emotion such as excitement rather than distress can also lead to suspension of belief. Truly delusional accounts are rare and are usually associated with other features of psychotic illness.

Referral

Some patients will prefer referral to a relative stranger, preferring to keep the general practitioner unaware of the details of the abuse. Many doctors and nurses will not want to be involved in therapy, or are aware that they lack the skills to do this work. It may be particularly difficult for the practice nurse or doctor to be the therapist when the perpetrator is also their patient. Some professionals will have memories of their own that prevent them remaining objective in their work.

Referral to a psychosexual problems clinic, individual psychotherapy, group psychotherapy, treatment by a clinical psychologist or full psychoanalysis are all options variably available in each region. Rape crisis organizations, Mind or other non-medical organizations often run support groups. Provided they are well supervised and advised, they can provide a useful lifeline for those who feel isolated and stigmatized by their experiences.

Confidentiality

This is often of paramount importance to those who are revealing abuse for the first time. The concern is, of course, tied up with the fear, shame and sense of responsibility for what happened. Absolute confidentiality cannot be promised when others may be at risk. For example, the knowledge that someone who abused the patient is applying to foster, or work with children, may precipitate disclosure. Usually it is possible for patients themselves to come to the decision that some authority must be told. In primary care the other members of the family involved, including the abuser, may also be patients. Recording of sensitive information must be considered in advance. Confidentiality is always extremely important (see Chapters 3 and 5c).

No choice

Health professionals have to deal with the survivors of childhood abuse whether they wish to or not. Some patients may present overtly. If the covert signs are missed, patients will not be helped and may suffer damage from overinvestigation and inappropriate treatment. An awareness of the possibility of abuse in childhood is essential for all who work with patients.

It is important to remain impartial and useful to the patient and not to become over-involved or overprotective. Professionals who do this work are in danger of becoming sexually or psychologically vulnerable themselves.[21] If they feel overburdened, they must seek professional support. This is something that doctors in particular have found difficult to access or accept in the past and practice nurses are often working alone. Better occupational health schemes for primary care are generally regarded as being overdue! Build up relationships with the local psychiatric and psychosexual services so that you have someone else to talk to that will understand the problem. They may be able to offer advice on the management of that patient, or help to share the burden.

References

1 **Arnold RP, Rogers D, Cook DAG.** Medical problems of adults who were sexually abused in childhood. *British Medical Journal* 1990; **300**: 705–8.

2 **Palmer RL, Coleman L, Chaloner D** *et al.* Childhood sexual experiences with adults. A comparison of reports by women psychiatric patients and general practice attenders. *British Journal of Psychiatry* 1993; **163**: 499–504.

3 **Walling MK, Reiter RC, O'Hara MW** *et al.* Abuse history and chronic pain in women: 1. Prevalence of sexual abuse and physical abuse. *Obstetrics and Gynaecology* 1994; **84**: 193–9.

4 **Kirkengen AL, Shei B, Steine S.** Indicators of childhood sexual abuse in gynaecological patients in a general practice. *Scandinavian Journal of Primary Health Care* 1993; **11** (4): 276–80.

5 **Salmon P, Calderbank S.** The relationship of childhood physical and sexual abuse to adult illness behaviour. *Journal of Psychosomatic Research* 1996; **40** (3): 329–36.

6 **Baker AW, Duncan SP.** Child sexual abuse—a study of prevalence in Great Britain. *Child Abuse and Neglect* 1985; **9**: 457–67.

7 **Halperin DS, Bouvier P, Jaffe PD** *et al.* Prevalence of child sexual abuse among adolescents in Geneva: results of a cross-sectional survey. *British Medical Journal* 1996; **312**: 1326.

8 **Hobbs CJ, Wynne JM.** Buggery in childhood, a common syndrome of child abuse. *Lancet* 1986; **ii**: 792–6.

9 **Wakley G.** Sexual health in the primary care consultation: using self-rating as an aid to identifying the training needs for general practitioners. *Sexual and Relationship Therapy* 2000; **15**: 171–81.

10 **Green R.** Taking a sexual history. In: Green R, ed. *Human Sexuality: a Health Practitioner's Text*, 2nd edn. Baltimore: Williams & Wilkins, 1979: 22–30.

11 **Jehu D.** *Beyond Sexual Abuse: Therapy with Women who were Childhood Victims.* London: John Wiley, 1989.

12 **Curtis H, Hoolaghan T, Jewitt C,** eds. *Sexual Health Promotion in General Practice.* Oxford: Radcliffe Medical Press, 1995.

13 Hooper PD. Psychological sequelae of sexual abuse in childhood. *British Journal of General Practice* 1990; 40: 29–31.

14 Wakley G. *Sexual Abuse and the Primary Care Doctor.* London: Chapman & Hall, 1991.

15 Skrine R. In: Lincoln R, ed. *Psychosexual Medicine: a Study of Underlying Themes.* London: Chapman & Hall, 1992.

16 Balint M. *The Doctor, his Patient and the Illness,* 2nd edn. London: Pitman, 1964.

17 Skrine R. Emotional contact and containment in psychosexual medicine. *Sexual and Marital Therapy* 1998; 13: 169–78.

18 www.ipm.org.uk

19 www.basrt.org.uk

20 Griffin M. Education and training in human sexuality. *International Review of Psychiatry* 1995; 7: 275–84.

21 Balakrishna B. Sexual abuse: how far do the ripples go? *Sexual and Marital Therapy* 1998; 13: 83–9.

Chapter 8b

Working with adult survivors of childhood abuse: the prevention and amelioration of psychological and physical problems

Jane M. Ussher

Introduction

Whilst the issue of childhood abuse is now an accepted part of the agenda of health professionals working with children and families, it has become increasingly clear that it is also of central concern for those working with adults. This follows growing empirical evidence that significant numbers of adult women and men have experienced either physical or sexual abuse as children, with studies variously reporting incidence rates of between 12 and 70 per cent.[1,2] This is coupled with the realization that childhood abuse can precipitate the development of long-term social, psychological and physical problems, including depression, anxiety, low self-esteem, difficulties in inter-personal relationships, self-destructive behaviour, substance abuse, post-traumatic stress disorder (PTSD), eating disorders, suicide attempts, sexual and reproductive problems, somatic disorders, and a tendency towards later victimization or acting out of abuse.[3-7]

Recognition of the role of childhood abuse in the aetiology of adult problems initially arose from the identification of high proportions in psychiatric populations of adults who had experienced childhood abuse, with rates of between 30 and 80 per cent being reported.[8,9] Comparisons of adults who have experienced childhood abuse with control groups[8] have found significantly higher rates of psychological and behavioural problems for those who have previously experienced abuse.

Preventing and ameliorating the long-term effects of childhood abuse

Professional intervention for childhood abuse

It is now widely acknowledged that long-term psychological, physical and behavioural problems can be prevented or ameliorated through a range of different therapeutic interventions.[10,11] Professional intervention to ameliorate the long-term effects of childhood abuse can take a number of different forms, and involve a range of health professionals. Due to the growing awareness of the need for intervention, specialized services for adults who have been abused in childhood are beginning to be developed, but these are still only available in a minority of geographical areas. The majority of professionals who work with survivors of abuse will be based in generic services, or in specialized services which focus on the particular presenting problem of the individual adult.

Whilst the GP will usually be the first person involved in the case, specialist referral is often necessary due to both time constraints, and the need for more specialized skills. Clinical psychologists, counsellors, psychiatrists, social workers and relevant specialist medical practitioners are the main groups involved in this care. Intervention can be offered on an individual, a group or a family basis, depending on the presenting problem, and the services available.

Self-help and survivors' groups for childhood abuse

In the last 20 years there has been a burgeoning of self-help groups for survivors of childhood abuse. These can be very effective in providing a context in which individuals can openly discuss childhood abuse, and experience a sense of empathy with others who have had similar experiences. Through providing support on an egalitarian basis, the pathologization or stigmatization of problems can be avoided, and a sense of community can develop. As these groups are not connected with statutory services, there is no need for disclosure to a health professional, and thus confidentiality can be assured. Self-help groups have also been said to offer a safer and more therapeutic environment than many professional services, which can be insensitive or destructive. They also offer a social or political analysis of personal problems, which is absent in many professional models of abuse.[2,12] Details of self-help groups in a particular area can be obtained through MIND.

Intervening with long-term problems associated with child abuse

Assessment of problems and appropriate referral

Appropriate and sensitive assessment is a key component to working with survivors of abuse. One of the most difficult steps for individuals in seeking help is disclosure. Many adult survivors of childhood abuse do not disclose the abuse unless directly asked, and reactions to disclosure can have a significant impact on both the subsequent course of problems, and the success of any treatment offered.

Assessment of problems invariably takes the form of a clinical interview. Psychometric instruments can be used to assist diagnosis, and help the clinician understand the presenting problem. Those commonly used include the General Health Questionnaire, the Beck Depression Inventory, The Hospital Anxiety Scale and a range of sexual health questionnaires.[13,14] However, it is recommended that a one-to-one discussion, examining women's subjective experiences, should accompany such inventories.

Possible treatment options should be discussed with the survivor, with individual preferences taken into account as much as is possible. Other factors which should be considered at the assessment stage in order to decide the priorities for treatment include the current danger, distress and incapacity the presenting problem entails for the survivor and others; the potential benefits of resolution of the problem for all concerned; whether problems are related and thus concurrent treatment is appropriate; whether treatment of specific problems should be prioritized; and whether significant others should be involved in treatment.[13,15]

Models of intervention

In the main, interventions will focus on both the abuse, and its original and compounded effects. In an analysis of therapy with adult survivors of child sexual abuse, Courtois[16] has argued that symptoms and defences are most appropriately conceptualized within a traumatic stress, a feminist or a family systems model, whereby the pathologization of presenting symptoms is avoided, and childhood abuse is recognized as potentially or even inevitably traumatic. Courtois has argued that if the impact of this trauma is not acknowledged, is unresolved or untreated, it will result in 'numbing symptomatology', or in compulsive repetitions or re-enactments of the trauma. These models view symptoms as secondary elaborations of the untreated original effects of the incest. The same argument could equally apply to other forms of childhood abuse, such as physical or emotional abuse, or neglect.

A range of treatment approaches can be effective in treating the long-term effects of abuse. These include crisis intervention which follows a stress response model; expressive cathartic therapy; psychodynamic therapy; cognitive behavioural therapy; or systems techniques. The decision about which model or technique to use will depend on the presenting problem, the preferences of the client and the services available. Regardless of the model of intervention adopted, it is important to individualize treatment in line with the specific history and personality of the client, as well as to foster the development of a safe therapeutic environment in which both the abuse and current problems can be explored.

Working with individual psychological or physical problems

Whilst presenting problems may differ across individuals, a common underlying issue is a low sense of self-worth, a repression of memories of abuse and an internalization of blame for distress.

Case

Cathy is a 32-year-old woman who was both physically and sexually abused by her father in childhood, and who as an adult has experienced a series of psychological problems, including depression, anorexia nervosa and chronic premenstrual syndrome. She was continuously told as a child that she was not good enough, both in terms of her performance at school, her general disposition, and her appearance. As an adult she blames herself for any difficulties in her life, and always expects the worst outcome in any situation. She believes that she was unlovable as a child, and that this was why her father mistreated her. She takes little pleasure in any of her achievements, continuously striving for success, but never being satisfied with what she produces. She always focuses on her own failings and faults, and not on her accomplishments. She has a deep sense of inadequacy about her body, and continuously tries to change it through drastic dieting and exercise. This gives her a sense of control, which is one of the things she strives for most in life.*

Arguably, treating the long-term effects of abuse is similar to treating any other stress response, involving exploration and integration of a difficult event, as well as the development of adaptational responses.[17] Courtois[16] has broken this down into a number of stages:

- acknowledging and accepting the occurrence of abuse;
- recounting the abuse;
- breaking the feelings of isolation and stigma;
- recognizing, labelling and expressing feelings; resolving responsibility and survival issues;

---

* All the case examples used in this chapter are composite cases, not based on any one individual woman, to protect client confidentiality.

- grieving;

- cognitive restructuring of distorted beliefs and stress responses;

- self-determination and behavioural change;

- education and self-building.

In the case of Cathy, this involved one-to-one therapy exploring the roots of her current distress in her early childhood experiences; acknowledging that it was not her fault, and that her reactions or symptoms were not uncommon; exploring her feelings of anger and betrayal towards both parents; looking at ways in which she could take responsibility for feelings and experiences in her adult life, and recognizing how she was now in a very different situation from the one she was in as a child; reinforcing her sense of self-worth through focusing on her achievements, not her self-perceived weaknesses; and finding more positive and adaptive ways of gaining a sense of autonomy and control in her life.

Working with interpersonal problems and preventing cycles of abuse

Interpersonal problems in adulthood are a common response to childhood abuse. These include insecurity, communication problems, difficulties with anger control, promiscuity or oversexualization and overdependency. Exploring and focusing on these issues in individual, couple or family therapy, or in groups, can allow the survivor to examine the effects of the abuse on current relationships, and to explore new ways of relating to others. This is an important part of breaking intergenerational patterns of abuse, where the survivor acts out the role of victim, or of abuser, in later relationships.[18]

Case

Anne coped with her abuse as a child by outwardly appearing to be happy, whilst inside she felt miserable. She repressed all anger or unhappiness, as displays of emotion served to increase the punishments meted out by her parents. As an adult she rarely felt upset in difficult situations, remaining stoical even when her husband hit her. As a child, her father frequently told her that the beatings were for her own good, and that they were a sign of his affection. He would often give her a treat the next day, so she believed him. As an adult, people found it easy to take advantage of her if they asked for things in a nice voice. Her husband's anger and violence was followed by abject contrition, so she told herself he didn't mean to hurt her. His overwhelming love on the 'good days' seemed to compensate for the beatings, and she gained some sense of strength through feeling that she could survive anything.

In treatment Anne explored the fact that whilst her psychological defences had allowed her to cope as a child, they led to problems in adulthood. She explored the way in which she had repressed all emotion and had adapted to the abuse through focusing on her survival strengths; her distorted perceptions of what was normal in a relationship, particularly the acceptability of violence; and her assumption that violence was a sign of love. Restructuring her feelings and thoughts allowed her to distinguish between acceptable and unacceptable behaviour, and to work towards developing relationships which met her needs, rather than repeated the cycle of abuse.

Anne's repetition of the role of victim in later life is not an uncommon pattern of behaviour for women who have been abused as children. Men are more likely to 'act out' their repressed distress, anger and rage, through perpetuating cycles of violence.[16,19] Those who act out the conflicts that were internalized in childhood through violence or abuse can be helped in a similar manner to those who only internalize it, although there is often greater resistance to recognizing cyclical patterns of behaviour.[14] Treatment programmes invariably start with teaching the abuser to recognize the effects of violence or abuse on the victim. Cognitive retraining has also been used extensively, including communication training, problem-solving skills, anger control, the modelling of non-sexist interactions, and parenting classes. In contrast, psychodynamic approaches will tend to focus on the underlying issues which drive the current abuse.

Conclusion

Childhood abuse can have considerable long-term effects on adult women and men. If psychological and physical symptoms go unrecognized and unacknowledged, symptoms can persist or worsen, and cycles of abuse may be perpetuated. There are currently very few specialist services available for survivors of childhood abuse; however, referral to generic services or the provision of information about self-help facilities has been shown to have positive benefits in improving subjective well-being and reducing physical and psychological symptoms.[20]

References

1 Finkelhor D. The international epidemiology of child sexual abuse. *Child Abuse and Neglect* 1996; **18** (5): 409–17.

2 Williams J, Watson G, Smith H, Copperman J, Wood D. *Purchasing Effective Mental Health Services for Women: a Framework for Action*. London: Mind Publications, 1993.

3 Browne A, Finkelhor D. Impact of child sexual abuse: a review of the research. *Psychological Bulletin* 1986; **99** (1): 66–77.

4 Beitchman JH, Zucker KJ, Hood JE, de Costa GA, Akman PA, Cassavia E. A review of the long-term effects of child sexual abuse. *Child Abuse and Neglect* 1992; **16** (1): 101–18.

5 Jumper SA. A meta-analysis of the relationship of child sexual abuse to adult psychological adjustment. *Child Abuse and Neglect* 1995; **19** (6): 715–28.

6 Finkelhor D. Early and long-term effects of child sexual abuse: an update. *Professional Psychology Research and Practice* 1991; **21** (5): 325–30.

7 Lyon C, de Cruz P. *Child Abuse Family Law*. London: Bristol Mind, 1993. (Kemp House, 152–160 City Road, London EC1 2NP.)

8 Palmer RL, Coleman L, Chaloner DA, Oppenheimer R, Smith J. Childhood sexual experiences with adults. A comparison of reports by female psychiatric patients and general practice attenders. *British Journal of Psychiatry* 1993; **163**: 499–504.

9 **Herman JL, Perry JC, van der Kolk BA.** Childhood trauma in borderline personality disorder. *American Journal of Psychiatry* 1989; **146** (4): 490–5.

10 **Ussher JM.** *Women's Madness: Misogyny of Mental Illness.* Hamel Hempstead: Harvester Wheatsheaf, 1991.

11 **Frosh S, Glaser D.** *Child Sexual Abuse,* 2nd edn. London: Macmillan, 1999.

12 **Herman JL.** *Father-daughter Incest.* Cambridge, Massachusetts: Harvard University Press, 1981.

13 **Jehu D.** *Beyond Sexual Abuse. Therapy with Women who were Childhood Victims.* London: Wiley, 1988.

14 **Viano EC.** *Intimate Violence: Interdisciplinary Perspectives.* Washington, DC: Hemisphere Publishing, 1992.

15 **Ussher JM.** *Women's Health: Contemporary International Perspectives.* Leicester: BPS Books, 2000.

16 **Courtois CA.** *Healing the Incest Wound: Adult Survivors in Therapy.* New York: Norton, 1996.

17 **Horowitz MJ.** *Stress Response Syndromes.* New York: Jason Aronson, 1986.

18 **Peled E, Jaffe PG, Edleson JL,** eds. *Ending the Cycle of Violence: Community Responses to Children of Battered Women.* London: Sage, l995.

19 **Dobash RE, Dobash R.** *Violence Against Wives. A Case Against the Patriarchy.* London: Open Books, 1979.

20 **Baker CD.** *Female survivors of Sexual Abuse.* London: Routledge, 2002.

Chapter 9

The future

Chapter 9a

Policy, empowerment and young people in primary health care

Christopher Cloke

Introduction

General practitioners and primary health care team members have a significant role to play in helping and supporting children and young people. This role derives not only from the provision of advice and health care but also from the *way* in which they treat and respect children, young people and their parents. Primary health care staff can promote the interests of children and young people by demonstrating to others, through their practice, how this group of patients should be treated and also, again drawing on their experience, by using their influence to change public policy. Of the 'caring professionals', primary health care workers are among the least stigmatizing, the most accessible, and the ones with whom most children and young people are familiar from a very young age and may even seek to emulate—how many children have played 'doctors and nurses' in their time?

Primary health care is a universal service, physically present in nearly all communities. Its members are also often held in high regard by professionals in other disciplines and also by many policy-makers and opinion formers. There is thus considerable potential for GPs and other members of the team to be a powerful force for change for the benefit of young people.

While many GPs and primary health care workers provide a service which goes some way to meeting these objectives, the potential has still to be realized in full. As with all professions, some members practice in ways which seem to be unsupportive of young people. The voluntary agency ChildLine[1] analysed a sample of the calls it received from children and young people in 1994/95 and in 1996/97 concerning health problems. Comments made by some callers indicate unhelpful responses from doctors: 'The doctor says I'm just lazy' or 'I feel as though the doctor isn't interested'.

The report of the study also describes some cases:

> Gordon had found a lump on his testicle. Before ringing ChildLine, he had made great efforts to find information about testicular cancer in his doctor's waiting room and in all the local chemist shops. Embarrassment made it hard for him to see a doctor or tell his parents.
>
> Helen, 13, said 'I've got a problem with spots. The boys call me names. I wish I was somewhere else.' Helen had been taunted to the point where she had kicked one of the bullies. She had been taken to the doctor. 'He didn't say much.'
>
> A very angry 14-year-old girl had been dismayed to find that her doctor had told her school that she had been to his surgery.

It could be argued that these somewhat negative responses from doctors are to be expected since our society in general, and its culture, is hostile towards children and it would be surprising if the attitudes held by most people were not found among health professionals too. The National Commission of Inquiry into the Prevention of Child Abuse[2] considered the position of children in society and concluded that as a society we do not recognize and make sufficient provision for children and many of our institutions and systems in fact operate against children's interests. Importantly, the Commission received considerable evidence which demonstrated another aspect of our culture: there is still a general reluctance to accept the fact that children suffer abuse or are harmed in such damaging ways and in such numbers. There is a very commonly held view that children must have provoked or in some way been responsible for their ill-treatment.

The Commission therefore concluded that 'such attitudes and blame, combined with a lack of understanding of children's behaviour, reflect and reinforce the widespread perception of children as the possessions of their parents and that no one but their parents is entitled to "interfere", except in extreme circumstances. One effect of this is to make the public reluctant to intervene in order to secure a child's well-being'. Over a thousand survivors of child abuse wrote to the Commission[3] and one graphically commented that

> Our culture and system of values has supported child abuse over the centuries simply by pretending it doesn't exist. General society would still not wish to have to acknowledge its existence. Not wanting to look, listen or believe, and finding it incomprehensible to understand.

That view was reflected in the submissions received by the Commission not only from other survivors but also from professionals and their representative organizations. It led the Commission to conclude that if we are to promote the well-being of children and young people there needs to be a fundamental change in our culture. While the Commission recognized the enormity of this task, it also felt that there were some grounds for optimism since it encountered everywhere 'a strong sense of what people want for all children not only for their own. They want all children to develop healthily and safely into adulthood. There is a personal, community and political responsibility widely accepted for trying to ensure this. It is this goodwill, allied to the principles already implicit in our legislation, that provides the solid ground on which to build a nationwide effort to prevent child abuse and neglect' and to ensure that children's needs are met.

General practitioners and other primary health care workers can and should be part of that nationwide effort. This chapter considers how that can be achieved, particularly addressing the professionals' role in empowering children and young people and in promoting public policy initiatives in order to change the culture and benefit this important section of the community.

Early identification of child abuse and neglect

Before addressing the role of primary health care staff in empowering children and promoting children's rights, consideration is given to their related and important role in the early identification of child abuse and neglect. In its evidence to the National Commission of Inquiry into the Prevention of Child Abuse, the Royal College of General Practitioners supported the view that GPs have an important part to play in health promotion and child health surveillance, but also pointed to the need for doctors to receive training and support in these activities. The Commission recommended that in order to prevent child abuse, children at risk must be identified at an early stage and their needs met. Drawing on the 'Hall 3' model,[4] the Commission proposed that child health surveillance programmes, which form part of wider child health promotion, should include checking for signs of possible abuse and providing preventative advice. Hall proposes the following checks: neonatal examination; a health visitor check when the baby is around 10–14 days old; a check within 6–8 weeks by a member of the primary health care team; immunization within 2–4 months; an examination between 6 and 9 months; a review at 18–24 months; a review at 39–42 months; and a medical at 54–66 months when the child enters school. These checks might be carried out by general practitioners, health visitors, primary health care team members or hospital staff. The Commission also emphasized the need to ensure that any missed appointments are followed up. It was felt that these checks should be part of a broader health promotion approach so that they are not viewed negatively by parents. If the specified health checks take account of child protection concerns, among other issues, and they are used as an opportunity to undertake preventative work and, where appropriate, mobilize family support, there is the potential to reach all vulnerable babies and young children. A revised 'Hall 4' model is likely to be introduced in 2003. This will suggest no universally scheduled checks between 8 weeks and school entry. Instead, a more opportunistic health and development review is encouraged, targeting vulnerable children in particular, whenever they attend. An interagency 'stocktake' at around 2 years is also envisaged: this may be particularly valuable in identifying precursors or early signs of abuse.

This is important, given that between one and two babies die each week following child abuse or neglect and infancy is the period in your life when you are most at risk of being killed. Babies and young children are thus particularly vulnerable to child abuse, so identification by primary health care workers at these stages is important. They are the main professionals who can have routine access to young children and can provide a full examination.

General practitioners, together with other primary health care workers, have a tradition of visiting young families in their homes. Home visiting services are generally seen as having a number of benefits for vulnerable families. A visit to the home is often considered by the parent to be preferable to having to contact external agencies and attending clinics or groups to which a stigma may be attached. The home visit also affords an opportunity for the 'visitor' to assess the home situation and observe parent–child interactions in a more relaxed environment. Support can be given to the family and parenting skills taught. Home visiting programmes have taken a number of forms involving health visitors, other paid workers, and also volunteers or members of the community who may be mothers themselves. GPs need to relate to such initiatives. In the UK, evaluations show that Homestart programmes have been highly valued by the users, who feel better equipped to care for their children. Gibbons and Thorpe[5] report that Homestart clients are more appreciative of the services received from their home visitors than are the clients of social services.

The Elmir Project in the USA is one of the most well-known initiatives that have shown the positive effects of a preventative home visiting service.[6] High-risk mothers receiving pre- and postnatal home visits had fewer reports of child maltreatment, were less punitive towards their children, had fewer subsequent pregnancies, and were more likely to be employed than a comparison group. A 15-year follow-up also found that they had fewer cases of reported abuse.

These studies indicate that home visiting has a general value. Primary health care workers are the main professions that have relatively easy access to the homes of young families. In this way GPs can make a critical contribution to ensuring that children are cared for and protected. GPs can make home visits themselves and ensure that they are undertaken by others.

The impact of more focused health screening in preventing child abuse has been much discussed and while the results of the studies are often inconclusive, research by Browne,[7] in Southend, Essex, evaluating health screening by health visitors, suggests that screening can be effective in identifying families at risk of abuse, in mobilizing support, and in reducing the number of children placed on child protection registers.

Similarly, Walter Barker and the Early Childhood Development Unit, University of Bristol, have developed a number of home visiting programmes using either specialist health visitors or 'community mothers'. The unit reports significant decreases in rates of substantiated cases of child abuse as a result of these programmes.[8]

Health visitors have a key role to play both in identifying children at risk and in mobilizing support for families under stress. There is substantial evidence that health visitors are much valued by parents as a non-stigmatizing service (compare submissions to the National Commission), not least because they are a universal service. There are, however, moves in a number of areas to target the service and reduce its universality. The National Commission was not alone, however, in arguing that such a development would have detrimental consequences for the prevention of child abuse. GPs can recognize at first hand the benefits of such health visiting services and should be powerful advocates for their continued provision.

The National Commission felt that once children enter school, the education service, including school nursing, should have a role in identifying children at risk of harm. At that stage the role of the primary health care team changes its emphasis in that it becomes less concerned with the *routine* examination of all children and instead is more concerned with ensuring that accessible, sensitive and supportive health care is provided to all children and young people when they need it and that those opportunities are used to address possible child protection concerns and related matters, as appropriate.

Children's rights and primary health care

General practitioners and primary health care professionals should also be strong advocates of children's rights. The 1990s saw an increased awareness of children's rights as an issue to which *all* practitioners working with children should respond. This has been a response to two instruments: the Children Act 1989 and the United Nations Convention on the Rights of the Child.[9] The then government argued that the Children Act reflected the Convention and provided in legislation a wide range of rights which children had not hitherto held. However, the legislation was enacted following the Cleveland child sexual abuse scandal, in a climate in which it was argued that parents' rights had been ignored or overridden by zealous professionals, particularly paediatricians. The government was therefore keen to strike a careful balance between children's rights and parents' rights in the legislation.

The United Nations Convention on the Rights of the Child is the first legally binding international human rights treaty to confer a wide range of rights specifically on children and young people. The Convention was adopted by the United Nations in 1989 and became law in September 1990, having been ratified by 20 nations. The UK government ratified the Convention in December 1991, 1 year after its adoption by the United Nations. Today all but two countries in the world have ratified the Convention.

Under international law, ratifying countries are legally bound to observe the children's rights principles contained in the Convention and to adopt laws, develop practice, and introduce any necessary regulations which will achieve these objectives. The Convention comprises 54 articles covering the social, civil, cultural and economic rights of *all* children and young people up to the age of 18. Together these articles provide a framework for assessing the extent to which the needs of children are met.

The relevance to health professionals of the UN Convention on the Rights of the Child is explicit in the NHS Executive guide to good practice *Child Health in the Community*[10] which states that 'purchasers and providers should take account of the provisions of the UN Convention, the principles of the Children Act and the Patients Charter.' In particular the NHS Executive points to rights relating to:

- the best interests of the child;
- respect for the child's privacy;
- the need to listen to the child's views;
- enabling children to have the highest attainable standard of health;
- access to treatment;
- special care for children with disabilities;
- protection against negligent treatment and abuse;
- a child's right to play and recreation.

A more comprehensive analysis of how the Convention can be implemented in primary health care has been provided by the British Association for Community Child Health (BACCH) in its guide[11] which seeks to translate the contents of the Convention into everyday examples of good practice and highlight the Convention's relevance to everyday health care.

The key article relating to the provision of health care is Article 24 which enshrines a commitment to recognize 'the right of the child to the enjoyment of the highest attainable standard of health and to facilities for the treatment of illness and rehabilitation of health. State parties shall ensure that no child is deprived of his or her right of access to such health care services.' The article continues to say that provision should be made to ensure the full implementation of this right, including in particular measures to:

- diminish infant and child mortality;
- ensure the provision of necessary medical assistance and health care to all children with emphasis on the development of primary health care;
- combat disease and malnutrition;
- ensure appropriate prenatal and postnatal health care for mothers;

- ensure that all segments of society, in particular parents and children, are informed, have access to education and are supported in the use of basic knowledge of child health and nutrition;
- develop preventative health care, guidance for parents and family planning education and services.

While some of the provisions of this article of the Convention may seem more appropriate to developing societies than to Western countries, they serve as an important reminder of the standards which need to be maintained in all states, as well as standards still to be attained.

Other articles contained in the Convention relevant to the delivery of health care for children are:

- *Article 3*: in all actions concerning children the best interests of the child shall be the primary consideration.
- *Article 12*: the right to express views and have them taken into account, in accordance with the child's age and maturity. This includes children having the right to express their view about the health care and treatment they receive.
- *Article 16*: the right to privacy and confidentiality.
- *Article 17*: the right of access to age-appropriate information, including materials relevant to the child's 'social, spiritual and moral well being and physical and mental health'.
- *Article 19*: the right to protection from 'all physical or mental violence, injury or abuse, neglect or negligent treatment, maltreatment or exploitation, including sexual abuse'. The right to protection through preventative programmes and procedures relating to the identification, reporting, referral, investigation, treatment and follow-up of cases of maltreatment.
- *Article 23*: the right of children with disabilities to enjoy a 'full and decent life' and to receive services to meet their individual needs and enable them to be as fully socially integrated as possible.
- *Article 25*: the right of children receiving treatment or long-term care to have that provision regularly reviewed and monitored.
- *Article 26*: the right to social security and benefit entitlements.
- *Article 30*: the right of children from black and minority ethnic groups to practise their own cultures, religions and languages.

These provisions have a number of implications for general practitioners and primary health care workers and there are a number of steps that can be taken. These include practical measures such as the ways in which health care is delivered, really listening to young people and allowing them to express their views, sharing information, enabling children and young people to exercise their rights to, for example, an adequate income, and participation in multiagency procedures that protect children and young people. Table 9.1 derives from the analysis carried out by the BACCH Working Group and describes the actions which can be taken to implement the Convention in primary health care.

Empowering children—why rights are important

The promotion of children's rights through both professional practice and policy development is a means of empowering children and young people. This should be an important part of any strategy for the prevention of child abuse. Children and young people who are listened to and respected by adults are more likely to turn to a trusted adult when they are experiencing problems or difficulties of any sort, including child abuse. Children and young people who are enabled to exercise their rights are more likely to be resilient and assertive and this will better equip them to take action to resist or stop abuse. It will also enable them to protect their peers and siblings.

The exercise of rights will also have an impact on our overall culture. With rights go responsibilities, and providing opportunities for children and young people to act responsibly will help change our culture, which, as has been argued, is generally hostile towards children. Providing children with a voice will also help influence professional practice and policies as adult practitioners and policy-makers are better able to understand children's needs and their view of services. An improved understanding of children's views and feelings will facilitate the development of child- and youth-friendly services and practices that are better able to respond to children's needs. In this way services which children and young people want and will use can be provided and some of the major obstacles of stigmatizing and irrelevant services may be overcome.

This also means that the promotion and implementation of children's rights benefits all of society, and not just young people. It will have the consequence of demonstrating that the exercise of their rights by children is not threatening to adults—something that will be apparent to anyone who has witnessed children acting in this way. Social disorder and unrest will not have ensued!

General practitioners and other members of the primary health care team, ideally working together, can promote the rights of children and young people through their professional practice in the ways described in Table 9.1. While few practitioners would reach the standards implicit in the Convention, it provides a goal to work towards. It is also undoubtedly the case that individual practitioners can use the Convention as a way of setting objectives for improving practice. Thus it is that policy and practice interrelate for the benefit of children and young people, practitioners and the wider society.

Table 9.1 Children's rights and primary health care: implications for intervention to prevent child abuse.

Article	Summary	Actions for GPs and health care teams	Implications for intervention
24	Child's right to highest quality health care Child's right to health services which prevent ill health and promote good health	• Health care must be available, accessible and acceptable to children and their carers • Surgery/health centre should be child and youth friendly: warm, welcoming and safe • Friendly, supportive reception and support staff • Provision of play area • Toilet provision • Provision for feeding and changing babies • Child-friendly consultation rooms • Provision of domiciliary services • Provision of preventative services including health checks and surveillance • Separate services to meet special needs • Promote/advertize services available to children and young people	• Parents, children and young people will only seek help if services are accessible, non-stigmatizing and appropriate to their needs • In order to provide quality health care to children and young people, special provision, including health surveillance, must be provided • Domiciliary visits help understanding of home circumstances
3	Best interest of the child should be prime consideration	• Professionals need to understand children's needs • Skills required in child care and communication • Understanding of children's rights	• Professionals need to recognize that the child or young person is the patient and not their parent • Avoidance of collusion with parents • Taining in child development
5/18	Support for parents and carers	• Understanding of stress factors which contribute to abuse • Provision of care and support to parents to enable them to look after their children • Understanding of support services and enabling access to them	• Identification of children at risk of abuse will be of limited value unless support services are provided • Support services can alleviate the stresses which can cause abuse • Value of community/self-help initiatives

Table 9.1 Continued.

12	Child's right to be consulted and have views taken into account	• Listen to what children and young people are saying • Facilitate involvement in decision-making • Patient participation initiatives to include children and young people—ask what services they want	• Children and young people who are listened to and consulted are more likely to seek help when they face problems • In developing services, the views of children and young people should be considered—only relevant services will be used
16	Child's right to privacy and confidentiality	• Respect child's/young person's right to confidentiality • Explain boundaries • Ensure young person understands how and why the practitioner will act	• Privacy and confidentiality are important to children and young people, including young parents • Services which fail to respect confidentiality will not be used • Implications for contraceptive advice
17	Child's right to access to information Protection from harmful information	• Develop and display Children' Health Charter • Provide information on services available to children and young people in child-friendly format • Display and provide leaflets on health and related matters and sources of help	• Many parents, children and young people are ignorant of what services are available • Information on helplines is valuable since they allow the individual to stay in control of his/her situation
19	Child's right to protection from violence, abuse and exploitation	• Identification of children at risk of abuse • Understanding of and participation in child protection procedures • Understanding of the role of child protection agencies and appropriate referrals • Provision and mobilization of support to families under stress	• Need for training in recognition and responding to child abuse in all its forms, including bullying • Health surveillance programmes • Follow up of missed appointments • Sharing information with other professionals • Participation in case conferences

Table 9.1 Continued.

Article	Summary	Actions for GPs and health care teams	Implications for intervention
23	Rights of disabled children to services enabling individual development and social integration	• Understanding and provision for the needs of children with disabilities • Recognition that children with disabilities are particularly vulnerable to abuse	• Professionals have attributed signs of abuse to a child's disability • Need to ensure effective methods of communication • Referral to appropriate specialists
30	Rights of minorities to practice their own cultures, religions and languages	• Understanding and response to the needs of minority group families • Understanding of the impact of racism on children and their families • Provision of translated materials • Access to interpreting services	• Black and minority ethnic families are discriminated against in the child protection system • Racism can constitute a form of abuse to children

This table derives from the work of the British Association of Community Child Health Working Group which produced *Child Health Rights: a Practitioner's Guide*.[11]

Promoting public policy for the benefit of children and young people

This discussion of children's rights may inadvertenty have created a view that children and young people are the sole players in promoting policies that will benefit them. While they should have a central role, as mandated by Article 12 of the Convention, the task of developing child-friendly policies should not be left to them alone, not least because they rarely have the power and authority to champion their cause. Obviously, this is particularly so with babies and young children. All adults and practitioners, including general practitioners and other primary health care workers, have a responsibility to contribute to policy formulation for the benefit of children.

Based on their understanding of children and young people, derived from consultation and careful listening, GPs are in a good position to influence policies for promoting the healthy development and well-being of children. Through their teams, organizational structures and professional groups, they can share their observations and experience in order to influence and change policy. Many GPs and other health professionals work in this way and are able to influence policy, and certainly such an approach could be seen as a key part of the public health role of health visitors. Nevertheless, it could be argued that general practitioners and their professional associations could do more to promote public policy objectives.

For example, there is now a strong body of opinion among a wide range of child welfare organizations that the law should be reformed so that children should be given the same protection from assaults as adults. Current UK law is based on an 1860 judgement, when Chief Justice Cockburn stated 'By the law of England, a parent . . . may for the purpose of correcting what is evil in the child inflict moderate and reasonable corporal punishment.' Today, a group of over 260 organizations and prominent individuals working with children, including the National Society for the Prevention of Cruelty to Children (NSPCC), the Royal College of General Practitioners, Barnardo's, Save the Children, the British Association for the Study and Prevention of Child Abuse and Neglect, the British Association of Community Child Health, and the Royal College of Paediatrics and Child Health, have come together to form the Children Are Unbeatable Alliance. It is campaigning for legal reform and for the promotion of positive, non-violent discipline. At the time of writing neither the British Medical Association nor the Royal College of Nursing have joined the alliance, despite the fact that many of their members must have seen or been aware of the severe injuries, including broken bones, that have been inflicted on children, sometimes using implements, under the pretence of 'reasonable chastisement'. As visitors to families, GPs and other primary health care workers must be aware that discipline based on physical punishment does not work and that 'light' or 'loving' smacks can easily escalate to serious forms of abuse. GPs are in a good position to influence the debate and policy on physical punishment but hitherto their voice has not been heard.

In January 2000, the Department of Health issued *Protecting Children, Supporting Parents: a Consultation Document on the Physical Punishment of Children*.[12] This paper represented the government's attempt to consult on how the law on physical punishment should be reformed following the Report of the European Commission of Human Rights in the case of 'A vs UK', which had stated that the law on parental discipline must be clarified to give children better protection. In the paper the government posed a number of questions seeking to define reasonable chastisement. It asked, for example, 'Should the law state that physical punishment which causes, or is likely to cause injuries to the head (including injuries to the brain, eyes, and ears) can never be defended as reasonable?' And, 'Should the law state that physical punishment using implements (e.g. canes, slippers, belts) can never be defended as reasonable?' The government also seemed to be proposing that the courts should only 'in some instances' consider the sex, age and state of health of the children who were being physically punished. Members of the Children Are Unbeatable Alliance found it extraordinary that the government should be asking these questions and considering that there might be circumstances in which hitting babies or children with disabilities could be judged reasonable. The Alliance argued that this approach was totally flawed and that a much clearer position was to reject any form of physical punishment.

Nearly all professional organizations responding to the consultation opposed all physical punishment of children. Seventy per cent of 'individual members of the public' who responded to the consultation apparently supported the *status quo*, however, although 76 per cent believed it should be illegal to smack a naughty child under the age of 2. The Department of Health's response, announced in November 2001,[13] stated that the government proposed no change in the law for England and Wales whatsoever, simply noting that now the Human Rights Act is in force, courts must take account of the judgement in the case of 'A vs UK'. The government says it will keep use of the 'reasonable chastisement' defence 'under review'. This contrasts with Scotland, which in September 2001[14] announced plans to ban all physical punishment of children up to their third birthday, all use of implements to hit children, shaking, and blows to the head.

Clearly, if the government were to reform the law so that 'reasonable chastisement' is more clearly defined along the lines suggested in their consultation, doctors and other health professionals might find themselves increasingly having to make judgements about the consequences of physical punishment on individual children. General practitioners are likely to have strong views on these matters and it would be interesting to know how many made representations to the government on the consultation paper. GPs and health visitors might also have an interest, given their potential role in providing advice to parents on positive parenting and alternatives to smacking.

There are many other examples of areas of policy in which general practitioners could make a significant policy contribution in relation to children, their welfare and their protection. They will know of the impact that poverty, homelessness and poor housing, unemployment and poor environments can have on children and their families. All these factors affect the health of patients and also impact upon the prevention of child abuse since they are stress factors that can precipitate abuse and neglect. GPs, as respected professionals, known in their communities, could influence the direction of policy in these areas. The role of GPs in Primary Care Trusts can be instrumental in this regard. These organizations, which bring together health professionals, local authorities and community representatives, can, through their contribution to local health improvement plans and their potential for joint policy-making and funding, make a significant contribution to the prevention of child abuse. The designation of certain especially deprived areas as health action zones will bring some extra funds: GPs can and should have a part to play in ensuring that some of these funds are deployed to benefit children and families.

The National Commission of Inquiry into the Prevention of Child Abuse concluded that most cases of child abuse and neglect could be prevented if there was the *will* to do so. Unfortunately, the Commission found that this will is often sadly lacking. The NSPCC's FULL STOP Campaign, launched in 1999, aims to stop cruelty to children within a 20-year period. That campaign is based on the premise that it is possible to end cruelty if the care and protection of children becomes *everyone's* responsibility. General practitioners can help stop cruelty both through their practice in response to individual patients and also, importantly, through helping to create the *will* to change how children are treated. That requires policy solutions as well as good professional practice. All professionals have an obligation to use their practice experience to influence policy. General practitioners are no exception and as valued supporters of families their chances for being successful are that much greater.

References

1 **ChildLine.** *I Know You're Not a Doctor but… Children calling ChildLine about Health.* London: ChildLine, 1998.

2 **National Commission of Inquiry into the Prevention of Child Abuse.** *Childhood Matters, Vol. 1. The Report.* London: Stationery Office, 1996.

3 **Wattam C, Woodward C.** *And do I abuse my children? …* In: National Commission of Inquiry into the Prevention of Child Abuse, ed. *Childhood Matters, Vol. 2. Background Papers.* London: Stationery Office, 1996: 43–148.

4 **Hall DMB.** *Heath for All Children: a Programme for Child Health Surveillance.* Oxford: Oxford Medical Publications, 1995.

5 **Gibbons J, Thorpe S.** Can voluntary support projects help vulnerable families? The work of Home-Start. *British Journal of Social Work* 1989; **19** (3): 189–202.

6 **Olds D, Kitzman H.** Review of research on home visiting for pregnant women and parents of young children. *The Future of Children* 1993; **3**: 53–92.

7 **Browne K.** Preventing child maltreatment through community nursing. *Journal of Advanced Nursing* 1995; **21** (2): 57–63.

8 **Barker W.** Practical and ethical doubts about screening for child abuse. *Health Visitor* 1990; **63** (1): 14–17.

9 **United Nations.** *UN Convention on the Rights of the Child.* New York: United Nations, 1989.

10 **National Health Service Executive.** *Child Health in the Community.* London: Department of Health, 1996.

11 **British Association of Community Child Health.** *Child Health Rights: a Practitioner's Guide.* London: British Association of Community Child Health, 1995.

12 **Department of Health.** *Protecting Children, Supporting Parents: a Consultation Document on the Physical Punishment of Children.* London: DOH, 2000.

13 http://tap.ccta.gov.uk/doh/intpress.nsf/page/2001-0524?OpenDocument

14 http://www.scotland.gov.uk/library3/justice/mssp-00.asp

Chapter 9b

Working with young sexual abusers

Eileen Vizard

Introduction

The sexual abuse of children by other children is a little understood topic which often causes anxiety and revulsion in the minds of public and professionals alike. However in recent years it has become apparent that a substantial minority of the sexual abuse of young children is perpetrated by their peers or older children: furthermore such early-onset sexually abusive behaviour links to undetected patterns of adult offending. This chapter suggests ways in which GPs can begin to recognize sexually coercive children, and find a way through the referral process towards an assessment of the young person, following which treatment and help can be offered.

Definitional issues

Research and clinical practice[1,2] confirm that a considerable number of descriptive labels have been given to sexually abusive children including sexually aggressive children, abuse-reactive children, sexual perpetrators, oversexualized children, sexually coercive children, sexual abusers and sexual offenders. Virtually all of these terms may be criticized on some basis or other, particularly when the attempt is to describe inappropriate or sexually abusive behaviour in very early childhood.

In England where the age of criminal responsibility is 10 years old, it is important to note that the term 'offender' does not have relevance for sexually abusive children under 10 years old who cannot be charged with a criminal offence. It is also the case that children and adolescents under the age of 16 years old cannot be given a psychiatric diagnosis of paedophilia within ICD-10 or DSM-IV (classification systems) since it is assumed that 'paedophile' interest in other children simply does not occur before that age. This assumption is not in line with existing Home Office criminal statistics on sexual offending against children by juveniles nor is it in line with clinical experience with sexually abusive children under 10 years old who fulfill many of the clinical criteria for adult paedophilia.[1]

Furthermore, there is a dearth of data available for comparison on 'normal' sexuality in childhood, a subject which remains controversial and subject to various religious and cultural interpretations. Normal childhood sexuality is virtually impossible to research[3] since there would be serious ethical implications involved in, for instance, testing reactions of normal children to sexually explicit material or allowing children to be involved in sexual behaviours which might be considered abusive, for the purposes of research observation.

Hank's 1997 discussion of normal sexual behaviour in childhood,[4] tabulated by age and developmental status, is helpful to clinicians working with sexualized young children, where a key question is often 'Is this abuse or is it "normal" childhood experimentation?' However, doubts about nomenclature for persistent, oversexualized behaviour in childhood and adolescence have led to procrastination in referral to existing services, with clinical evidence of worsening of behaviour over time.[1]

Research findings

UK estimates[5] suggest a 1-year prevalence rate of 1.5 juvenile sexual offenders per 1000 males aged 12–17 years i.e. 0.85 per 1000 12–17 year olds overall. In a cross-sectional study of the prevalence of child sexual abuse among adolescents ($n = 1116$) in Geneva, Halperin et al.[6] found that 35 per cent of the 201 abusers described in the study were adolescents under 18 years of age. This is in line with the prevalence rates reported in most studies[7–9] and reviews,[3] which have concluded that between 30 and 50 per cent of all child sexual abuse is perpetrated by young people under 21 years of age. Such estimates of around one-third of sexual abuse against children having been perpetrated by other young people are likely to underestimate the problem since it is currently unusual for the younger child, age 10–14 years old, to be prosecuted for sexual offences.

Notwithstanding the publication of an influential National Children's Home report in 1992,[10] and the above evidence, the problem of young sexual abusers of other children remains largely unrecognized today, with most research into sexually abusive behaviour focusing on findings from work with adult sex offenders.[11]

Research with adult sex offenders has destroyed the myth that child sexual abuse is perpetrated on a 'one off' basis by offenders of previously good character. Research with convicted sex offenders indicates that large numbers of undetected sexually abusive actions against children over months and years are the norm rather than the exception.[12] The research literature[3] indicates that many adult sex offenders begin to fantasize about prospective child victims and to commit undetected crimes during their adolescence or even earlier. Research with adolescent sexual offenders[13] confirms these findings and indicates that many but not all adolescent sexual offenders have histories of their own child sexual abuse, physical abuse or neglect, or other childhood experiences which have caused trauma and lasting emotional damage.

Conclusive treatment outcome results are not yet available for juvenile sexual offenders but it is known that recidivism is less during the treatment process and during follow-up by professionals[14,15] and that recidivism rises when follow-up stops.[16]

Clinical experience strongly suggests that the outcome is better when children start in treatment at a young age, preferably before puberty. However, follow-up research data on these young children is not yet available.

More recently, research findings from the field of brain biochemistry[17] suggest that there are significant neurobiological sequelae of childhood trauma, i.e. their own history of child abuse resulting in the clinical signs of post-traumatic stress disorder which, it is hypothesized, may have a longstanding physiological basis. In reviewing this literature Hawkes *et al.*[18] have suggested a link between such disturbances in the brain biochemistry of child sexual abuse victims and the later development (in a minority of boy victims) of compulsive sexually aroused behaviour towards other children.

Overall the research literature indicates that sexually abusive behaviour towards other children often starts in adolescence or younger, may be a sequel to sexual or other trauma (such as bullying) in childhood, links directly with later patterns of adult sexually abusive behaviour and suggests that such sexual arousal towards children may be reinforced at a number of levels including physiological, emotional and behavioural.

Recognition

The recognition of sexually aroused and coercive children, and of young sexual abusers of other children, requires the same approach as the diagnosis of any other type of child abuse. In other words, no one type of emotional disturbance or behavioural pattern is diagnostic of the problem but all aspects of the child's psycho-social functioning need to be taken into account. Additionally, in younger children and in older learning disabled children, there are major definitional and ethical issues to be addressed,[3] in terms of what constitutes intentionally abusive behaviour as opposed to the sexualized sequelae of earlier abuse.

GPs and others in the primary health care team (PHCT) should be alert to sexualized behaviour in younger children that moves on from self-stimulating masturbatory behaviour (which is quite normal for a short while in very young children), to more compulsive masturbation and then on to attempts to involve other children in sexualized acts. Young children who threaten other children or physically force themselves upon other children in order to attain sexual contact with, or penetration of, another child, should be seen as having the beginning of a sexually aroused and coercive attitude towards other children that merits assessment. Any verbally or physically coercive sexualized behaviours by young children towards other children should not, therefore, be written off as 'boys will be boys' or as child's play, particularly if it is persistent and does not respond to the normal social disapproval which eventually extinguishes more ordinary childhood sexual experimentation.

Strategies used by young sexual abusers

Research and clinical experience now suggest that such coercive sexual behaviour will usually be the outcome of:

- a preceding period of *fantasizing* about possible abuse;
- *targeting* a suitable, vulnerable victim;
- *isolating* this victim from their carers;
- engaging in *grooming*, a softening up process preparing the victim for abuse;
- before finally *committing the abuse.*

Since this sort of pattern is also the natural history of sexually abusive behaviour as described in many studies dealing with adult and adolescent sex offenders, professional intervention at this point with children will be essential if an escalation into more serious abusing is to be stopped.

Listed below are some of the behaviours which should alert professionals to the need for assessment:

- compulsive masturbation with attempts to involve other children in the behaviour;
- persistent sexualized talk or obscenities directed at other children or adults;
- coercive verbal or physical sexual overtures towards other children;
- persistent touching of the genitals of other children or adults;
- showing obscene drawings or pornographic material to other children or adults as an inducement into sexual behaviour;
- repeated acts of physical violence towards selected children or adults accompanied by a sense of sexual arousal;
- attempted or successful sexual penetration of another child by fingers, penis or object;

- oral, anal or vaginal rape of another child;

- sexualized behaviour with, or penetration of, animals;

- evidence of persisting bizarre sadistic or sexual fantasies about vulnerable human beings or about animals, or serious cruelty to animals;

- the use of objects such as pens, broom handles, etc. to sexually assault victims;

- the use of weapons such as knives or guns to threaten or subdue victims;

- the use of restraints such as gags, hoods, ropes, handcuffs, etc. to control victims;

- preoccupation with scenes of damage to bodies, sadistic violence or death.

In listing such individual factors, it is important to emphasize that *none of these behaviours should be taken in isolation* but should be assessed as part of a carefully gathered health, developmental, family and school-based history. In terms of assessing dangerousness and risk, it will be apparent that specialist assessment (see below) is needed. However, it should also be obvious that a young child starting out on a process of targeting and abusing other children will pose a less serious risk than the 15-year-old adolescent with fixed masturbatory patterns involving sadistic rape fantasies where there is a history of known sexual assaults.

Assessment

Since work with young sexual abusers involves serious child protection issues, it is essential that recommended child protection procedures are followed. Government guidance[19] makes it clear that there should be a child protection conference in respect of the alleged abuser, something which is often avoided in relation to young sexualized children but may happen occasionally with older overtly dangerous boys. No matter what the level of sexual arousal or sexually abusive behaviour may be, it is essential that a properly conducted child protection conference occurs since failure to do so may allow continued significant harm to be inflicted upon other children. It has been noted[1] that 'it is vital to create a full inter-agency systemic context around each referred case of a child as a young abuser since there is then a better chance that the (inevitable) inter-agency conflicts will be survived and a supportive network emerge'. This means that GPs or other professionals should *never* undertake exploratory, assessment or counselling interviews with young sexual abusers or their families without the active involvement of a named child protection social worker.

Specialized assessment of the mental state, offending patterns and risk posed by the young abuser should be undertaken following referral to a specialist resource. The model described by the Young Abusers Project[1] comprises four components, including a preliminary *professionals' meeting*, *psychiatric* assessment interviews, *psychological* assessment and a production of a comprehensive *report*. Assessment of young abusers should always include a full consideration of the family background, the child or young person's school performance, mental state issues and relationship with peers. Within such an assessment, the sexually abusive behaviour should be neither ignored or minimized nor should it be overstated or seen as the only assessment issue.

Management

As mentioned above, cases involving an alleged or known young sexual abuser of young children should be managed like other child abuse cases with careful attention to existing procedures and a fully systematic interagency approach which results in an agreed care plan being produced.

The age of criminal responsibility in England and Wales is 10 years old and therefore young children above this age threshold can be prosecuted and convicted for sexual offences: if found guilty, such a child can be put on the sex offender's register. Human rights issues do arise from the prosecution of very young children within the adult court context[20] and it remains to be seen if this is the best way to deal with very young child defendants. Nevertheless, it is also the case that a conviction within the criminal court, if coupled with a criminal supervision order to a named clinician, can be extremely helpful in providing a clear legal mandate for treatment with a very resistant client group.

Many children and young people who sexually abuse other children are also children in need in terms of the Children Act 1989 and may therefore be said to be 'dual status' children whose welfare needs should also be considered. Given the many developmental, health, educational and psychiatric problems experienced by this group of child defendants,[3] it is essential that assessments are made of the child's fitness to plead in any criminal proceedings and that an opinion is given about the psychiatric disorder, learning disability and likely response to treatment.

Young child defendants charged with serious sexual offences should always have psychiatric assessments to exclude psychiatric disorders and psychological assessments to exclude learning difficulty and other cognitive (thinking) problems. It is essential that agencies such as the local YOTs (Youth Offending Teams), under the auspices of the Youth Justice Board (YJB) with their multiagency, multidisciplinary brief to prevent youth offending, are involved in the care planning for the young person at the earliest possible stage.

Treatment

Treatment for young sexual abusers of other children must begin by removing the sexually aroused young person from any contact with other children that could fuel his fantasies and exacerbate the problem. Once placed in a neutral but containing environment, and following a full assessment, a young sexual abuser may enter into *individual psychotherapy, group work* with other young sexual abusers, *family therapy* or a *combination* of all three approaches.

Since rather different theoretical models will be used to inform each different type of therapy, there needs to be careful overall coordination of the therapeutic programme. In practice, group work with young sexual abusers supported by concurrent group work for their carers[21] appears to offer a satisfactory way of dealing with young sexual abusers in a community setting. With certain young sexual abusers, individual psychotherapy will be the treatment of choice[22] but must also be arranged within a child protection context so that the therapist can be in touch with the local authority should any child protection issues emerge during sessions. Family work with the family of origin or with a foster family may be necessary with younger children, but many teenage sexual abusers are already separated from parents and living in care.

Role of the GP

The GP has several important functions in relation to young sexual abusers:

- To be alert to behavioural indicators (see above) which could suggest a known or emerging pattern of sexual arousal to children.

- To refer promptly a child who appears to have such a problem both to the child protection services (social services) and to a local specialist resource (such as a child psychiatrist).

- To make available to a case conference or for other colleagues' perusal all relevant health documents in relation to the known or suspected young abuser, since the developmental and health history in these cases is often of crucial importance. The GP must not feel constrained by notions of spurious confidentiality between him or herself and the known or suspected young abuser or their family. Young people can and do inflict very serious emotional and physical harm on other children and the GP's duty of care extends beyond one child and family to the welfare of the other children in the area.[23]

- To support and follow up the physical and emotional welfare of children suspected of abusing others. Long-term follow-up studies of these children are urgently needed in order to track which of them may ultimately progress to adult sex offending. GP records of all health and social matters are of direct assistance in relation to this issue.

Practice implications

There are a number of practice implications for GPs and other disciplines. First, a fresh approach to *identifying young sexual abusers* needs to be taken: persistently sexualized or coercive behaviour towards other children should no longer be seen simply as sequelae of earlier sexual abuse, but should be noted as a possible indicator of sexual arousal towards other children.

Second, there is a real need for the *provision of local specialist resources* to assess and offer treatment to this worrying subgroup of child abuse perpetrators. GPs can play a role in local discussions to set up multidisciplinary advisory panels which may help to identify the problem, as well as by supporting initiatives to set up local treatment programmes, via their commissioning input to Primary Care Trusts (PCTs) and equivalent bodies. Within such locally based treatment resources, it is essential that health professionals, such as child psychiatrists, child psychologists and child psychotherapists work along with local authority or NSPCC social workers. Sexually abusive children and young people have a range of physical and mental health care needs,[24] which require specialist health assessment in addition to their sexualized behaviour problems. In planning for such specialist services, GPs should push for the earliest possible (prepubertal) identification of oversexualized children at risk of later abusing behaviour.

Primary prevention may mean very different things to different care groups, but in the context of young sexual abusers primary prevention should mean preventing the youthful sexual abuser from abusing in the first place and certainly from progressing into a career path of adult sexual offending against children. The GP's role in this process of primary prevention is absolutely vital.

References

1 Vizard E, Wynick S, Hawkes C, Woods J, Jenkins J. Juvenile sexual offenders assessment issues. *British Journal of Psychiatry* 1996; **168**: 259–62.

2 Calder M. *Children who Sexually Abuse.* Lyme Regis, Dorset: Russell House Publishing, 1997.

3 Vizard E, Monck E, Misch P. Child and adolescent sex abuse perpetrators: a review of the research literature. *Journal of Child Psychology and Psychiatry* 1995; **36** (5): 731–56.

4 Hanks H. 'Normal' psycho-sexual development and knowledge. In: Calder MC, ed. *Children who Sexually Abuse.* Lyme Regis, Dorset: Russel House Publishing, 1997.

5 James AC, Neil P. Juvenile sexual offending: one year period prevalence study within Oxfordshire. *Child Abuse and Neglect* 1996; **13**: 571–85.

6 Halperin DS, Bouvier P, Jaffe PD *et al.* Prevalence of child sexual abuse among adolescents in Geneva: results of a cross sectional survey. *British Medical Journal* 1996; **312**: 1326–9.

7 Horne L, Glasgow D, Cox A, Calam R. Sexual abuse of children by children. *Journal of Child Law* 1991; **3**: 147–51.

8 Davis G, Leitenberg H. Adolescent sex offenders. *Psychological Bulletin* 1987; **101**: 417–27.

9 Kelly L, Regan L, Burton S. *An Exploratory Study of the Prevalence of Sexual Abuse in a Sample of 16–21 year olds. Report for the ESRC.* London: Child Abuse Studies Unit, University of North London, 1991.

10 National Children's Home. *Children who Abuse Other Children.* London: National Children's Home, 1992 (85 Highbury Park, London N5 1UD, UK).

11 Hollin CR, Howell K. *Clinical Approaches to Sex Offenders and their Victims.* Chichester: Wiley, 1991.

12 Abel G, Becker JV, Mittelman MS *et al.* Self-reported sex crimes of non incarcerated paraphiliacs. *Journal of Interpersonal Violence* 1987; **2**: 3–25.

13 Becker JV, Cunningham-Rathner J, Kaplan MS, Kavoussi R. Adolescent sexual offenders, demographics, criminal and sexual histories and recommendations for reducing future offences. Special issue: the prediction and control of violent behaviour: II. *Journal of Interpersonal Violence* 1986; **1**: 431–45.

14 Smith WR, Monastersky C. Assessing juvenile sex offender risk for re-offending. *Criminal Justice and Behaviour* 1986; **13**: 115–40.

15 Bremer JF. Addressing the serious juvenile sex offender: components of residential treatment. In: Darquis A, ed. *State of Corrections.* Proceedings of ACA Annual Conferences. Laurel, MD: The American Correctional Association, 1989.

16 Groth AN, Longo RE, McFadin JB. Undetected recidivism among rapists and child molesters. *Crime and Delinquency* 1982; **28** (3): 450–8.

17 Perry BD. Neurobiological sequelae of childhood trauma: post traumatic stress disorder in children. In: Murray M, ed. *Catecholamines in Post-traumatic Stress Disorder: Emerging Concepts.* Washington, DC: American Psychiatric Press, 1994: 253–76.

18 Hawkes C, Jenkins J, Vizard E. Roots of sexual violence in children and adolescents. In: Varma V, ed. *Violence in Children and Adolescents.* London: Jessica Kingsley, 1997: 84–102.

19 Department of Health, Home Office, Department of Education and Employment, the National Assembly for Wales. *Working Together to Safeguard Children: a Guide for Interagency Working to Safeguard and Promote the Welfare of Children.* London: Department of Health, 1999.

20 JUSTICE. *Children and Homicide. Appropriate Procedures for Juveniles in Murder and Manslaughter Cases.* London: JUSTICE. 1996 (59 Carter Lane, London EC4V 5AQ).

21 Griffin S, Williams M, Hawkes C, Vizard E. The Professionals Carers Group: supporting group work for young sexual abusers. *Child Abuse and Neglect* 1997; **21** (7): 681–90.

22 Vizard E, Usiskin J. Providing individual psychotherapy for young sexual abusers of children. In: Erooga M, Masson H, eds. *Children and Young People who Sexually Abuse Others.* London: Routledge, 1999: 104–23.

23 General Medical Council. *Confidentiality.* London: General Medical Council, 2000.

24 Vizard E. Adolescents who sexually abuse. In: Welldon EV, Van Velsen C, eds. *A Practical Guide to Forensic Psychotherapy.* London: Jessica Kingsley, 1997: 48–55.

Chapter 9c

Organizing the primary care team: practice-based training in child protection

Deborah T. Hodes and Amy B. Weir

Hobbs and Heywood[1] suggest doctors should play a key role in the identification of children at risk given the prevalence of abuse,[2] although child protection is not necessarily seen as one of their core responsibilities.[3] There is a growing interest in seeking to involve GPs in identifying parenting difficulties and children in need of protection; many of the constraints to the work have been discussed in the literature. It is often a low priority because of the small number of children on the child protection register on a GP's list. Some GPs avoid such families, comparing them to opening a 'can of worms'. There is evidence that GPs have been unable to commit much dedicated time to this area of activity.[4,5] Finally all doctors may be reluctant to share information with others because of the confidential nature of the consultation.

A survey by Goodhart,[6] looking at GPs' training needs, found they wanted to learn more about child abuse and have the opportunity to acquire practical experience. They also expressed a need for practice-based training in which the whole team could be involved. We designed our training to take account of the issues raised by local GPs in Goodhart's study and the preference for 'informal' learning centred on clinical cases along with easy access to telephone advice rather than formal lectures.[7]

By adopting a multiprofessional approach by virtue of our own different backgrounds and experience, we demonstrated some of the potential and actual tensions which may exist organizationally and professionally.

The training coordinator (AW) initially contacted all the GPs by letter describing the aims of the training, explaining that there would be two training sessions on their premises, each lasting approximately 2 hours over the lunchtime period. She asked what they wanted from the training and booked sessions immediately. The GPs were encouraged to invite other practice staff: health visitors, practice nurses, district nurses, midwives, practice managers and receptionists.

In the introductory session, AW covered the legislative basis for child protection including a brief look at the major principles of the Children Act (1989, updated in 1999).[8] The medical practitioners' guide *Medical Responsibilities*[9] was discussed and copies of this and the *ABC of Child Abuse*[10] were left at every practice. Further sessions included case studies with reference to the interprofessional and interagency basis of child protection. An appreciation of the context of the daily work of a general practitioner enabled the trainers to advise on the delicate balance between legislative and professional requirements and a realistic outcome. The general practitioner's dilemma of having to consider the paramountcy of a child's welfare over and above that of their parents, who may also be patients at the practice, was a key element of the training.

We emphasized the availability of consultancy, using either the consultant community paediatrician for immediate advice via his or her mobile phone, known as the 'child protection hotline' or by a referral to the 'community children's clinic'. We encouraged GPs to seek information and advice from health colleagues and local social services managers. We also held topic-based workshops covering adult mental health issues and child protection, signs and symptoms in child abuse and female genital mutilation.

The training reached more than 70 per cent of the general practitioners in the City and Hackney. Our evaluation showed that the vast majority of GPs found the information and the case studies valuable and contributed to interesting discussions. One participant commented that the training was 'very salient to our concerns' and others mentioned the advantages of practice-based training. There has been a steady increase in both patient referrals and telephone enquiries to the consultant community paediatrician.

This training model and our experience of using it for more than 4 years has high-lighted several issues. 'Selling the training' and a broadly based open and non-critical approach were essential; arranging a visit often included several phone calls and once a date was finalized there were some cancellations. We found it essential not to be put off by any reluctance or hesitation on the part of the GPs, otherwise we may have found ourselves only accessing practices with an interest in child protection. The involvement of the consultant community paediatrician was important, for arranging follow-up visits and during case discussions.

Many GPs were reluctant to participate in discussion, commenting at the beginning of the session that there were no such problems amongst their practice patients. It was noticeable how much they used case examples from their own list as the session continued. They discussed particular families causing concern in an open and self-critical way. The description of the Children Act principles and the concept of significant harm enabled them to consider cases in a new light and with an increased awareness and understanding. Explaining and discussing the social work perspective allowed them to think more about interagency working.

This model overcame the problems of having standardized training packs[12] by allow-ing the GPs and their practice staff to set the agenda with us. The GPs' time limits were accommodated and their need for short intensive training appreciated.

Working relationships within the practice varied. One GP described how difficult she had found dealing with a family within which there was a high probability of incestuous relationships between adults and children over many years. Another practice discussed a family with a disabled child and previous concerns about physical abuse. They explained that they tagged the computer screen of such children but during our discussion noted they had not tagged the mother's partner. The practice then made a decision to tag all relatives in future.

Carter[13] has discussed how the issue of confidentiality presents moral and ethical dilemmas for GPs, particularly when a practitioner has to deal with a conflict of interest between a child's safety and maintaining confidentiality. One GP in our study asked what she should have done about a 7-year-old girl who presented with vaginal bleeding and tears to the hymen on examination. She thought that the girl had been raped and suspected the mother was a prostitute. The mother did not want the police informed and the GP did not refer the girl. In another practice, a GP referred a 9-year-old girl who had a vaginal discharge to a consultant gynaecologist; 6 months later he received notification that she had been treated for gonorrhoea. By that stage, he did not know what further action to take. It is clear from these and other cases that GPs need considerable open support to deal with such dilemmas. It appeared to us that a substantial degree of child abuse goes unreported by GPs.

There were examples of excellent practice. One GP described her concerns about a young pregnant woman with learning difficulties who told her GP that the father was a man whom the GP knew had previously been convicted of sexually abusing his daughter from a previous relationship. The GP identified the issues and sought appropriate advice about how to deal with this and to ensure that the new baby would be protected. In another practice, the GPs recognized that their concerns about a 7-year-old girl living with an alcohol and substance-abusing mother, had reached the point where they decided to put the child's interests first and refer to social services.

Many GPs have negative attitudes to social services and fear the consequences for the child, the family and themselves once they make a referral. This was clearly illustrated by an anonymous GP, writing to the *British Medical Journal* in 1996.[14] The writer described the rapid deterioration in his relationships with a pregnant teenager, her stepfather who had fathered the child and her mother, after informing social services of the situation. Interestingly neither the commentary nor the letters that followed[15–17] discuss the bene-fits of interagency working in such difficult cases. A referral to a paediatrician with an an interest in child protection or even an obstetrician would have allowed one of them to inform social services, leaving the GP available, without blame, to continue his sup-port of his three patients. It may also be that some bridge building with the local social services team is required to prevent such difficulties whilst there is still an opportunity for working together more positively.

We encouraged GPs to talk about difficulties they have in interagency working and this was enhanced by the presence of a social worker. In one practice, we arranged a meeting with the local team and set about successfully specifying what would constitute the 'ideal social worker' and the 'ideal GP'.

The whole primary care team was often involved and we found this an effective means of initiating discussions and encouraging collaboration. Bhrolchain *et al.*[18] have recently described the benefits of this approach, which it was felt may have an advantage over multiagency training as it is shorter and concentrates on discussions relevant to GP practice.

There is strong evidence that much child abuse goes undetected within the UK. Almost all children and their families are registered with a GP and their practice provides that critical window of opportunity for both making and keeping children safe.

References

1 **Hobbs CJ, Heywood PL.** Childhood matters. *British Medical Journal* 1997; **314**: 622.

2 **National Commission of Inquiry into the Prevention of Child Abuse.** Childhood matters. *Report of the National Commission of Inquiry into the Prevention of Child Abuse*, Vols 1 and 2. London: Stationery Office, 1996.

3 **General Medical Services Committee, BMA.** *Core Services—Taking the Initiative.* London: British Medical Association, 1996.

4 **Lea-Cox C, Hall A.** Attendance of GPs at child protection case conferences. *British Medical Journal* 1991; **302**: 1378–9.

5 **Simpson CM, Simpson RJ, Power KG, Salter A, Williams GJ.** GPs' and health visitors' participation in child protection case conferences. *Child Abuse Review* 1994; **3**: 211–30.

6 **Goodhart LC.** General practitioner training needs for child health surveillance. *Archives of Disease in Childhood* 1991; **66**: 728–30.

7 **Marshall MN.** Qualitative study of educational interaction between general practitioners and specialists. *British Medical Journal* 1998; **316**: 442–5.

8 **Department of Health, Home Office, Department of Education and Employment, the National Assembly for Wales.** *Working Together to Safeguard Children: a Guide for Interagency Working to Safeguard and Promote the Welfare of Children.* London: Department of Health, 1999.

9 **Department of Health, British Medical Association, Conferences of Medical Royal Colleges.** *Child Protection: Medical Responsibilities.* London: HMSO, 1994.

10 **Meadows R.** *ABC of Child Abuse.* London: British Medical Association, 1994.

11 **Burton K.** *Child Protection Issues in General Practice: an Action Research Project to Improve Interprofessional Practice.* Essex, 1996.

12 **Payne H, Smail S, Sibert J.** *Child Protection Training Manual for Primary Health Care Teams.* Cardiff: Department of Postgraduate Studies and Department of Child Health, University of Wales College of Medicine, 1997.

13 **Carter YH.** *Abuse: a Dilemma for General Practice.* In Update: the Journal of Continuing Education for General Practitioners. London: Reed Business Information, 15 January, 1995.

14 **Anonymous.** An ethical debate. Child protection: medical responsibilities. *British Medical Journal* 1996; **313**: 671–2.

15 **Fish D.** Child protection: referrals to social services may be damaging. *British Medical Journal* 1996; **313**: 1548–9.

16 **Mellon AF.** Child's needs should be central. *British Medical Journal* 1996; **313**: 1549.

17 **Butler V.** Girl should have been offered a chance of safety. *British Medical Journal* 1996; **313**: 1549.

18 **Bhrolchain C, Shribman S, Hales V.** Training the practice healthcare team. *Child Abuse Review* 1995; **4**: 83.

Chapter 9d

Training issues in child protection

Enid Hendry

Introduction

> Effective child protection depends not only on reliable and accepted systems of co-operation, but also on the skills, knowledge and judgment of all staff working with children in relation to child protection matters. Sound training therefore underpins effective working practices.[1]

Child Protection: Medical Responsibilities[1] goes on to make clear that a sound foundation of knowledge in relation to child abuse needs to be developed at the undergraduate stage, to be maintained and developed at the postgraduate stage and to continue in practice. It argues the case for the participation of doctors in multidisciplinary training once an initial grounding has been achieved. *Working Together to Safeguard Children*[2] reinforces the requirement that:

> GPs should take part in child protection training and have regular updates as part of their postgraduate educational programmes. As employers, GPs are responsible for their staff and therefore should ensure practice nurses, practice managers, receptionists and any other staff, are given the opportunity to attend local child protection courses, or undergo such training within the practice team (para. 3.30).[2]

A survey by Hallett[3] of a sample of professionals with involvement in child protection cases showed that half the doctors interviewed had had no input on child abuse in their basic qualifying training. While recently qualified general practitioners may have benefited from some initial undergraduate training on abuse, there are many practising GPs who have had little or no formal training in this area. There are also those whose training preceded the introduction of the Children Act 1989, and who have not had the opportunity to become familiar with the developing knowledge base in relation to abuse, to keep up-to-date with changes in the way enquiries into possible abuse are to be handled, or to learn the costly and painful lessons from the various inquiries into the deaths of children as a result of abuse.

Training needs

Bannon and Carter,[4] in their study using both focus groups and questionnaires, showed that child protection is certainly seen as a source of considerable anxiety and uncertainty by many GPs. This was especially so in relation to how their role was defined, the process for referring concerns and the potential for damage to their relationship with families when they initiated child protection procedures. The three most commonly identified needs were accurate diagnosis, appropriate referral and legal issues.

The remainder of this chapter will consider the essential areas of knowledge, skill and judgement to be covered in training GPs if they are to make an informed and effective contribution to the protection of children. Alternative approaches to the engagement of GPs in child protection training, which take account of some of the barriers to engagement, will be considered, and the strengths and problems of multidisciplinary programmes will also be explored.

Key areas to be covered by training

> Everybody who works with children, parents and other adults in contact with children should be able to recognise possible indicators of abuse or neglect, and how to act upon indicators that a child's welfare or safety may be at risk (para. 5.2).[2]

GPs need to be aware of the predisposing factors, the presentation and identification of abuse. This should include an emphasis on early indications that a child's health and development are being impaired, either as a result of abuse or neglect or parenting that does not respond to the child's essential developmental needs. Because they work with patients of all ages they also need an appreciation of the interrelationship between domestic violence and child abuse and an understanding of how drug and alcohol abuse and mental health problems can increase the likelihood of abuse. Training must cover the GP's own role and that of others in responding to concerns as well as providing up-to-date understanding of how concerns will be dealt with once raised.

GPs need to be able to carefully weigh and evaluate the worrying information they may have about risk to a child, so that they know when the 'critical threshold of professional concern' has been crossed and their concerns need to be shared with others. Training should provide an opportunity to consider the circumstances in which breaching the confidentiality of one patient is necessary and justified in order to safeguard the interests of a child. This involves not only ensuring familiarity with the guidance to the medical profession on this issue, but also exploring ethical dilemmas faced by GPs, the consequences of withholding information and the impact of disclosing information on patient–doctor relationships. In addition, GPs need to have an understanding of the purpose and processes of child protection conferences and to have considered any implications for their own contribution arising from the participation of parents and children.

Training for GPs should not only cover procedural and legal knowledge, technical skills and the development of professional judgement in this complex and sensitive area of work. It should also allow for the exploration of values and attitudes and the development of the skills needed for cooperative work with people from other disciplines.

Effective collaboration to protect children is unlikely without a recognition of the dangers of 'going it alone' and an understanding, not only of roles, but of the particular contribution and limitations of other professionals, and an understanding and respect for differences and skills in conflict resolution.

Bannon and Carter[4] summarize the key training objectives for GPs in child protection as follows:

1. A clear appreciation of their role and that of others in the child protection process.

2. An attitudinal change with respect to the paramountcy principle that the safety and welfare of children is the overriding consideration.

3. A reduction in levels of anxiety and uncertainty.

4. An awareness of relevant legal issues including advice on confidentiality, preparation for court appearances and the Children Act 1989.

5. An adequate knowledge of clinical indicators of abuse within the setting of primary care.

6. An awareness of local child protection procedures and sources of advice and support.

7. Strategies for maintaining relationships with families.

8. Case conference preparation and participation.

Engaging GPs in the training process

Anecdotal evidence abounds on the difficulty of engaging GPs in training on child protection. The factors that contribute to this difficulty have to be understood and addressed if the learning needs identified above are to be met. Four contributory factors will be considered.

Conflicting priorities and demands

It seems that the number of situations involving abuse that come to the attention of GPs is relatively low, and constitutes a small proportion of the workload of most family doctors.[3] This is likely to influence choices about priorities for training; however, choices are also influenced by our values and, in this instance, the value placed on sound child protection.

Time and availability

A doctor's continuing duty to his or her patients and the need to be available on call, makes participation in any formal training problematic. This can be a particular problem in small and single GP practices. Locum cover can be obtained in many situations when resources are available and are prioritized for this purpose. In Suffolk, when it was recognized that many GPs were not up to date with procedural guidance, the health authority allocated a budget to cover costs for participation in an accredited programme of training, which was then delivered in the workplace, either at lunch-time, or as early morning sessions. While this overcame some of the problems, the training was still subject, on occasion, to postponements and to interruptions; however, the trainers concerned understood the very real constraints on the availability of GPs and were able to be flexible.

Motivation and felt need

Exhortations to training by the Department of Health, British Medical Association and others, cannot compel compliance. There has to be a perceived need by GPs who recognize the importance of improving their practice in this area. All good training starts with a thorough needs analysis which engages those concerned. There will, however, be those doctors who continue not to recognize any need for training. For them, alternative methods of providing the absolutely essential information have to be found, and examples will be given below.

Appropriateness and relevance

Timing, content, style, methods and choice of trainer all need to be appropriate to the family doctor if they are to be engaged. A 2-day workshop on case conference participation using role play exercises may well be relevant, but given the difficulties doctors experience attending child protection conferences for relatively short periods of time, it is questionable whether this particular training approach is appropriate to GPs. The opportunity for expert coaching prior to attendance; for debriefing following participation and for observing professionally made videos of conferences are likely to be much more appropriate approaches.

Alternative approaches

In addition to the use of coaching and debriefing by colleagues, or designated specialists in child protection, three alternative approaches will be considered which are being used successfully in different parts of the country.

Provision of materials for self-directed learning

These can be short, punchy, information sheets, which highlight key things to remember and think about, which can be displayed on notice boards for ease of reference; alternatively, fuller resource and reference packs can be provided. An example of the latter is the resource pack developed for Camden and Islington GP practices by their health authority. This is designed to help readers to get the information they require in emergency situations quickly, as well as to allow them to review their practice in more depth. It includes information on local contact points and makes provision for periodic updates. This approach has the advantage of being locally tailored and easily accessible. It addresses the need for procedural, legal and technical knowledge, but is not designed for skills development, or for the improvement of processes of collaborative working.

Flexible training packs for primary health care teams

Some training packs have been developed to assist people with a responsibility for training health professionals. Generally these packs include all the materials and information needed to deliver training and can be used flexibly, for example in practice meetings. One such pack[5] has been developed for use in primary care teams by Area Child Protection Committee (ACPC) interagency trainers, a GP tutor and a primary care facilitator in Oxfordshire. The pack was piloted in 1995 in a number of GP practices with very positive responses. This pack includes trainer notes and guidance, exercises, case studies, short information papers/handouts and contact points. Another pack, *A Safer Practice: a Child Protection Guide for GPs and the Primary Health Care Team* was developed by Helen Armstrong[6] in 1996. This approach has twin advantages of flexibility, as programmes can be adapted to meet needs, and of focusing on the primary health care team as a whole. The exercises encourage discussion and the development of collaborative working practices.

Problem-solving seminars using 'real' material

The use of case material, issues and dilemmas that have arisen and are current to a particular practice as the basis for workplace seminars has proved successful in some areas. For instance, a situation where a fretful child had been presented to a GP, a practice nurse and a health visitor at different times over a 2-week period, was used to explore the importance of sharing information. The case had a particularly powerful impact as the child had been seen in casualty shortly afterwards with multiple fractures which had taken place over the course of several weeks. Such material obviously requires sensitive handling as well as local knowledge.

Polnay and Blair[7] describe how, following the death of Leanne White in Nottinghamshire in 1993, a training package was designed to maximize the take up of training by GPs. This consisted of a 2-hour interactive training session which was recognized for postgraduate education purposes and received health authority funding. It began with an audiotaped extract of an adult survivor of physical abuse describing her experiences as a child, and moved on to consider the particular concerns of participants and four key themes of recognition, communication, child protection procedures and record keeping.

The second half of the workshop was case based and included practical information about sources of advice and contact numbers. The above training had excellent take-up rates resulting in 53 per cent of practices in Nottingham having at least one GP attending. The authors attribute the success of this model to 'the pairing of a locally known general practitioner and community paediatrician which helped to establish "street credibility" for this programme' and on the time spent telephoning practices on a personal basis (see also Chapter 9c).

Interdisciplinary training for GPs?

While involvement in multidisciplinary training in the primary health care team may be valued, the participation of GPs in interagency child protection training organized through ACPCs is generally low. Some of the reasons for this relate to the factors identified earlier, but in addition there seem to be some attitudinal blocks to participation and some substantive difficulties in ensuring that interagency training adds value and is time well spent. GPs can be characterized by their independence and autonomy. Hallett and Stevenson[8] noted in 1980 that after qualification, doctors show very little interest in joint training, or in the dynamics of collaboration.

Interagency training can be problematic. It needs to take full account of the differences of those involved—differences, for instance, of professional socialization and education, of language, of preferred learning style, of practical issues such as availability, as well as differences of power and status. In taking account of these differences, interagency training may risk meeting no-one's particular needs.

If interagency training is to be effective and relevant, it is essential that someone who is familiar with the needs and context of family doctors is fully involved in the planning and design stages and, if possible, in the delivery of the training. If GPs are to be assisted to get cover to attend such training, the organizers need to ensure the programmes are either paediatric accredited, or accredited in relation to postgraduate education. Again, a practice-based approach involving members of a primary health care team who are already familiar with each other can overcome some of these educational/learning difficulties and lessen time and cover constraints.

When interagency training works well it can provide a thorough knowledge and appreciation of the skills of others and of their working context and this in turn can provide a sound basis for developing joint working. In some parts of the country this has been achieved through the establishment of locality-based training. Representatives from different agencies who are working with children and their families in a relatively small local area, come together forming core groups, which identify their local training needs and provide or commission training. These sometimes take the form of lunch-time sessions on specific topics. Locality-based interagency training has the advantage of bringing people together who are likely to be working together, and so serves the dual purpose of training and relationship/network building.

Some 90 per cent of GPs are accredited to carry out preschool health surveillance. In some districts training on child protection is seen as a prerequisite for taking on this role. Whether it be in a multidisciplinary setting or in specially targeted programmes, one way forward would be for child protection training to be compulsory for those undertaking child health surveillance. While GPs are expected to undertake 30 hours postgraduate training each year, there is currently no obligation for individual practitioners to choose child protection, in contrast to the situation in the USA.[9]

Conclusion

Children have a right to expect that their doctors will be able to help protect them from the harm that results from abuse. GPs' involvement with children and their families at different stages of their lives puts them in a unique position to contribute to the protection of children. Experience alone is unlikely to be sufficient to equip doctors with the knowledge and skills this complex area of practice requires. For effective working practices that recognize that the welfare of the child is paramount, the provision and use of relevant, accessible and flexible learning opportunities is essential, as is the commitment to continued training.

References

1 **Department of Health, British Medical Association, Conference of Medical Royal Colleges.** *Child Protection: Medical Responsibilities.* London: HMSO, 1994.

2 **Department of Health, Home Office, Department of Education and Employment, the National Assembly for Wales.** *Working Together to Safeguard Children: a Guide for Interagency Working to Safeguard and Promote the Welfare of Children.* London: Department of Health, 1999.

3 Hallett C. *Inter-agency Co-ordination in Child Protection.* London: HMSO, 1995.

4 **Bannon M, Carter YH.** *An Evaluation of the Training Needs of General Practitioners in England in Child Protection: Management Summary.* London: Queen Mary and Westfield College, 1998.

5 **Oxfordshire Area Child Protection Committee, National Society for the Prevention of Cruelty to Children (NSPCC) Training Project.** *Child Protection in Practice: an Introduction to Child Abuse and Child Protection.* London: NSPCC, 1995.

6 **Armstrong H.** *A Safer Practice: a Child Protection Guide for GPs and the Primary Health Care Team.* Leicester: Community Education Development Centre, 1996.

7 **Polnay J, Blair M.** A model programme for busy learners. *Child Abuse Review* 1999; **8**: 284–8.

8 **Hallet C, Stevenson O.** *Child Abuse: Aspects of Inter-professional Co-operation.* London: Alien & Unwin, 1980.

9 **Gordon M, Paivski VJ.** Physician training in the recognition and reporting of child abuse, maltreatment and neglect. *New York State Journal* 1991; **91**: 1–2.

Part 3

Violence against women by known men

Chapter 10

The context

Jalna Hanmer

Historical overview

Violence against women from men they know **and with whom they often live is** common. In the past two decades, social knowledge of this widespread behaviour has increased, but not for the first time. Historically, public **awareness of violence against** women is associated with agitation for women's rights.[1,2] In our times the special events that created a climate where violence against women began to become socially visible once again arose when the Women's Liberation Movement took up this issue in the early 1970s.[3,4] After a long period of neglect women began to provide advice, counselling and accommodation services for other women who turned to the movement for assistance with problems of violence from known men.

While there are parallels between approaches and understandings, each wave of recognition of the problem has had its own interpretation and ways of responding. For example, the second half of the nineteenth century was a time of widespread knowledge about the abuse of women, when campaigns and concern focused particularly on the vulnerability of women in or accused of prostitution, on domestic service as an occupation, and on relations within marriage. The physical and sexual abuse that women were enduring in all three of these situations were seen to result from their social and legal status **and was not seen as a problem** suffered by a few inadequate or abnormal individuals. Considerable effort went into effecting legislative changes from the Married Women's Property Acts, to legislation on divorce, maintenance, custody and guardianship of children, and raising the age of consent to 16 years. Securing the vote for women after the First World War was seen as a way of achieving many aims, including the control of male violence, as it was believed that a fully enfranchized female population would ensure the legislation needed to enable all women to have a decent life.

Public knowledge of violence towards women then declined, reaching its lowest point in the period immediately after the Second World War: but even at its lowest ebb a residual knowledge of violence towards women remained among professional workers in certain occupations such as community health services, the law and social work. During this period when conscious knowledge was at its most restricted, the social aspect of the problem was lost and violence was redefined as the problem of a few individual deviant people, and possibly the problem of certain social groups. As the problem became located in the personalities of women, few professional workers saw the abuse of women as requiring that they take action to protect the victim. They thought women should learn to stop precipitating the violence.

While these attitudes are still with us today, victim-blaming approaches are more widely contested with each passing year and in a variety of ways. As well as voluntary sector provision of refuges, advice and counselling, improvements have been made in professional education and in-service training,[5,6] in the development of agency policies and through interagency initiatives and working practices,[7,8] and in public education, for example, through Zero Tolerance poster campaigns that seek to promote the unacceptability of physical and sexual violence against women and girls.[9] These activities are a culmination of 30 years of women's agitation for recognition and for new responses that will protect the victim from continuing attacks and assist her and her children to gain control over their lives.

The rediscovery of home-based violence from husbands, cohabitees and boyfriends began in the UK and by 1974 there was a network of refuges in England, Northern Ireland, Scotland and Wales.[10–13] Recognition of different types of violence continued to develop through women's disclosures to each other.[14] Women who contacted rape crisis centres, first established in England in 1976, helped in the identification of incest and other sexual assaults on children and the development of new services from 1980 onwards.[15] The concept of 'victim' with its implied passivity was rejected by women who 'discovered' childhood sexual abuse in favour of the more dynamic word, 'survivor'. Around the same time equal opportunity legislation began to recognize sexual harassment at work.[16,17] Reclaim the Night marches held throughout the UK raised issues of women's safety and the influence of pornography. The homicide of women by men and the refusal of the courts to recognize the relevance of repeated violence to wives in their killing of husbands have led to further campaigns through Justice for Women.[18] The close relationship between violence against women and violence against children by men in the family is of increasing concern.[19] These issues subsequently have been taken up worldwide by women's groups and by governmental and international organizations. Eliminating all forms of violence against women, for example, is part of the global platform to achieve women's equality agreed at the United Nations Conference on Women in Beijing in 1995.[20]

Sociological overview

Parallel with these changes in consciousness and public awareness is an upsurge of interest in understanding violence against women. Explanations of violence concentrate on four areas: (i) biology and personality, (ii) interpersonal relations, (iii) culture or ideology, and (iv) institutional and structural factors. Embedded in the literature is the moral question, 'who is responsible?' and this question leads to another, 'is the aggressor or the victim to blame?' Almost all the literature that attempts to explore why men abuse women incorporates commonsense understandings and is responsive to current developments in intellectual thought. Theoretical perspectives have a profound impact on the professional responses deemed to be appropriate and, therefore, require close attention.

A major issue that has provided a backdrop for the construction of theory generally concerns the relative importance given to nature and nurture. For example, in the nineteenth century, men's behaviour was thought to be dominated by biology so the control of male vice and excesses in and out of marriage resulted in demands for male self-control. The militant suffragette Christobel Pankhurt's famous slogan 'votes for women', contained a second demand, 'and chastity for men'. The Purity Movement, as it became known, like society generally, understood sexual passion to be a biological attribute with men having more and women less. Moral development and will power were the means of overcoming social evils that were thought to have their origin in biology. Today the concern is with human agency and the development of theory that can account for both social and individual factors.[21,22]

An early study of professional workers, including doctors and health visitors, found that professionals tended to locate explanations either in individual personalities or in factors they believed provoked stress and frustration.[23] Further, the personality of the woman was consistently rated as more important than that of the man in explaining violence. Holding the victim responsible is not only a question of professional practice, it is also one strand of the explanation in the academic and clinical literature that is gradually becoming less acceptable. For example, Erin Pizzey described some battered women as 'violence prone' and, as in the work of the psychiatrist Gayford, argued that women may seek violent relationships.[24,25] This approach can be based on biological or personality theories.

Other explanations of the causes of violence place the emphasis on immediate situations that cause stress for the aggressor. These are often social factors, such as poverty, unemployment and housing—aspects of social life that impinge on individuals, but do not originate within them. Illness, handicap and mental disorder are defined as stress factors. Aggressors can be seen to have blocked goals, to be underachieving or to be unable to fulfil roles seen as primary for the male; i.e. as a result of work difficulties, inadequate income or unemployment.[26] Violence to women is then a secondary response, deflected from the true source of conflict. Unable to achieve personal autonomy, authority and respect in the economic and public world, the man is thought to vent his frustration in the home on his wife and children or in public on unknown women. The most interesting aspect of this perspective, however, is that victims are never described as having problems of stress or blocked goals, only the male aggressors—which raises an issue of the gendered nature of this concept. The distinction between stress and personality factors seems to be the degree to which specific variables are thought to be within the control of the individual. By implication, there is less moral culpability with stress factors than with those associated with personality.

Questions about the importance of an individual's past in his or her family of origin give rise to an explanation for violent behaviour based on childhood socialization. This view suggests that observing or experiencing violence as a child predisposes one to violent behaviour when an adult if male, and to becoming a victim if female; i.e. establishing a cycle of violence.[27] Violence is seen as learned behaviour and the family as a primary training ground. This view is widely held and part of its attractiveness is that, while implying responsibility for violence is socially located, it is neither the fault of the aggressor nor the victim. Responsibility conveniently lies in the preceding generation, in a past that is beyond reach. This explanation can be criticized for overdetermining the behaviour of people. The link between past learning and present behaviour may not be obvious and direct. An individual may consciously reject the lesson, moulding behaviour on another set of values and experiences.

Other explanations focus on learning gendered behaviour, in particular patterns of masculinity that conflate sexuality with violence. Denying their violence or minimizing its seriousness is a common characteristic of men.[28] By and large, men do not perceive their violent behaviour to women or children to be a personal psychological problem. There is little demand from men themselves for treatment that promotes insight or alternative social learning, but they are motivated to take part in re-education programmes if these are presented as an alternative to prison.[29]

The current wave of consciousness about violence to women from men whom they know raises questions such as, is violence to women an aspect of a system of social relations in which men dominate? An affirmative answer to the latter leads inexorably to the question of who then benefits from male violence towards women? How do they benefit? And is there a relationship between violence and sexuality, particularly heterosexuality? How important are cultural representations, particularly pornography, in increasing or decreasing actual violence? What is the role of the state through its various agencies in maintaining or curtailing male violence to women? These major questions constitute the backdrop against which current studies are framed and findings interpreted.

The first of the new research studies on violence against women shifted the analysis from an individual problem caused by the personal failure of the victim, to structural explanations of male domination and patriarchal social relations in the family and society.[30,31] This work followed an analysis begun by the Women's Liberation Movement, elaborating key insights. In this analysis the family is conceived as the locus of male dominance and female subordination and violence as the outcome of unequal relations. Further, violence and its threat is conceived as the underpinning of all hierarchical systems; it is equally applicable to an analysis of social class, 'race', imperialism and gender relations. This explanation is both individual and social.

The state is an important source of the power of men over women in families as it defines the family as located in the private rather than in the public domain. The argument is that legitimated violence and its threat is regulated and exercised by the state and the state can both exercise its power through what it does and what it does not do. By not intervening in any serious way in the exercise of violence and threat by individual men against individual women, the state gives legitimacy to the maintenance of hierarchical relations between women and men in families and in society generally.[21,32,33,50] Important differences between women are created and maintained by the state, for example, a woman who enters the UK to marry a UK citizen may not leave him for a year no matter how he treats her unless she is prepared to be returned to her country of origin.[34] Through informal practices, statutory agencies respond differentially to women from different ethnic communities, which creates differences in how women experience violence and its resolution.[35,36] While this may be unintended, none the less women are receiving differential services.

With attention directed to sexual violence and to male power the question of the relationship between heterosexuality as a sexual practice and as a system of social relations then arises. Is heterosexuality violent? Or is violence an aberration or extreme end of heterosexuality? One solution is to define all violence as sexual in recognition of its largely heterosexual location, while another is to elaborate the forms violence may take and to explore women's violence to men and to each other. This is both an empirical and theoretical response to issues of individual agency, differences between women, the concepts of power and subordination, social domination and oppression.[37]

For professional responses it is of great importance whether the victimized woman is seen *to be the problem* or seen *as someone with a problem*. Even if seen as someone with a problem, the way that problem is understood is also important in shaping professional practice.

With some exceptions, particularly amongst health visitors, health-related professionals have been amongst the last to recognize the relevance of violence against women to their work.[38] The growing emphasis on health promotion, however, is creating a more aware approach as the concept of the prevention of disease includes psychosocioenvironmental–epidemiological models.[39] A health promotion model recognizes that illness and disease are caused by many factors, both social and biological. The overall economic costs of violence against women are also beginning to be studied.[40,41]

Epidemiological overview

While the incidence (the number of violent acts per head of population) and prevalence (the number of victims per head of population) of violence against women is not accurately known, certain findings are replicated by research studies and/or by criminal justice statistics.[43] Notably, violence to women is largely perpetrated by men whom women know and the closer the relationship the more likely there is to be violence and the repetition of violence. Stranger assault is much less frequent and much less likely to be repeated on the same women. Women may be responded to with violence when children, when adults and in old age and, while some women have a more or less continuous personal history of living with violence, younger women are more likely to be victimized. The significance of age is associated with the greater dependency of women on men when pregnant and when their children are very young. Age is the one variable consistently found to be associated with variations in the incidence and prevalence of home-based violence against women, unlike social class, ethnicity and 'race'. There are numerous methodological problems with incidence and prevalence studies, but the overall conclusion is that violence and violent crime against women are major social problems.

Victimization surveys involving large samples began to be undertaken by the Home Office in 1982. Until these surveys the only data on incidence was provided by criminal justices statistics, which suggested[53] then as today that 25 per cent of violent crime is wife assault[30] and that the reporting rate to police for assault, battery and breach of the peace offences varied between 2 and 14.5 per cent.[30,31,42] Later work suggests that women are more likely to report physical than sexual assaults.[44,45] Comparisons between surveys is limited as definitions and methods or research vary, but even so trends can be observed. The British Crime Surveys have become progressively better at obtaining data from the approximately 11 000 person household surveys in England and Wales conducted every 2 or 3 years in the past two decades. Results suggest that violence against women by partners, ex-partners and relatives is the most common form of physical interpersonal crime, exceeding even that of assaults on males. The location of assaults is gender-related as eight out of 10 women were assaulted at home, while eight out of 10 men were assaulted in public places. Men are much less likely to be the recipients of domestic violence, and when they are, their assailants are often other men—just as they are in public places. Assaults by women on men are infrequent. The 1992 British Crime Survey found that the total number of domestic assaults was just over 500 000 in the previous 12 months.[46] The 1996 British Crime Survey found that 4.2% of women between 16 and 59 years were assaulted by a current or former partner in the past year.[52]

Women define violence more broadly than do men. If women's understandings are accepted for research, then over a lifetime women experience the following: mental cruelty behaviours of verbal abuse, being deprived of money, clothes and sleep, and prevented from going out (37 per cent); actual physical violence (32 per cent); threats of violence (27 per cent); rape or non-consensual sex (23 per cent).[44] A significant proportion of incidents occurred to women who had separated from partners or who had never lived with them. One in 16 women received broken bones and one in 10 experienced attempted strangulation, the most common method used in the killing of women by known men. The Islington survey[44] used a bodily harm definition of violence to create a composite violence rate of 30 per cent. Over women's lifetimes this results in numbers running into the millions.

Prevalence is always lower than incidence as some women are victims more than once over time. This is true of all types of crime, and particularly so with domestic violence. The British Crime Survey of 1992 found that 35 per cent of victims of domestic violence generated 66 per cent of the total number of incidents and of 1996 that 45% experienced repeated violence. Half the women who reported domestic violence incidents experienced more than one offence within the survey period of 1 year. Surveys agree that victims perceive domestic violence as serious even though they do not report it to the police or other agencies, and women are likely to assume responsibility for domestic violence attacks upon them.

Doctors and other health professionals are amongst those most likely to have contact with women in violent, sexually and emotionally abusive domestic situations.[47,51] The British Crime Survey found that 25 per cent of women subject to domestic assault saw a doctor; however, only a small proportion are likely to have explained the origin of their injuries or more general complaints. Being able to recognize domestic violence as the cause of emotional and physical distress is the first step in improved professional practice.[48,49] Knowing which local agencies can also help women through advice, counselling and emergency accommodation are vital preventative health measures and require medical and other health professionals to take an interagency approach to their work.

References

1 Clark A. *Women's Silence, Men's Violence Sexual Assault in England 1770–1845*. London: Pandora, 1988.

2 Cobbe FP. Wife torture in England. In: Jeffreys S, ed. *The Sexuality Debates*. London: Routledge & Kegan Paul, 1987 (first published in 1878).

3 Kantor H, Lefanu S, Shah S, Spedding C, eds. *Sweeping Statements: Writings from the Women's Liberation Movement 1981–83*. London: Women's Press, 1984.

4 Dobash RE, Dobash R. *Women Violencce and Social Change*. London: Routledge, 1992.

5 Hanmer J, Statham D. *Women and Social Work: Towards a Women-centred Practice*, 2nd edn. Basingstoke: Macmillan, 1999.

6 Mullender A. *Rethinking Domestic Violence: the Social Work and Probation Response*. London: Routledge, 1996.

7 Hague G, Malos E, Dear W. *Multi-agency Work and Domestic Violence: a National Study of Inter-agency Initiatives*. Bristol: Policy Press, 1996.

8 Home Office, Welsh Office. *Inter-Agency Circular: Inter-Agency Co-ordination to Tackle Domestic Violence*. London: Home Office Public Relations Board, 1995.

9 Zero Tolerance. *Zero Tolerance Bulletin* and other campaign material. Zero Tolerance Charitable Trust, 25 Rutland Street, Edinburgh EH1 2AE.

10 Welsh Women's Aid. *Annual Report*. Cardiff: Welsh Women's Aid, 1998.

11 **Women's Aid Federation of England.** *Annual Report.* Bristol: Women's Aid Federation of England, 1998.

12 **Nothern Women's Aid.** *Annual Report.* Belfast: Northern Women's Aid, 1998.

13 **Scottish Women's Aid.** *Annual Report.* Edinburgh: Scottish Women's Aid, 1998.

14 **Painter K, Farrington D.** Marital violence in Great Britain and its relationship to marital and non-marital rape. *International Review of Victimology* 1998; 5 (3/4): 257–76.

15 **Kelly L.** *Surviving Sexual Violence.* Cambridge: Polity Press, 1988.

16 **UNISON, Primary Health Office.** *Violence in GP Surgeries—Results of UNISON Survey.* London: UNISON, 1996 (Mabledon Place, London WC1H 9AJ).

17 **National Audit Office.** *Report by the Comptroller and Auditor, General Health and Safety in the NHS Acute Hospital Trusts in England.* London: Stationary Office, 1996.

18 **Radford J, Russell DEH.** *Femicide: the Politics of Woman Killing.* Buckingham: Open University Press, 1992.

19 **Mullender A, Morley R,** eds. *Children Living with Domestic Violence: Putting Men's Abuse of Women on the Child Care Agenda.* London: Whiting & Birch, 1994.

20 **United Nations.** *Beijing Declaration and Platform for Action, Adopted by the Fourth World Conference on Women: Action for Equality, Development and Peace.* United Nations, 1995 (available from Women's National Commission, Level 4, Caxton House, Tothill Street, London SW1H 9NF, http://www.undp.org/fwcw/daw1.htm).

21 **Hester M, Kelly L, Radford J,** eds. *Women, Violence and Male Power.* Buckingham: Open University Press, 1996.

22 **Maynard M, Winn J.** Women, violence and male power. In: Robinson V, Richardson D, eds. *Introducing Women's Studies,* 2nd edn. Basingstoke: Macmillan, 1997: 175–97.

23 **Borkowski M, Murch M, Walker V.** *Marital Violence: the Community Response.* London: Tavistock, 1983.

24 **Gayford JJ.** Ten types of battered wives. *Welfare Officer,* 1976; 1: 5–9.

25 **Pizzey E, Shapiro J.** Choosing a violent relationship. *New Society* 1981; 23 April: 133–5.

26 **Gelles RJ.** *The Violent Home.* Beverley Hills, CA: Sage, 1974.

27 **Byron E.** A history of abuse is a major risk factor for abusing the next generation. In: Gelles R, Loseko D, eds. *Current Controversy on Violence.* Newbury Park, CA: Sage, 1993: 00.

28 **Hearn J.** Men's violence to known women: historical everyday theoretical contradiction by men. In: Fawcett B, Featherstone B, Hearn J, Toft C, eds. *Violence and Gender Relations: Theories and Interventions.* London: Sage, 1996: 22–37.

29 **Dobash R.** *Re-education Programmes for Violent Men: an Evaluation.* Research Findings No. 46. London: Home Office, 1996.

30 **Dobash RE, Dobash R.** *Violence Against Wives: a Case Against the Patriarchy.* New York: Free Press, 1979 (reprinted by Open Books, Shepton Mallet, UK 1980).

31 **Hanmer J, Saunders S.** *Well-founded Fear: a Community Study of Violence to Women.* London: Hutchinson, 1984.

32 **Hester M, Pearson C, Radford L.** *Domestic Violence: a National Survey of Court Welfare and Voluntary Sector Mediation Practice.* Bristol: Policy Press, 1996.

33 **Hanmer J. Maynard M.** *Women, Violence and Social Control.* London: Macmillan, 1987.

34 **European Womens's Lobby.** *Confronting the Fortress: Black and Migrant Women in the European Community.* Luxembourg: European Parliament, 1993.

35 **Mama A.** *The Hidden Struggle: Statutory and Voluntary Sector Responses to Violence Against Black Women in the Home.* London: Runnymede Trust, 1989.

36 **Hanmer J.** *Policy Development and Implementation Seminar Patterns of Agency Contact with Women.* Occasional Paper No. 12. Leeds: Leeds Metropolitan University, 1994.

37 **Richardson D,** ed. *Theorising Heterosexuality: Telling it Straight.* Buckingham Open University Press, 1996.

38 **Department of Health.** *On the State of the Public Health: the Annual Report of the Chief Medical Officer of the Department of Health for the Year 1997.* London: Stationery Office, 1998.

39 **Nettleton S.** Women and the new paradigm of health and medicine. *Critical Social Policy* 1996; **16** (3): 33–53.

40 **Stanko EA, Crisp D, Hale C, Lucraft H.** *Counting the Costs.* Swindon: Crime Concern, 1998.

41 **Heise L, Pitnaguy J, Germain A.** *Violence Against Women: the Hidden Burden.* World Bank Discussion Paper 255. Washington, DC: World Bank, 1994.

42 **Dutton DG.** *The Domestic Assault of Women: Psychological and Criminal Justice Perspectives.* Boston: Allyn & Bacon, 1988.

43 **ESRC Violence Research Programme.** *Taking Stock: What do We Know About Interpersonal Violence?* UK Royal Holloway University of London, 2002.

44 **Mooney J.** *The Hidden Figure: Domestic Violence in North London.* London: Middlesex University, 1993.

45 **Canadian Panel on Violence Against Women Changing the Landscape: Ending Violence—Achieving Equality.** Ottawa: Ministry of Supply and Services. Cananda, 1993.

46 **Mayhew P, Ave Maung N, Mirrless-Black M.** *The 1992 British Crime Survey.* Home Office Research Study 132. London: HMSO, 1993.

47 **Mezey G, Khan M, MacClintock T.** Victims of violence and the general practioner. *British Journal of General Practice* 1998; **48**: 906–8.

48 **Stark E, Flitcraft A.** *Women at Risk: Domestic Violence and Women's Health.* Thousand Oak, CA: Sage, 1996.

49 **Bewley S, Friend J, Mezey G.** *Violence Against Women.* London: RCOG Press, 1997.

50 **Hanmer J, Itzin C.** eds. *Home Truths about Domestic Violence Feminist influences on Policy and Practice, a Reader.* London: Routledge, 2000.

51 **Davidson LL, King V, Garia J, Marchant S.** What role can health services play? In: Taylor-Browne J, ed. *What works in Reducing Domestic Violence.* London: Whitnig and Birch, 2001.

52 **Home Office.** *Domestic Violence: Findings from a New British Crime Survey Self-completion Questionnaire* London: Home Office Research Studies, 1999.

53 **Home Office.** *The 1998 British Crime Survey, England and Wales.* London: HMSO.

Chapter 11

The meaning of domestic violence

Iona Heath

Introduction

In 1990 a *Home Office Circular* to police forces, advising on their role in responding to violence in the home, declared:

> Violent assaults, or brutal or threatening behaviour over a period of time by a person to whom the victim is married or with whom the victim lives, are no less serious than a violent assault by a stranger.[1]

In September 1991, speaking 1 year after the issuing of the circular, John Patten, the then Home Office Minister, said:

> We wish to dispel for good any lingering notion that a man who attacks a woman in the home is somehow automatically less deserving of society's censure than one who assaults a woman he doesn't know in the street. I hope that approach has been consigned to the dustbin of social attitudes.

Yet in 1996, when, in a blaze of publicity, the footballer Paul Gascoigne assaulted his wife causing severe bruising and dislocated fingers, Sir Donald Finlay was reported as saying:

> Let he who has never had a bust-up with his wife cast the first stone.... That is the man's private life and that is how it will remain unless he wants to talk.

Sir Donald was, at the time, vice-chairman of Glasgow Rangers Football Club. However he is also a QC and one of Scotland's foremost criminal lawyers. That one of such standing should continue to peddle such attitudes is profoundly shocking but serves to illustrate the faltering process 'by which behaviours or social conditions, which may have been long experienced as private pains or sorrows, become defined as public ills'.[2]

The scale and severity of domestic violence

Domestic violence is the cause of a terrifying amount of private pain and sorrow. The 1992 British Crime Survey showed that violence against women by partners, ex-partners and relatives is the most common form of physical interpersonal crime.[3] The total number of domestic assaults as the 12 months covered by the survey was estimated at just over 500 000. As many of 25 per cent of women are estimated to have been exposed to domestic violence at some point in their lives.[4–6] The 1996 British Crime Survey reported that 46 per cent of all violent incidents against women were domestic, and that four out of five incidents of domestic violence against women took place at home.[7] Any woman is at risk of domestic violence, regardless of race, ethnic or religious group, class, age, sexuality, disability or lifestyle.[8] Apart from the police and the military, the family is the most violent grouping and the home the most violent setting in society.[9] Nor does the break-up of the family necessarily bring relief. Divorced and separated women risk violence as much as, and probably more than,[10] married women; once married, the risk of abuse falls significantly only for the widowed.

Domestic violence usually escalates in frequency and severity. By the time a woman's injuries are visible, violence may be a long-established pattern. On average, a woman will be assaulted by her partner or ex-partner 35 times before actually reporting it to the police.[11] In a consecutive-sample survey study of 62 episodes of domestic assault to which police had been called, 68 per cent involved weapons and 15 per cent involved serious injury. In 89 per cent of episodes there had been previous assaults by the current assailant, 35 per cent of them on a daily basis.[12] For some women the escalation is fatal. One in five of all murder victims is a woman killed by a partner or ex-partner; almost half of all murders of women are killings by a partner or ex-partner.[13] Thirty per cent of men charged with the murder of their spouse admit previously being violent, and 80 per cent describe chronic marital problems, recent divorce, separation or threats of separation.[14]

The nature of commonly inflicted injuries

Injuries resulting from domestic violence range from bruises, abrasions, cuts, fractures and miscarriages to permanent injuries including damaged vision or hearing, and scars from burns, bites or knife wounds.[15] Women suffering injury as a result of domestic violence are much more likely to have multiple injuries than those injured in accidents. Abused women are more likely to sustain injuries to the face, neck, breast, chest and abdomen, as opposed to accident victims who are more likely to have injuries to the extremities. Indeed, in one study those injured as a result of domestic violence were 13 times more likely to have injuries to the breast, chest or abdomen than those injured in accidents.[16] One in four domestic violence incidents reported to police in the London Borough of Hackney involved serious injury such as strangulation, stabbing, fractures or attempts to kill or set fire to the victim. One in 10 abused women presenting to a GP surgery had been knocked unconscious and 7 per cent had sustained fractures.[17] Domestic violence is often accompanied by sexual abuse and rape.

The sequelae

Women seem to be at particular risk of domestic violence during pregnancy with between 4 and 17 per cent of women reporting abuse in the current pregnancy.[18] Violence is associated with increased rates of miscarriage, premature birth, low birth weight, fetal injury and fetal death.[19] There is a strong association between living in a physically abusive relationship and one or more episodes of pelvic inflammatory disease,[20] chronic pelvic pain and a wide range of other gynaecological symptoms.

Finding oneself a repeated victim of someone else's violence is intensely demeaning and demoralizing. Victims tend to lose their self-esteem and begin to accept the counteraccusation that they themselves are somehow to blame.[21]

> I said Make your own fuckin' tea. That was what happened. Exactly what happened. I provoked him. I always provoked him. I was always to blame. I should have kept my mouth shut. But that didn't work either. I could provoke him that way as well. Not talking. Talking. Looking at him. Not looking at him. Looking at him that way. Not looking at him that way. Looking and talking. Sitting, standing. Being in the room. Being. What happened? I don't know. [22]

Evidence suggests that these processes take a profound toll of the psychological well-being of those who are subjected to repeated abuse. Women who have experienced domestic violence suffer a high incidence of psychiatric disorders, particularly depression and various self-damaging behaviours including drug and alcohol abuse, suicide and parasuicide. However, it is essential to understand that these present after the first exposure to violence and must therefore be viewed as consequences of the violence rather than causes of it, or even excuses for it. In Stark and Flitcraft's study,[16] one in every four battered women attempted suicide at least once, one in seven abused alcohol and one in 10 abused drugs. One in three were referred to emergency psychiatric services and one in seven were eventually institutionalized. The toll on these women's health is horrifying, yet these hugely damaging consequences can serve to distract attention from the underlying cause. The processes of medicalization focus attention on the consequences of violence rather than women's experience of the reality of the violence itself and the imperative for society to address the causes of this violence.[16]

A chronic, long-term condition

For less than 10 per cent of abused women is domestic violence an isolated event followed by effective resolution or permanent separation from the abuser. For the vast majority domestic violence is endured as a chronic long-term condition which escalates over time. Hope that the violence will stop is very persistent and this probably explains the usually extended time which elapses between the start of the violence and the woman seeking help. If she is to extract herself from an abusive situation, a woman must often pay a high price in terms of loneliness and, perhaps, disrupting her children's relationship with their father. The violent relationship may be the only intimate relationship that she has and this is a lot to lose. For many women, there is also an economic price to pay, with the decision to leave a violent home resulting in a substantial fall in income. Worse, a woman may have been threatened by her partner and may fear that she will be killed if she tries to leave. In these circumstances, staying may seem the only way to protect herself from something even worse.[8]

All this helps to explain why so many women return again and again to face the risk of repeated violence, to the amazement and sometimes the exasperation of the police, doctors and others trying to help. Effective help must be directed towards enabling the woman to retake control of her own life, to offer her realistic choices while accepting that the decisions are hers alone and are always valid in her particular situation. No woman should be condemned for a decision to return to her abuser. It can take a very long time for a woman, demoralized by years of violence, to find the confidence and courage to choose a different life for herself and her children.

> The wonder is not that women find it hard to leave the scene of the violence but that so many find the courage to do so. It is often only when violence is directed at the children that women will summon up the courage to take a decision to do something about it and seek help.[23]

The effects on children

The abuse of women and the abuse of children are intimately connected. In 90 per cent of incidents of violence within families that include children, those children are in the same or the next room at the time.[24] In a study of 62 episodes of domestic assault to which police had been called, 85 per cent of assaults were directly witnessed by children.[23]

> What did I do in the 80s? I walked into doors. I got up off the floor. I became an alcoholic. I discovered that I was poor, that I'd no right to the hope I'd started out with. I was going nowhere, straight there. Trapped in a house that would never be mine. With a husband who fed on my pain. Watching my children going nowhere with me; the cruellest thing of the lot. No hope to give them. They saw him throw me across the kitchen. They saw him put a knife to my throat. Their father; my husband.[22]

The effects of this on the children can be imagined but is poorly documented. They may blame themselves for the violence or being unable to prevent it happening. They may try to intervene and be injured themselves. The Women's Aid Federation (England) (WAFE) report a wide range of effects on children that have been noted by refuge workers. These include confused and torn loyalties, lack of trust, unnaturally good behaviour, taking on the mother's role, guilt, isolation, shame, anger, lack of confidence, and fear of a repeat or return to violence.[16] Children may also present with symptoms suggestive of post-traumatic stress disorder.[26]

Battered women are 10 times more likely than non-battered women to report child abuse or to fear it.[16] More than half of those men who use violence against their partners also abuse their children.[27] Children whose mothers are battered are more than twice as likely to be physically abused as children whose mothers are not battered. In an American study, at least 45 per cent of the mothers of abused children were found to be themselves battered, and these women had already presented an average of four injury episodes to the hospital. However, the battering clearly predated the child abuse, and the children of battered mothers are significantly more likely to be physically abused than neglected.[28] Similar findings are now reported from the UK and the National Society for the Prevention of Cruelty to Children (NSPCC) has found similar levels of domestic violence towards the mothers of children who are known to have been abused. In another UK study, 27 per cent of abused mothers reported that their partners had also abused the children.[28]

Despite these correlations, many general practitioners will have experience of women who have been held responsible by social services departments for their inability to protect their children from violence to which they are also being subjected.

> In contrast to battering, where sexist interpretations and practices confront a grass-roots political movement, in the child abuse field, stereotypic and patronizing imagery of women goes unchallenged. One result is that men are invisible. Another is that 'mothers' are held responsible for child abuse, even when the mother and child are being battered by an identifiable man. . . . the best way to prevent child abuse is to protect women's physical integrity and support their empowerment.[28]

For just these reasons, WAFE's statement of aims and principles defines domestic violence as 'the emotional, sexual or physical abuse of women and children in their homes by partners or known others, usually men'. Their explicit guiding principle is that the safety and empowerment of the non-abusing parent (usually the mother) is the most effective form of child protection.

Male violence against women from ethnic minority communities

Women from ethnic minority communities face particular difficulties which include racism, language barriers and worries about what will happen to their immigration status if they attempt to leave their violent partner. The enduring pervasiveness of racism within British society and the stereotyping of members of some communities means that black women may be very reluctant to call the police or involve them in any way, feeling that by doing so they are betraying their whole community. Some women may be subjected to enormous pressure from their extended families to stay with a violent partner because of the stigma which is attached to the breakdown of family structures. Some whose first language is not English may have insurmountable problems in communicating their predicament to professionals or agencies who might be able to offer help. Other women may fear deportation if they leave a violent partner within 12 months of coming to the UK.[8]

Male violence against women with disabilities

> In attempting to address the specific problem of male violence against women with disability it is necessary to take into account the fact that all people with disability face a range of oppressive and discriminatory factors in their lives.[30]

There is some evidence to suggest that disabled women are at increased risk of violence[31] and certainly the relatively increased dependency and isolation, which so often accompanies disability, can make it harder for disabled women to extricate themselves from violent situations. The abuser may be the woman's sole carer, and fears of continuing violence may be balanced by fears of being unable to cope alone, fears of becoming dependent on the inadequacies of statutory services, and, perhaps at worst, fears of being obliged to accept institutional care. Others, including relatives and friends, may be unwilling to accept that the partner who seems willingly to accept the additional burden of caring for a disabled partner, could be capable of violence. Health care professionals should be aware that the confidentiality of a disabled person may be much more easily compromised because of the, sometimes accustomed, presence of a carer.

Violence within other domestic relationships

Domestic violence is not exclusively male assaults of women, although there is little doubt that this accounts for the major proportion of such violence, particularly violence which results in serious injury. Even at the ultimate extreme of domestic violence, approximately 15 women in Britain kill their partners each year, as compared with 100 men. Significantly, there is a paradoxical gender bias in the response of the legal system, in that 40 per cent of the women are convicted of murder, but only 25 per cent of the men.

Very little is known about the extent of violence within other domestic relationships, and more research is needed into the extent and nature of violence directed against men by their female partners, violence directed against parents, particularly single mothers, by adolescent children, and violence within gay relationships, both male and female. While paying particular attention to the vulnerability of women and children, general practitioners need to retain an awareness of the potential for violence within any relationship, and the damaging health consequences of such violence.

> Domestic violence remains a major health issue affecting the lives of thousands of women and their families. The health community has a responsibility to intervene in this escalating spiral of violence which results ultimately in the homicide of many women and, indeed, of some men, when women kill in self-preservation and self-defence.[32]

References

1 **Home Office.** *Home Office Circular (60/1990)*. London: Home Office, 1990.
2 **Hallett C.** Child abuse: an academic overview. In: Kingston P, Penhale B, eds. *Family Violence and the Caring Professions*. Basingstoke: Macmillan, 1995.

3 Mayhew P, Maung NA, Mirlees-Black C. *The 1992 British Crime Survey*. London: HMSO, 1993.

4 Jones T, Maclean B, Young R. *The Islington Crime Survey*. Aldershot: Gower, 1986.

5 Mooney J. T *The Hidden Figure: Domestic Violence in North London*. London: Islington Council, 1994.

6 McWilliams M, McKiernan J. *Bringing it Out in the Open: Domestic Violence in Northern Ireland*. Belfast: HMSO, 1993.

7 Mirrlees-Black C, Mayhew P, Percy A. *The 1996 British Crime Survey: England and Wales*. London: Stationary Office, 1996.

8 Women's Aid Federation of England. *Domestic Violence. Memoranda of Evidence*. Memorandum 22 to the Home Affairs Committee. London: HMSO, 1992.

9 Gelles R, Straus M. Violence in the American family. *Journal of Social Issues* 1979; **35** (2): 15–39.

10 Feldhaus KM, Koziol-McLain J, Amsbury HL *et al.* Accuracy of 3 brief screening questions for detecting partner violence in the emergency department. *JAMA* 1997; **277**: 1357–61.

11 Yearnshire S. Analysis of cohort. In: Bewley S, Friend J, Mezey G, eds. *Violence Against Women*. London: RCOG Press, 1997: 45.

12 Brookoff D, O'Brien KK, Cook CS, Thompson TD, Williams C. Characteristics of participants in domestic violence: assessment at the scene of domestic assault. *JAMA* 1997; **277**: 1369–73.

13 Home Office. *Criminal Statistics*. London: Home Office Research and Statistics Department, 1992.

14 Kay T, Kent JH. Women victims of domestic violence. *BMJ* 1989; **299**: 1339.

15 Council of Scientific Affairs, American Medical Association. Violence against women—relevance for medical practitioners. *JAMA* 1992; **267**: 3184–9.

16 Stark E, Flitcraft A, Frazier W. Medicine and patriarchal violence: the social construction of a 'private' event. *International Journal of Health Services* 1979; **9**: 461–93.

17 Stanko E, Crisp D, Hale C, Lucraft H. *Counting the Costs: Estimating the Impact of Domestic Violence in the London Borough of Hackney*. London: Hackney Safer Cities, 1997.

18 Mezey GC, Bewley S. Domestic violence and pregnancy. *BMJ* 1997; **314**: 1295.

19 Webster J, Chandler J, Battistutta D. Pregnancy outcomes and health care use—effects of abuse. *American Journal of Obstetrics and Gynecology* 1996; **174**: 760–7.

20 Schei B. Physically abusive spouse—a risk factor of pelvic inflammatory disease? *Scandinavian Journal of primary Care* 1991; **9**: 41–5.

21 Harwin N. Domestic violence: understanding women's experiences of abuse. In: Bewley S, Friend J, Mezey G, eds. *Violence Against Women*. London: RCOG Press, 1997: 63.

22 Doyle R. *The Woman Who Walked into Doors*. London: Jonathan Cape, 1996.

23 Victim Support. *Report of a National Inter-Agency Working Party on Domestic Violence*. London: Victim Support, 1992.

24 British Medical Association. *Domestic Violence: a Health Care Issue?* London: British Medical Association, 1998.

25 Gulbenkian Foundation Commission. *Children and Violence: Report of the Commission on Children and Violence Convened by the Gulbenkian Foundation*. London: Calouste Gulbenkian Foundation, 1995.

26 Kilpatrick KL, Williams LM. Post-traumatic stress disorder in child witnesses to domestic violence. *American Journal of Orthopsychiatry* 1997; **67** (4): 639–44.

27 Gayford JJ. Wife battering: a preliminary survey of 100 cases. *BMJ* 1975; **1**: 194–7.

28 Stark E, Flitcraft A. Women and children at risk: a feminist perspective on child abuse. *International Journal of Health Services* 1988; **18**: 97–118.

29 **NCH Action for Children.** *The Hidden Victims: Children and Domestic Violence.* London: NCH Action for Children, 1994.

30 **Strathclyde Regional Council.** *Male Violence Against Women with Disability: a Report for the Zero Tolerance Campaign.* Glasgow: Strathclyde Regional Council, 1995.

31 **Doucette J.** *Violent Acts Against Disabled People.* Toronto: DisAbled Women's Network (DAWN), 1986.

32 **Edwards SSM.** The law and domestic violence. In: Bewley S, Friend J, Mezey G, eds. *Violence Against Women.* London: RCOG Press, 1997: 105.

Chapter 12

The presentation and diagnosis of domestic violence

Iona Heath

Introduction

> That was my life. Getting hit, waiting to get hit, recovering; forgetting. Starting all over again.[1]

General practice has enormous potential to offer help to women enduring domestic violence.[2] The general practice surgery is freely accessible to all and there is no stigma attached to a visit to the general practitioner, the practice nurse or the health visitor, as there might be for a visit to the police domestic violence unit or the offices of the local social services department. Despite this, many general practitioners and other primary health care professionals have been slow to exploit the potential of their situation.

> Although woman abuse is second only to male–male assault as a source of serious injury to adults ... clinicians rarely identify the problem, minimize its significance, inappropriately medicate and label abused women, provide them with perfunctory or punitive care, refer them for secondary psychosocial problems but not for protection from violence, and emphasize family maintenance and compliance with traditional role expectations rather than personal safety.[3]

In many cases of domestic violence, general practice is the first formal agency to which victims present for help. However, the possibility of violence is seldom raised directly,[4,5] and it has been estimated that only a quarter of women seeking medical help actually disclose the fact that they have been beaten.[6] Many use the 'calling card' of an apparently unimportant physical symptom to test the attitudes and sensitivity of the doctor, and so begin the processes of seeking help diffidently and indirectly. In the past, general practitioners have often failed to respond, accepting the 'calling card' at face value, because of lack of confidence in their ability to intervene effectively,[7] and sharing the sense of helplessness of the victims in the face of society's apparent ambivalence.[8] Yet, the manner in which the general practitioner responds to a woman's first tentative· attempt to seek help to change her situation can make an immense difference to that woman's life and those of her children.[9]

Once established, domestic violence usually continues and escalates in both frequency and severity. A study of women living in Women's Aid refuges showed that some women had suffered abuse for more than 30 years, while the average duration of abuse was 7 years.[10] Early detection and appropriate intervention can help to prevent future violent incidents and the consequent psychiatric morbidity, and can help to save and salvage lives.[11] As with much else in general practice, the most important aid to diagnosis is a high index of suspicion. To ignore the offered 'calling card' is to collude with the continuing concealment of domestic violence behind closed doors.

Consider the possibility

The possibility of domestic violence should be considered in *any* general practice consultation and particularly in the following situations:

- The patient reports past or present abuse.
- The patient presents with unexplained bruises, whiplash injuries consistent with shaking, areas of erythema consistent with slap injuries, lacerations, burns or multiple injuries in various stages of healing.
- The patient has injuries to areas hidden by clothing which may be found inadvertently while, for example, doing a routine cervical smear.[5]
- The patient has injuries to the head, face, neck,[12] chest, breast and/or abdomen.[13]
- The patient has symptoms or signs suggestive of sexual trauma.
- The extent or type of injury does not seem to match the explanation given by the patient.
- There is a substantial delay between the time of injury and the presentation for treatment.
- The patient describes an 'accident' in a hesitant, embarrassed or evasive manner.
- Review of the medical record reveals that the patient has presented with repeated 'accidental' injuries.
- The patient presents repeatedly with physical symptoms for which no explanation can be found.[14] This presentation may be particularly common among women whose first language is not English, and who therefore may find it difficult to express their feelings and suffering.[15]
- The partner accompanies the patient, insists on staying close to her and/or seems very attentive but is reluctant to allow her to speak for herself.
- The patient is pregnant.[16] Domestic violence often begins with the first pregnancy, and injuries are most commonly to the breasts or abdomen.[17]

- The patient has a history of miscarriage. Women experiencing domestic violence are 15 times more likely to have suffered a miscarriage.[18]

- The patient or her partner has a history of psychiatric illness, or alcohol or drug dependence.[14,19]

- The patient has a history of attempted suicide.[13,20] In the USA, domestic violence accounts for one in four suicide attempts by women.

- The patient has a history of depression, anxiety, feeling unable to cope, social withdrawal or an underlying sense of helplessness.

- There is a history of behaviour problems or unexplained injuries to children.[21]

Emphasize confidentiality

The family is meant to be a place of love, warmth, support and intimacy. The difficulty of admitting that the family is also a source of violent abuse should never be under-estimated. Many women will feel distressed and ashamed of their predicament, and it is essential that the patient feels that her account is respected and believed. If at all possible, the women should be offered the chance to talk to a woman health care professional if she prefers to do so. She should always be enabled to consult on her own, and she should be reminded that anything she chooses to talk about is confidential. The only exception to this will arise if the doctor becomes aware that a dependent child is also at risk.[22,23]

The concept of medical confidentiality may be unfamiliar to many first-generation immigrant women and the protection it offers will need to be very carefully explained and emphasized. Provided the patient gives consent, the involvement of translators, advocacy workers or ethnic community link-workers can be very helpful to both patient and doctor.

Ask the question

This is more easily said than done; it is always difficult to confront a patient with the possibility that her injuries have been caused by domestic violence. Practitioners fear that the question will cause offence and jeopardize the mutual respect of the doctor–patient relationship. They also feel inadequate to deal with the problems presented, having neither sufficient time nor sufficient information at their disposal[7]. Yet 'if you do not ask a direct question, you do not even have the possibility of a direct answer',[24] and the evidence suggests that women who are being subjected to violence want to be asked, and that women who are not, do not mind being asked.[25]

> —I fell down the stairs again, I told her.—Sorry. No questions asked. What about the burn on my hand? The missing hair? The teeth? I waited to be asked. Ask me. Ask me. Ask me. I'd tell her. I'd tell them everything. Look at the burn. Ask me about it. Ask.[1]

It is important to ask direct questions in a gentle, non-threatening and non-judgemental manner.

> The doctor never looked at me. He studied parts of me but he never saw all of me. He never looked at my eyes. Drink, he said to himself. I could see his nose moving, taking in the smell, deciding.[1]

Practitioners will need to try out various forms of words and identify those that feel most comfortable. Possibilities include:

- I have noticed you have a number of bruises. Could you tell me how they happened? Did someone hit you?

- Did someone at home do this to you?[26]

- You seem frightened of your partner. Has he ever hurt you?

- Many patients tell me they have been hurt by someone close to them. Could this be happening to you?

- You mention your partner loses his temper with the children. Does he ever lose his temper with you? What happens when he loses his temper?

- Have you ever been in a relationship where you have been hit, punched, kicked or hurt in any way? Are you in such a relationship now?

- You mentioned your partner uses drugs/alcohol. How does he act when drinking or on drugs?

- Does your partner sometimes try to put you down or control your actions?

- Sometimes, when others are overprotective and as jealous as you describe, they react strongly and use physical force. Is this happening in your situation?

- Your partner seems very concerned and anxious. That can mean he feels guilty. Did he hurt you?

- I notice that you have been drinking. Sometimes desperate situations demand desperate measures. Are you in a desperate situation?

In an American study[27] of women using emergency departments, 27 per cent had a history of physical or non-physical partner violence in the previous year. Seventy per cent of these were detected by the answers to any of the following three questions:

- Have you been hit, kicked, punched or otherwise physically hurt by someone in the past year? If so, by whom?

- Do you feel safe in your current relationship?

- Is there a partner from a previous relationship, who is making you feel unsafe now?

In the study, 25.5 per cent reported having been physically hurt in the previous year, 19 per cent by a current or past partner; 11.5 per cent felt unsafe in their current relationship; and 13 per cent felt threatened by a partner from a previous relationship.[27]

> I'd get worked up waiting. I believed it was just a matter of luck. Maybe this time. A nurse would look at me and know. A doctor would look past his nose. He'd ask the question. He'd ask the right question and I'd answer it and it would be over. Charlo was always with me. He was always there. Behind the curtain was the only time I was alone. His shadow on the curtain. A few minutes. One question. One question. I'd answer; I'd tell them everything if they asked. Ask me.[1]

Many argue that all women presenting for health care should be asked routinely about their exposure to domestic violence, and that such an approach is justified by the estimated prevalence of domestic violence and by the toll it takes of the physical and psychological health of so many women.[28] This proposal may well prove to be appropriate in such settings as antenatal clinics, but it will be important to establish through systematic research that the intervention is effective before advocating its widespread introduction.[33] It seems unlikely that routine screening questions will ever be appropriate in the very diverse setting of ordinary general practice consultations, where formulaic, protocol-driven approaches can so easily dominate the patient's own, often carefully planned, agenda for the consultation. None the less, it is essential that all practitioners retain a high index of suspicion within all consultations, and are prepared to act on those suspicions as soon as they arise.

Examination

If there is any suggestion of physical injury, the patient should be carefully examined. Any examination should be both sensitive and thorough. The practitioner should bear in mind that the injuries characteristic of domestic violence are often to areas hidden by clothing, including the chest, breasts, abdomen and perineum. It can be very easy to find an excuse, in the context of a busy surgery, not to examine a patient properly. Women from certain ethnic minority groups may be at particular risk of inadequate examination because of the excuse offered to the practitioner by the woman's apparent shyness and the sometimes unfamiliar nature of her clothing.

Documentation

Accurate documentation of the patient's history and her injuries, at successive consultations over time, may provide cumulative evidence of abuse, and is essential for use as evidence in court, should the need arise. Proper records may also be needed to prove a right to rehousing.

The practitioner should make clear notes which include the following:

1. Any data from the previous medical record which is suggestive of prior abuse.

2. The time, date and place of, and any witnesses to, the assault or accident.

3. The whereabouts of any children at the time of the assault or accident.

4. If the patient states that the injury was caused by abuse, preface the patient's explanation by writing: 'Patient states . . . '.

5. Any subjective data that might be used against the patient should be avoided (for example, 'It was my fault he hit me because I didn't have the kids in bed on time').

6. If the patient denies being assaulted, write: 'The patient's explanation of the injuries is inconsistent with the physical findings' and/or 'The injuries are suggestive of battering'.

7. Record the size, pattern, approximate age, description and location of all the injuries. A record of 'Multiple contusions and lacerations' will not convey a clear picture to a judge or jury, but 'Contusions and lacerations of the throat' will back up allegations of attempted strangling. If possible and appropriate, make a body map of the injuries, and include any signs of sexual abuse.

8. Record any non-bodily evidence of abuse, such as torn clothing, or damage to the home if the patient is seen on a home visit.

Photography

Whenever possible, photographs should be taken of all patients with visible injuries. If the practitioner is not equipped to do this, the patient should be advised to have photographs taken by a professional photographer or at the police station.

Protocol for handling photographic evidence

1. Explain to the patient that photographs will be very useful as evidence if she decides to prosecute the abuser either now or in the future.

2. Explain to the patient that the photographs will become part of her medical record and, as such, can only be released with the her explicit, written permission.

3. Obtain the patient's written consent to take photographs. Such written, informed consent should include the statement, 'These photographs will only be released if and when the undersigned gives written permission to release the medical records'.

4. Use a good Polaroid camera with colour film flash bulbs.

5. Photograph in the brightest light possible.

6. Attempt to take a close-up photograph of the injury, but try to include an identifiable feature of the patient. If this is not possible, a long shot should be followed by a close up.

7. The photographer should sign and date the back of each photograph.

8. Place the photographs in a sealed envelope and attach securely to the patient's record. Mark the envelope with the date and the notation 'Photographs of patient's [give name] injuries'.

9. Bruising is often more obvious 2 or 3 days after the injury. If this is likely to be the case, the patient should be advised to return at a later date, or to have more photographs taken elsewhere.

Assess, the present situation

The patient must be enabled and given time to tell her story.

—in order to understand the extent of the impact of violence on women, it is important not to pre-determine the meaning of the term. The starting point is to hear from women themselves and the meaning they attach to their experiences.[29]

It is important to gather as much information as possible, and to try to include the following:

1. Any past history of abuse (including past and present physical, emotional and/or sexual abuse).

2. Any attempts the patient has made to remedy her situation (for example, through police, courts, separation, refuges, and so on).

3. Any sources of emotional support available to her.

4. Details of her current living situation. Is there some place, other than home, where she can go to recover and take stock, if it is dangerous for her to return home?

5. The degree of immediate danger to herself, her children and the professionals involved with her:
   - Is the abuser verbally threatening her?
   - Is the abuser frightening her friends and relatives?
   - Is the abuser threatening to use weapons?
   - Is the abuser intoxicated?
   - Does the abuser have a criminal record?
   - Are the children in danger? Where are they at the moment?
   - Is there any perceived threat to the professionals involved? Has the abuser any history of violence to those outside the home?

Provide information[30]

All general practitioners and other primary health care professionals should assemble sufficient information about local resources and agencies so that they are able and prepared to inform the woman's choice of action, both immediately and in the future.

1. Explain to the patient that violence in the home is as illegal as violence on the street and that she is the victim of a crime and has legal rights.[28]

2. Explain the physical and emotional consequences of chronic battering.

3. Provide written information[31] about legal options and help offered by:

    - police domestic violence units;

    - Women's Aid National Helpline (Tel.: 08457 023468), Women's Aid refuges (Asian women's refuges and services available for women from other ethnic minorities can usually be contacted through Women's Aid);

    - local authority social services departments;

    - local authority housing departments;

    - the Benefit's Agency

4. Offer help in making contact with other agencies.

Devise a safety plan

In the context of a history of violence, often extending over many years, which erodes and destroys self-esteem, self-determination and autonomy, it is essential to understand that effective help must be directed towards enabling the woman to retake control of her own life. The aim should be to offer her realistic choices, while accepting that the decisions are hers alone and are always valid in her particular situation. No patient should ever be pressurized into following any particular course of action. Her individual autonomy, self-esteem and self-determination should be encouraged and respected. Even if the patient decides to return to the violent situation, she is not likely to forget the information and care given and, in time, this may help her to break out of the cycle of abuse. Beware of the danger of the needs of some ethnic minority patients being ignored under the guise of 'respect' for different cultures.

1. If she does not wish to return to the abuser, agree a plan of action and make an appropriate referral.

2. If she chooses to return to the abuser, discuss the following:[32]

    - a *protection plan*:
      (i)   when abuse is occurring, curl up into a ball to protect abdomen and head;

      (ii) remove potential weapons from the home;

      (iii) shout and scream loudly and continuously while being hit;

      (iv) if possible, arrange with a sympathetic neighbour that, if screams are heard, the neighbour will call 999;

      (v)   teach the children how to dial 999 if they feel unsafe;

- an *escape plan*:
    (i) encourage her to plan ahead for what she will do the next time abuse occurs; where will she go? how will she get there? what will she take?

    (ii) give her the phone number of the local women's refuge;

    (iii) Advise her to keep some money and important financial and legal documents hidden in a safe place, in case of emergency.

3. If children are likely to be at risk, seriously consider referral to social services, if possible with the patient's consent.

References

1 Doyle R. *The Woman Who Walked into Doors*. London: Jonathan Cape, 1996.

2 Heath I. *Domestic Violence: the General Practitioner's Role*. London: Royal College of General Practitioners, 1998.

3 Stark E, Flitcraft A. Women and children at risk: a feminist perspective on child abuse. *International Journal of Health Services* 1988; **18**; 97–118.

4 Pahl J. The general practitioner and the problems of battered women. *Journal of Medical Ethics* 1979; 5:117–23.

5 Mehta P, Dandrea L. The battered woman. *American Family Physician* 1988; **37**: 193–9.

6 Dobash RE, Dobash RP. *Violence Against Wives*. New York: Free Press, 1979.

7 Sugg NK, Inui T. Primary care physicians' response to domestic violence. Opening Pandora's box. *JAMA* 1992; **267**: 3157–60.

8 McWilliams M, McKiernan J. *Bringing it Out in the Open: Domestic Violence in Northern Ireland*. Belfast: HMSO, 1993.

9 Richardson J, Feder G. How can we help?—the role of general practice. In Bewley S, Friend J, Mezey G, eds. *Violence Against Women*. London: RCOG Press, 1997: 157–67.

10 Binney V, Harkell G, Nixon J. *Leaving Violent Men: a Study of Refuges and Housing for Battered Women*. Bristol: Women's Aid Federation (England), 1981.

11 Pahl J. Health professionals and violence against women. In: Kingston P, Penhale B, eds. *Family Violence and the Caring Professions*. Basingstoke: Macmillan Press, 1995: 00

12 Ochs HA, Neuenschwander MC, Dodson TB. Are head, neck and facial injuries markers of domestic violence? *Journal of the American Dental Association* 1996; **127** (6): 757–61.

13 Stark E, Flitcraft A, Frazier W. Medicine and patriarchal violence: the social construction of a 'private' event. *International Journal of Health Services* 1979; **9**: 461—93.

14 Jaffe P, Wolfe DA, Wilson S *et al.* Emotional and physical health problems of battered women. *Canadian Journal of Psychiatry* 1986; **31**: 625–9.

15 Fenton S, Sadiq A, eds. *The Sorrow in My Heart . . . Sixteen Asian Women Speak about Depression*. London: Commission for Racial Equality, 1993.

16 Mezey GC, Bewley S. Domestic violence and pregnancy. *BMJ* 1997; **314**: 1295.

17 Lent B, ed. *Reports on Wife Assault*. Ontario: Ontario Medical Association Committee on Wife Assault, 1991.

18 Stark E, Flitcraft A. *Women at Risk*. London: Sage, 1996.

19 Andrews B, Brown GW. Marital violence in the community. *British Journal of Psychiatry* 1988; **153**: 305–12.

20 Gayford JJ. Wife battering: a preliminary survey of 100 cases. *BMJ* 1975; **1**: 194–7

21 Abrahams C. *The Hidden Victims: Children and Domestic Violence.* London: NCH Action for Children, 1994.

22 British Medical Association. *Domestic Violence: a Health Care Issue?* London: British Medical Association, 1998.

23 Wilson P. Careless talk costs: the limits of confidentiality in histories of violence. In: Bewley S, Friend J, Mezey G, eds. *Violence Against Women.* London: RCOG Press, 1997: 291–301.

24 Stanko EA. Models of understanding violence against women. In: Bewley S, Friend J, Mezey G, eds. *Violence Against Women.* London: RCOG Press, 1997: 13–26.

25 Friedman LS, Samet JH, Roberts MS, Hudlin M, Hans P. Inquiry about victimization experiences. A survey of patient preferences and physician practices. *Archives of Internal Medicine* 1992; **152**: 1186–90.

26 Jones III RF. The abused woman. In: Bewley S, Friend J, Mezey G, eds. *Violence Against Women.* London: RCOG Press, 1997: 83–4.

27 Feldhaus KM, Koziol-McLain J, Amsbury HL *et al.* Accuracy of 3 brief screening questions for detecting partner violence in the emergency department. *JAMA* 1997; **277**:1357–61.

28 Jones III RF. Domestic violence—a physician's perspective. In: Bewley S, Friend J, Mezey G, eds. *Violence Against Women.* London: RCOG Press, 1997: 76–82.

29 Lloyd S. Defining violence against women. In: Bewley S, Friend J, Mezey G, eds. *Violence Against Women.* London: RCOG Press, 1997: 3–12.

30 Department of Health. Domestic violence: a resource manual for health care professionals. London: Department of Health Publications, 2000. (www.doh.gov.uk/domestic.htm)

31 Osborne J. *Domestic Violence Fact Pack.* London: HMSO, 1990.

32 Pahl J. Health professionals and violence against women. In: Kingston P, Penhale B, eds. *Family Violence and the Caring Professions.* Basingstoke: Macmillan Press, 1995.

33 Ransay J, Richardson J, Carter YH, Davidson LL, Feder G. Should health professionals screen women for domestic violence? Systemic review. *BMJ* 2002; **325**: 314–18.

Chapter 13

Onward referral

Chapter 13a

Introduction

Iona Heath

While, as detailed in the preceding chapter, there is much that the general practitioner can and should do for a woman presenting with a history of having been subjected to domestic violence, there is little scope for direct intervention (Fig. 13.1). Perhaps this is appropriate, because the medical profession is notorious for taking action on behalf of patients, whereas the key to escaping from domestic violence is through promoting the autonomy and self-determination of women themselves. None the less, however limited the practitioner's scope for providing direct help, members of the primary health care team are very well placed to provide information and to refer on to other agencies.

Depending on the circumstances, these agencies will include the local police domestic violence unit, Women's Aid (including those groups working with women from ethnic minority communities), local authority housing and social services departments, and solicitors and law centres. Every primary health care professional has a responsibility to obtain information about the relevant local agencies and to have up-to-date contact telephone numbers readily available.

The following subsections of Chapter 13 have been written by representatives of each of the major agencies, detailing the expertise, help and support they are able to offer to a woman experiencing domestic violence who presents in a general practitioner's surgery. Each has been asked to explain:

- what general practitioners need to know about the work their agency does in order to be able to work effectively and cooperatively with them;
- what general practitioners can expect of their agency in the context of domestic violence; and
- what general practitioners can do to help the work of the agency.

INADEQUATE
GENERAL PRACTITIONER
RESPONSE

HELPING FACTORS	HINDERING FACTORS
Desire to offer a high standard of service to all patients whatever their health need	Time constraints within general practitioner service
Long-term relationship of general practitioner and patient	Hidden presentation that offers the general practitioner the opportunity of collusion
Accessibility, acceptability and lack of stigma of the general practice consultation	Fear of revealing a problem that is difficult and time-consuming to tackle
Increasing 'partnership of experts' within general practice allowing empowerment of the patient	Sense of helplessness about being able to improve the situation combined with a fear of making things worse
Changing attitude towards domestic violence within society with lessening of stigma	Relationship between the general practitioner and the extended family
Services and information offered by Women's Aid	Difficulty of asking the question
Increased availability of information about services which can offer appropriate help	Inadequate record-keeping
Increasing presence of police domestic violence units	Lack of availability of information at the moment of the consultation
Heightened awareness of the prevalence of domestic violence	
Increasing understanding that domestic violence causes other health problems	

EFFECTIVE AND ENABLING
GENERAL PRACTITIONER
RESPONSE

Fig. 13.1 Forcefield analysis of general practitioner role in domestic violence.

Very occasionally, men will present to general practitioners, acknowledging their violence and asking for help in controlling their anger, or in altering a pattern of behaviour which they have recognized as destructive. Unfortunately, there are very few agencies offering specific help in such circumstances:

- the probation service is now working with men who are referred through the courts, and it may be worth seeking the advice of the Domestic Violence Intervention Project on 020 8563 7983;

- CHANGE based at 4–6 South Lumley Street, Grangemouth, FK3 8BT, telephone 01324 485595, has compiled a directory of organisations and agencies working with men who are violent to women (www.changeweb.org.uk);
- conventional psychiatry and psychology services may be able to offer help and advice.

However, general practitioners need to be aware of the dangers of offering a medical explanation for the crime of violence against women. Such an explanation would seem to require a medical solution and a way of avoiding the judicial consequences of criminal behaviour.

Much must and can be done for those who seek help both as survivors and, occasionally, as perpetrators, of domestic violence, but the recurring patterns which underpin the terrifying prevalence of domestic violence within our society will be altered only by fundamental changes in the social and economic structures which maintain the subordination of women.[1]

Health professionals may not feel in a position to alter the social and economic structures which support male dominance, but they should recognise that this is the context in which abused women approach them for help.[2]

References

1 **United Nations.** *Violence Against Women in the Family.* Vienna: Centre for Social Development and Humanitarian Affairs, United Nations, 1989.
2 **Pahl J.** Health professionals and violence against women. In: Kingston P, Penhale B, eds. *Family Violence and the Caring Professions.* Basingstoke: Macmillan Press, 1995.

Chapter 13b

The role of the police

Susan Reed

The police service is committed to taking positive action to assist victims of domestic violence.

Definition of domestic violence for police purposes

Domestic violence is defined in the Home Office *Interagency Circular* as including any form of physical, sexual or emotional abuse between people in a close relationship. It can take a number of forms such as physical assault, sexual abuse, rape and intimidation. It may be accompanied by other kinds of intimidation such as degradation, mental and verbal abuse, humiliation, depravation, systematic criticism and belittling.

The offender or victim may be of either gender and regardless of this the victim will be provided with the correct referrals and support by police. The relationship between the parties include husband and wife, boyfriend and girlfriend, gay relationships and any parent–offspring combinations. Disabled persons cared for by a relative or partner are particularly vulnerable because their carer may be the only person on whom they depend, and making an allegation against their carer could result in the victim being placed in a community home. Domestic violence can affect any individual regardless of their social standing, culture or environment.

Police objectives

In order to offer victims support, dedicated units were introduced into the Metropolitan police service from 1987. Every London borough now has domestic violence services incorporated within a Community Safety Unit and county forces operate similar schemes.

The work of the units incorporates:

1. Ensuring that every allegation of domestic violence is properly investigated.

2. Ensuring that incidents are not treated in isolation but are considered in the light of any previous history.

3. Maintaining records of the civil remedies, including injunctions with power of arrest.

4. Establishing links with other agencies so that victims can be made aware of the full range of services that may assist them.

The police role is to provide a gateway to other services and does not seek to take on the responsibilities and functions of other agencies involved in the field.

Aims of the community safety unit

The unit provides support and relevant options to the victim and aims to reduce crime and repeat victimization. Early intervention is the key; we actively encourage the public to seek advice at the earliest opportunity, even if the incident appears only minor.

The victim may have a multitude of options available, dependent on the circumstances. Where criminal offences have been committed an arrest of the aggressor is only one option and this may not be the solution sought by the victim.

Referral options

Referral options can range from solicitors regarding applications made under civil law, to liaison with housing departments or social services. The police, together with the victim, attempt to identify the cause of the problems and to seek appropriate solutions.

In many of the cases alcohol features strongly and if this is determined as the cause then referral would be made to some form of alcohol management counselling. Referrals may be appropriate for the victim, aggressor or for both parties.

Contacting victims

Victims contact the unit in various ways, some have seen local literature and contact the unit directly for advice, others have been referred by police officers or external agencies.

A report compiled by the officer attending the incident will be forwarded to the unit. Contact with the victim is made by telephone where possible, or alternatively by letter. Once contact has been established officers from the unit will arrange to meet the victim at a location suitable to them, e.g. a local park or cafe. The officers in the units do not generally wear uniform, which facilitates their ability to meet victims in any surrounding.

Prosecution cases

The case will be followed through by the unit and the victim is kept informed at each stage of the investigation. If the matter is one in which a charge has been preferred and the case is in the process of going to court, the victim will have each step of the procedure explained and will be provided with ongoing support.

After the charge, police will actively seek bail conditions to be imposed on the aggressor; this would mean that the victim would be offered some protection from the aggressor pressurizing them to withdraw allegations. The conditions may vary but in the main it would consist of the following type of restrictions, where the aggressor would be forbidden from:

- attending the home address;
- contacting the victim directly or indirectly.

There may also be a condition stating that the aggressor resides at a stated alternative address.

If the victim is required to give evidence at the trial then arrangements can be made for them to be met at the court by either an officer or a member of the victim support service, depending on the style of the trial. Attendance at court for the victim is always stressful, particularly as this may be the first occasion since the incident that they have seen their aggressor. Support for the victim is offered until police involvement is no longer appropriate or necessary.

The following are some examples of the types of cases dealt with by the police units.

Case study 1

Case

Mrs Green was the main carer for her husband. Mr Green suffered from multiple sclerosis and was confined to a wheel chair. They lived in a private address in an exclusive area. Mrs Green had been looking after her husband's needs for about 5 years and this included bathing, dressing and feeding him. Friends became alarmed when they received phone calls from Mr Green stating that his wife had been ill-treating him. The friends would call at the address but found that Mrs Green was reluctant to let them in and often gave weak excuses as to why their visit was inconvenient. In desperation the friends turned to the domestic violence unit for guidance.

The unit made sensitive enquiries, working closely with social services. The investigation revealed that Mrs Green, due to the stress of caring for her husband 24 hours a day, had developed the condition obsessive compulsive disorder. This had the effect that Mrs Green would clean excessively. Mrs Green's reluctance to admit visitors was mainly because their presence aggravated her condition. It also transpired that Mr Green had suffered assaults from his wife as she had frequently used a brillo pad to wash him. This behaviour was linked directly to her obsessive disorder.

Conclusion

There was evidence of assault by Mrs Green on her husband. Realistically arrest would not have been a suitable option. Following a case conference with social services, immediate arrangements were made for Mr and Mrs Green to receive respite. The situation is now continually monitored and the couple have the support of social services.

Case study 2

Case

The unit received a request by a head teacher of a local primary school to meet with a parent who needed advice. Officers attended and met privately with Miss Blue, a young parent. She was in a distressed state and nervously she relayed her story. Miss Blue stated that her partner was insecure and possessive to the extreme. She was, however, quick to state there had never been any violence in their relationship. Mr Brown's insecurities had manifested themselves in his not allowing his partner to bathe, change her clothes or wear make-up. When Miss Blue went shopping her partner would not only give her the exact monies required but also timed her. Her partner would threaten to take the youngest child if she failed to return within the allotted time. Mr Brown ensured that Miss Blue had no financial means of her own—all part of his controlling behaviour.

The victim wanted to know what choices and resources were available to her. Miss Blue stated that she feared for the safety of the children and was concerned that where ever she went they would be found by her partner.

Conclusion

Arrangements were made for Miss Blue to meet us at the school the following day. This was the only legitimate time she could be away from her partner. Miss Blue was advised to bring with her the child benefit books, cheque book, birth certificates and rent book. The amount of clothing she could conceal was limited to essentials only. At the agreed time we transported the victim and children to a refuge outside the locality. The arrangements for her accommodation had already been made and the staff at the refuge were appraised of her situation.

Miss Blue remained within the refuge system for a few weeks before being rehoused by another borough. No further police intervention has been necessary.

Case study 3

Case

Mrs White had been separated from her husband for 5 years and divorced for the last 3 years. It had been alleged that Mr White had cut the telephone wire at the address of his ex-wife. He regularly called at the address to visit their youngest son aged 10 years. Mrs White was contacted by an officer from the unit but the victim declined any offer of advice or support.

Several weeks later Mrs White contacted the unit and asked to meet us. When she arrived at the station we noted excessive bruising to her face around both eyes. Mrs White stated that Mr White had punched her in the face causing the blackened eyes and fractured nose and eventually related her account of the incident. Mrs White stated that since the divorce her ex-husband still had control over her and she was in fear of him. Mr White visited her address regularly and forced her to have sex with him; her consent was not given freely. Mrs White told us that when her ex-husband wanted sex he would grab her around the neck and squeeze until she would lose consciousness, when she came round she would find her clothes dishevelled and she knew he had had sex with her. On this occasion as he placed his hands around her neck she fought back—something in her mind had snapped. For years she had accepted that this was a part of her life but at that moment she decided that she could capitulate no more. The victim struggled with him and he lashed out with his fists causing the injuries to her face. Mrs White, although quite badly injured, told us that she thought that she had got off lightly this time.

Conclusion

All the options—both criminal and civil—were explained to the victim. After careful consideration she decided to provide police with a statement regarding the assault but did not pursue the allegations of rape. Mr White was subsequently arrested and charged with the assault and received a fine imposed by the court, a suspended sentence and was ordered to pay the victim compensation.

The penalty imposed by the court is not as important as the two messages that it sends, firstly that a court of law had decided that this behaviour is unacceptable and secondly that the victim regains control of her life and starts to value herself as a person.

Often victims comment that something in them suddenly gives them the courage and strength to stop the violence. For some victims the first assault would promote the need to take action, but for others the violence continues for years. The decision is an individual one and not everyone finds a solution, but it is vital the necessary support is in place should they seek help.

Case study 4

Case

Mrs Grey contacted the unit and requested that officers visited her home address. It was ascertained that Mr Grey was away at a conference and there was no likelihood of him returning unexpectedly. Mrs Grey was nervous and reluctant to enter into conversation. Throughout the visit Mrs Grey kept looking over to a small, patterned, plastic food mat which was positioned on the floor next to the back door. Mrs Grey stated that she had married young and that her life had been dominated and controlled by her husband. For years he had assaulted her if she did not do things exactly the way he wanted. Mr Grey was a professional, articulate man and Mrs Grey thought no-one would believe her if she reported the assaults. Mrs Grey later revealed to us that the mat on the floor was where she ate her meals as her husband would not allow her to eat at the table.

Conclusion

After considering her options and with the support of the unit, Mrs Grey left the relationship. Mrs Grey later divorced her husband on the grounds of unreasonable behaviour. Although Mrs Grey decided not to pursue any criminal allegations against her husband she did obtain an injunction to keep her husband away.

Children

Children are also the victims of domestic violence or abuse. Often it is the children who witness these assaults and the effect can be detrimental to their development. In cases where there are children involved or present, and it is believed that they are either in danger themselves or there are concerns for their welfare, a referral report will be submitted to social services.

Why would someone stay in a violent relationship?

There are many diverse reasons given for parties remaining together, such as: financial, housing, children, families, loyalty and love. Often the victim either still loves or has feelings for their aggressor. It is because of this that this type of crime is so unique. With the abuse comes the constant erosion of a person's self-worth and confidence; it is this more than anything that prevents the victim from seeking the help they so desperately need.

What can the general practitioner offer?

A sympathetic and non-judgemental approach is the first step to helping someone along the road from victim to survivor. Most police areas have some type of domestic violence unit and these can be contacted either directly or via the local station. It would be beneficial for general practitioners to acquaint themselves with the resources that are available to them locally.

It would be impossible to cover every aspect of the unit's work, but as a general rule if the matter is of a domestic nature, within the definition given, then consideration should be given to referring the patient to the domestic unit. If a GP requires any advice regarding this subject they should contact their local police station. All enquires are dealt with in confidence.

If a patient informs their GP that they have been assaulted, the injuries should be recorded fully, as the patient may wish to subsequently use this for evidential purposes. Police will often make requests for statements by doctors in relation to their examination of particular patients. For certain categories of assault it is unlikely that an aggressor will be charged without the necessary medical evidence, therefore the GP's cooperation in expediently dealing with any requests will facilitate the investigation and provide the victim and their family with the immediate protection of the courts.

Chapter 13c

The role of Women's Aid and refuge support services

Nicola Harwin

Introduction

For over 25 years, Women's Aid refuge services throughout the UK have given practical and emotional support to women and children living with violence and abuse. In the absence of legal or statutory provision, the first refuges were set up in response to women's desperate need for a place to stay with their children, where their violent partners could not find them. Since those early days, Women's Aid has continued to be the key support agency for women and children experiencing physical, emotional and sexual violence and abuse in their homes, and has continued to expand the range of services and improve the quality of refuge provision.

Women's Aid is the national organization that supports and resources the English network of over 250 local refuge projects. There are also sister organizations in Wales, Scotland and Northern Ireland. We offer a unique national network of safe accommodation, specialist help, advocacy and residential and outreach support.

In England alone 53 000 women and children use refuges each year, and there are over 150 000 calls to Women's Aid services for advice and help.[1] Research shows that refuges are the only services which are consistently praised by women who have experienced violence.[2] Refuges are not just a resource for 'when all else fails', but an integral part of the process of obtaining protection under the criminal and civil justice systems, a role clearly recognized by the Inter-Agency Working Party report[3] and the *Home Affairs Select Committee Report into Domestic Violence.*[4]

The Women's Aid approach

The main values and principles of the Women's Aid approach are:

- To believe women and children's experience of abuse, and make their safety a priority.
- To support and empower women to take control of their own lives.
- To recognize and care for the needs of children affected by domestic violence.
- To promote equal opportunities and antidiscrimination in all our work and services.

The work and standards of local member groups are informed by these principles and by other policy statements and good practice guidelines. The majority of our members are local refuges and agencies that run support services for women and children. Refuges offer a safe breathing space for women and children escaping domestic violence.

Local Women's Aid organisations provide a range of services that benefit women and children, including:

- 24-hour access to emergency refuge;
- information, advice and support;
- outreach support to women who may not want refuge;
- advocacy: legal and welfare rights;
- specialized services for children;
- aftercare and follow-up;
- education and public awareness.

Prioritizing women and children's safety

A key role of refuge services has been to offer women safe confidential help and safe emergency accommodation. A crucial part of this is protecting the secrecy of refuges and the confidentiality of telephone numbers and addresses. This safety can be threatened if agencies fail to understand the realities of abused women's experiences, and how charming and devious abusive men can be in order to find women.

The concern of Women's Aid organisations to protect the safety of women and children escaping domestic violence is an important feature of the *Women's Aid refuge network*. It offers safety and security to women and children who may need to move out of their local area to another part of England, or elsewhere in the United Kingdom, where they cannot easily be found by their partners. If a woman's whereabouts is discovered, she can very quickly be moved to another refuge, and will be given support in settling herself and her children in the new area. For this reason telephone numbers and addresses of refuges are kept confidential, although many organisations can be contacted through a dedicated public line.

Women's Aid nationally has clear guidelines on *confidentiality* including confidentiality in relation to female service users (whether or not they are resident in the refuge), children, employees, management committee members, etc. Women's Aid organisations groups do not disclose information to other agencies without the woman's knowledge and consent. If confidentiality has to be limited or breached then this is made clear to the woman, but the limits to confidentiality are primarily in relation to children and child abuse issues, and this is made clear from the outset.

Women's Aid also operates an '*open door*' policy, which means that no woman or child needing refuge will be turned away without assistance. Women can refer themselves to a refuge, rather than having to be reliant on an official organization, and Women's Aid refuge services do not require women to offer proof of physical violence. This does not mean that refuges will accept all referrals however full they are; but it does mean that Women's Aid will not turn women away without assistance, and will either offer emergency overnight accommodation, will find another refuge place or will help women obtain other emergency accommodation, e.g. bed and breakfast.

Working with abused women: promoting empowerment

Being in a refuge, or in contact with other women survivors, allows women to get a breathing space from an abusive situation and reflect on their own needs, and to overcome their isolation and sense of shame, which many women feel at being abused by a partner, ex-partner or family member. A vital aspect of ending an abusive relationship can be the opportunity to share experiences with other survivors—through talking and discussion, and through mutual support with dealing with day to day problems and practical tasks. Many women who use refuge services have stayed involved with Women's Aid and have later become volunteers or paid staff themselves.

For women who have been in abusive relationships with men, becoming empowered means taking control back from the abuser. They are able to gain self-esteem, self-confidence and the financial, material and emotional resources to control their own lives, rather than living under the influence or control of a violent man. For this reason, the principle of the women-only group—women helping women—can support this process by providing powerful role modelling. Many women also prefer to receive services from female staff in helping agencies.[5] Finally, refuge services run by women for women can contribute to maintaining safety and security procedures within the refuge or advice centre. This need not compromise interagency working or the individual support needs of users as male professionals such as solicitors or doctors can visit or be involved by prior arrangement.

The range of services offered by Women's Aid

The refuge

A refuge is the basic building block of provision—safe emergency accommodation is one of the most vital needs of women and children escaping violence. Women can stay in a refuge from one night to 2 years, and many women will use refuges more than once as part of the process of ending an abusive relationship. However, if refuge security has been breached, and the address becomes known to the violent partner of a woman wishing to re-enter the refuge, she may have to be referred elsewhere. Individual refuge policies on this issue will vary.

Refuge provision varies enormously from purpose-built or renovated houses for five or more families, to three bedroom accommodation, let on short-term lease from a local authority, although the latter are now relatively rare. In recognition of institutional racism as well as the specific cultural or practical needs of some women, there are a number of specialist refuges. There are specialist refuge services for black women (African women, Asian women), as well as other specific ethnic groups (e.g. Turkish women, Latin American women).

Although refuges have to operate as safe emergency accommodation for many women, often with a high turnover, Women's Aid refuges try to create a home-like atmosphere for families. In practice this also means supporting women to learn to live cooperatively with other women and children and to share responsibility for the management of the house on a day-to-day basis. Staff facilitate regular weekly house meetings to air problems and discuss issues, as well as to agree rotas for cleaning and other tasks. In some refuges, children's support workers facilitate similar meetings for children, to help empower them and to encourage non-aggressive resolution of problems and conflicts.

Advocacy and support with all aspects of legal, welfare and housing rights

A key element of all our work is providing support for women and children and advocating on their behalf with all the agencies with which they have to interact as part of the process of ending the violence. Emotional and practical help and support is offered with all aspects of legal, welfare, housing and financial matters. A refuge is often used a safe place from which to apply for legal protection, or as a last resort when injunctions fail (as they do so often). Access to safe alternative accommodation is often the only way to live free from abuse, and Women's Aid has worked for many years to improve public housing policy and local authority responses to women and children homeless because of violence.

Day-to-day experience of the ineffectiveness of legal protection for abused women and children under both the civil and criminal law has meant that Women's Aid has consistently lobbied for better provision and enforcement. From the beginning we have also been 'institutional advocates', lobbying for improvements to law, policies and practice in relation to domestic violence, and working with other agencies and practitioners to initiate and implement changes in criminal justice, social welfare and housing responses to violence against women and children in their homes.

Outreach

There has always been a demand for help and support from women who, for whatever reason, do not want to use refuges, as well as from women in temporary accommodation such as bed and breakfast or local authority hostels, where no support or help is provided. In practice this has often been difficult to meet, because of the disjuncture between our resources and the level of demand. Women's Aid offers both aftercare to ex-residents and outreach to non-residents. On average, refuge organisations give aftercare support to 24 families per year, although only 10 per cent have specific staff for this work.[6] The demand on for Women's Aid outreach services has also significantly increased since the improvement of responses by some other agencies, notably the police.

The range of outreach work undertaken locally has expanded through a number of recent initiatives: for example, the development of separate advice centres, specialist projects for Asian women, and a number of rural initiatives. Outreach work in conjunction with primary health care professionals such as health visitors and GPs is also being developed in some areas. The success of mutual support systems in refuges provides a model for the development of support groups of women survivors within the community. In some areas these groups have operated from Women's Aid drop-in centres and have been run for both non-residents and ex-residents of refuges.

Work with children in Women's Aid

Many children coming into refuges have themselves been abused; some may have been forced to watch or take part in abuse of their mothers; some will have tried to intervene and stop the violence; most will also have suffered indirectly from the abuse their mother have experienced. Research into work with children in refuges has shown, however, that the effects of witnessing or experiencing domestic violence can be alleviated or reversed if child-centred activities and adequate support and resources are available.[7]

All refuge organisations provide specific services and resources for children and over 75 per cent have children's support workers. These staff are not just 'play workers' but also do one-to-one work, group work and run holiday schemes, as well as providing advocacy for children to outside agencies and liaison with schools, education and welfare departments, health visitors, etc.

Over the last 10 years, Women's Aid has developed a national training programme for refuge staff and external agencies to improve policy development and service provision to abused women and children. Underlying all work with children, both in and after their stay in refuges, is a recognition of the need to promote non-violent relationships, to support women and children to develop non-violent strategies for managing family life, as well as to challenge traditional sex-role stereotyping which can reinforce and support abusive relationships.

Over the last 25 years, refuge services have often had a key role in identifying child abuse, as children may disclose for the first time to childworkers. Many Women's Aid organisations in England are jointly developing child protection policies and procedures with their local social services departments. These aim to satisfy both the needs of social services to protect children, and our commitment to protecting and empowering both women and children. Our guiding principle is that the safety and empowerment of the non-abusing parent (usually the mother) is the most effective form of child protection. Women's Aid has a national child protection policy and has issued detailed guidance on working with children.

Education, public awareness and interagency work

Education and public awareness have always been a key focus of local and national activity, as the biggest problem we encounter are the prevailing attitudes to domestic violence. Unhelpful stereotypes abound about 'types' of women, 'types' of families, alcohol, drugs and poverty as being the cause of violence. All of these are discounted by research[2] and the practical experience of the Women's Aid movement over the past 25 years. Local services have for many years tried to raise awareness of the extent of the problem through local talks, media contact and joint initiatives with specific local voluntary and statutory agencies. More recently, Women's Aid has been in the forefront of multiagency initiatives to tackle domestic violence, although their development has not been unproblematic, given the differences in status and knowledge of participating agencies.[5] The specific expertise of Women's Aid, and our unique status as the only agency to offer independent advocacy for women and children escaping domestic violence, makes our participation vital. The Home Office Interagency Circular of August 95 recommends that statutory agencies, with more resources, should look at how they can enable this.

Referral and contact

Referral procedures vary locally. Many local services now have separate public numbers, but the addresses and phone numbers of the refuges themselves are confidential and may only be given out to specific agencies or individuals, when it is made clear that they must not be passed on without permission, or given out to violent partners or other family members in any circumstances. Women frequently self-refer via word of mouth, and Women's Aid refuges rarely require women to offer proof of violence.

Many groups also have separate public telephone numbers and can be found in the telephone directory. Out of normal working hours, some groups have 24-hour contact via telephone switch-over systems or pagers; others organize out of hours referrals through other 24-hour services like the police, the Samaritans or the emergency duty team of social services who then contact the refuge; some groups only have resources to have answerphones at night with the telephone number for the police and some other agencies on them. However, over 50 per cent of groups do provide 24-hour contact systems or helplines, using rotas of staff and voluntary members.

Thirty per cent of refuge projects have separate offices or advice centres that offer a public drop-in point for face to face help and advice; others will arrange to meet women in safe locations if they just want to talk.

If the local refuge is full, then staff or volunteers will either support the woman in applying to the local housing department for emergency accommodation, or find her a place in a refuge out of the area until space becomes available. For some women referral on to another refuge is the preferred option if they have friends or family elsewhere or feel it is too dangerous to stay in their local area.

To support this national network of provision, the national office of Women's Aid publishes and regularly updates the only UK-wide directory of refuge and helpline services 'The GoldBook'. This is available online on the Women's Aid Website at www.womensaid.org.uk. Access to local services and support is also facilitated by the *Women's Aid National Helpline* (tel: 08457 023 468) and by other regional and locally based helplines.

Any agency or practitioner is advised to contact their local refuge service to find out their local referral procedures, or for more information on specific policy aspects of referrals. Admissions policies will vary; although member groups within the Women's Aid Federation strive to operate an 'open door' policy, which means that no woman or child needing refuge will be turned away without assistance to find some safe accommodation. However project guidelines may vary—some refuges have admissions policies that limit access for families with teenage boys, or women with substance dependencies. 'Open door' may be limited in practice by access for women with disabilities or by lack of provision for women with specific language or cultural requirements.

How can GPs and health care services support the work of Women's Aid by responding more effectively to women experiencing domestic violence?

The recent publication of reports on domestic violence by professional medical bodies such as the British Medical Association and the Royal College of Obstetricians and Gynaecologists have begun to indicate the challenge facing the medical profession and health service providers. Some of the practical ways that we can improve options for abused women, and develop common ground for joint working with Women's Aid, are indicated below.

Developing a proactive approach

- Acknowledge the extent of domestic violence: between 10 and 47 per cent of female patients may have a history of domestic violence and be at risk.[8]

- Recognize that active intervention is beneficial, reducing the risk of death, suicide or serious injury to women, as well as reducing the risk of harm to children; the financial costs of non-intervention are also significant.

- Develop a policy and practice approach that can promote women's safety and choice.

- Develop an understanding of the dynamics of abuse in order to develop appropriate responses, and to overcome feelings of embarrassment, powerlessness and frustration. Recognize that ending a violent relationship can be a very lengthy and traumatic process, and that a woman may see reconciliation as the safest course for her immediate survival when legal and social systems are not effective.

- Break the 'chasm of silence' that can exist between doctors and women experiencing domestic violence.

Practical steps

- Insist that you see women separately at some point in the consultation.

- Assure confidentiality and clarify any limits to this (i.e. where risks to children may be involved).

- Ask questions directly and routinely.

- Give clear messages about the unacceptability of domestic violence, both in the surgery and in waiting areas.

- Give information directly about sources of help and ensure that this is also clearly displayed in waiting areas, examination rooms and women's toilets.

- Make informed referrals to Women's Aid and other agencies as appropriate.

- Support women to take control (e.g. by offering access to a telephone to contact help agencies).

- Offer women opportunities to talk at more length if specialist counselling or support group services are available in your practice.

- Help your patient draw up an escape plan if she is not yet ready to leave: emergency clothes, money, important documents, addresses and telephone numbers could be stored with a family member or neighbour; plan how she can contact help at any time.

- Document evidence of abuse and its effects on the woman for use in legal proceedings.

Take a clear position on perpetrators

- Do not condone statements that try to place the blame on the woman.

- Do not confront the abuser without asking the woman or making sure she is safe.

- Do not give any information or hints that will lead him to her.

- Do not be 'charmed'—abusive men are not monsters, they can seem very nice people—but they are dangerous to 'their' women.

- Remember, abusers avoid taking responsibility for their actions: they deny, minimize, lie and justify.

Enabling health care for women and children staying in refuges

In many areas, refuge services have reported problems in accessing GP services for women and children living in the refuge, including situations where women had to register with a doctor several kilometres away because local practices would not take them on. Direct reasons are frequently not given, but are likely to relate to attitudes to domestic violence and refuge occupants as well as to the nature of the health care demands. In multioccupation, the effects of domestic violence impact on the already exacerbated health problems of several families, resulting in high level of health care needs. The presence of many young children, and the cumulative effect in terms of out of hours calls and home visits, must also be understood in the context of the risks women may face when going outside the refuge. In the USA, shelters routinely offer in-house health services of all kinds, but so far there are only relatively few designated health visitors in some areas of the UK.

GPs urgently need to lobby for funding allocations by primary care organizations to reflect the higher per capita costs involved, so that abused women and children are not once again penalized for a situation that is not of their making.

Joint work with Women's Aid

As a first step it is important to clarify the range of services provided by your local refuge organisation including local contact and referral systems (see above). This might be best achieved by asking the local service to meet with practice staff or to run a training session. It is also important to give feedback where systems are not working effectively in order that improvements can be made.

There may also be opportunities to develop specialist advice and support services within local health centres, provided by Women's Aid staff in conjunction with health professionals, as a potential solution to the problem of the busy GP, and the need for further counselling or practical support. Women identified through other contacts, e.g., antenatal clinics or specialist interpreting services, where they exist, could also be referred on. Lack of resources is a current problem; Women's Aid organisations have very limited resources as the core service is often already dependent on the support of committed volunteers. If, however, resources could be found to set up advice surgeries or to run support groups within the aegis of the health centre, this could provide a crucial safe access point for women.

Such developments are likely to depend on the whether individuals within the health service are prepared to advocate on the issue of domestic violence, and to press health care trusts and government for the resources needed to meet this problem. Despite the growth of multiagency work to tackle domestic violence in the last few years, there are currently very few health professionals involved directly and this absence needs to be rectified. GPs, like professionals and activists in other parts of the welfare and criminal justice system, need to use their expert status in the public interest, to press for changes to the laws, policy and practice that restrict abused women and children of access to full human rights.

References

1 **Women's Aid.** *Women's Aid Annual Report, 1996–1997.* Bristol: Women's Aid Federation of England, 1997.

2 **Smith L.** *Domestic Violence.* Working Paper No. 107. London: HMSO, 1989.

3 **Victim Support.** *Domestic Violence: Report of a National Inter-Agency Working Party.* London: Victim Support, 1992.

4 **Home Affairs Select Committee.** *Home Affairs Select Committee Report into Domestic Violence.* London: HMSO, 1993.

5 **Malos E, Hague G, Dear W.** *Multi-agency Work and Domestic Violence.* Bristol: Policy Press, 1996.

6 **Ball M.** *Funding Refuge Services.* Bristol: Women's Aid Federation of England, 1994.

7 **Ball M.** Children's Workers in Women's Aid Refuges: a report on the experience of nine refugees in England. London: National Council of Voluntary Child Care Organisations, 1990.

8 **Warshaw C, Ganley AL.** *Improving the Health Care Response to Domestic Violence: a Resources Manual for Health Care Providers.* San Francisco: Family Violence Prevention Fund, 1995.

Chapter 13d

Local authority housing departments

Sarah Edwards

Introduction

Interagency working at strategic and operational level is essential to make the link between health and housing services. Practitioners working in primary health care are often the first professionals to whom a victim of domestic violence presents their problem. Therefore, effective joint working arrangements between general practitioners and housing professionals must be in place to help anyone fleeing from actual or threatened domestic violence.

The statutory joint consultative committee and joint care planning teams should provide a central framework for coordinating strategy and service delivery. However, it is helpful for general practitioners to understand how their local housing authority works, and to establish contact with housing practitioners. This will help to break down professional barriers and facilitate the development of local protocols for confidential onward referrals for women patients fleeing domestic violence.

How local authority housing departments work

Over the last decade local authorities have experienced a period of great change. They have been encouraged to take on a more strategic role and to commission others to provide new social housing. As a result, fewer and fewer authorities are developing new rented housing. Instead, they are working in partnership with housing associations, private sector developers and the voluntary sector. Some local authorities have competitively tendered their housing services and others have transferred all or part of their housing stock to other housing organizations. Many local authorities have also streamlined access to social housing through common housing registers. However, despite these changes, local authorities still own and manage about 60 per cent of social rented housing and they retain ultimate responsibility in relation to homelessness.

Local authority housing advice and homelessness services

The way local authorities operate their advisory and homeless persons housing services varies from area to area. Historically, provision was often linked into local factors such as the geography, population and demand for services.

Many local housing authorities have a separate homeless persons unit, which operates in office hours, and an emergency contact number is made available for use outside office hours. They usually offer access to a range of temporary accommodation, which may include women's refuges, hostels and other supported accommodation, unsupported accommodation or, as a last resort, bed and breakfast.

Local authority statutory responsibilities

The Housing Act 1996 gave all local authorities a new responsibility to make sure that advice and information about homelessness and the prevention of homelessness is available free of charge to any person in their area (Section 179). Local authorities can meet this duty by providing the service themselves; securing the service from some other organization; or working in partnership with another organization.

Although this is a new statutory duty, some authorities had already provided appropriate advisory services whilst others are developing new or existing services. The Act provides an impetus for authorities to look at their existing housing advice services and to take the opportunity to rethink their housing advice strategies.

The Chartered Institute of Housing (CIH) advises authorities to provide comprehensive housing advisory services.[1] It also recommends that services should cover a range of functions including: information, advice, assistance, advocacy, policy development, training, education and publicity services; and that 'Housing advice strategies should be developed in partnership with a range of local bodies, including housing associations, private landlords, mortgage lenders, voluntary agencies, social services departments, health authorities and local users of services'.

Joint planning and operational cooperation between housing and health

Many of the provisions of the Housing Act 1996 (Part VI and VII) require joint planning and operational cooperation between local housing authorities and health authorities. The Department of the Environment and Department of Health (DOE/DOH) *Code of Guidance on Parts VI and VII of the Housing Act 1996*[2] emphasizes the importance of joint working, stating that a joint approach should be agreed between local housing and social services and health authorities to include:

- Mechanisms and triggers for referral between housing, health and social services in relation to housing and community care issues, and alerting relevant agencies of any difficulties.

- The assessment of individuals who require emergency accommodation.
- The identification of clients with interdependent health, housing and social services needs.

In the context of domestic violence, it is essential for GPs to have effective links for the onward referral of patients to local housing authorities and appropriate voluntary agencies.

Domestic disputes and homelessness

The Housing Act 1996 provides some helpful clarification of the definition of domestic violence as meaning:

- *violence from a person with whom s/he is associated*; or
- *threats of violence from such a person which are likely to be carried out.*

In some cases of domestic dispute, threatened or actual homelessness may arise and authorities should be ready to assist where household members are at risk of violence or abuse.

The DOE/DOH 1996 code recommends that in assessing homelessness, local authorities should consider whether it is reasonable for a person to continue to occupy accommodation if s/he would be subject to domestic violence. Section 177 of the Housing Act 1996 provides that it is not reasonable for a person to continue to occupy accommodation if it is probable that this will lead to domestic violence against him/her.

The Code also clarifies the following:

- the violence or threat of violence is not confined to the home but extends to violence outside the home;
- it should not be assumed that the violence is unlikely to occur because it has not yet occurred; and
- no applicant for assistance under the homelessness provisions due to domestic violence should be obliged to take out an injunction if s/he thinks it would be ineffective.

Working effectively with local authority housing departments

In 1992, the report of the Victim Support Working Party on Domestic Violence[3] recommended the formation of local, multiagency domestic violence forums. This was also supported by the Home Office, when it issued a circular in 1995, on behalf of the Inter-Departmental Group on Domestic Violence which emphasized that interagency coordination is one of the principal planks of government policy on domestic violence.[4]

However, although many local authority housing departments have historically developed excellent interagency links with social services, police and voluntary agencies, links with health have often been much poorer. Indeed a recent national study[5] of interagency initiatives as responses to domestic violence found that although there are at least 200 forums nationally, 'health services were very frequently absent and the research found evidence that their greater involvement would be widely welcomed'.

An example of a local authority domestic violence policy procedure

The London Borough of Greenwich has a comprehensive domestic violence policy[6] produced to promote good practice amongst frontline staff who deal with issues arising from domestic violence. The policy procedure contains details of its homeless services, options and support, tenancy issues, action against perpetrators, and interpreting services; it also emphasizes the importance of confidentiality and security.

It has a multiagency domestic violence forum, which includes representatives from the voluntary sector, health, the refuges and the police. Copies of the policy have been sent to all general practitioners in Greenwich and direct referrals will be taken from them.

How general practitioners can cooperate with local authorities

The CIH's recent publication *Housing and Health: A Good Practice Briefing*[7] provides many examples of effective joint working between housing and health. One of these if the East Surrey Housing Strategy Group, which brings together senior staff from district councils, social services, the health authority and health trusts. It has regular meetings that provide networking benefits and a chance to share experiences and problems. The group also works on joint projects such as a referral service for all special needs groups in East Surrey.

The CIH *Housing Management Standards Manual*[8] recommends that social housing landlords should treat women who are homeless because of violence or threats of violence sympathetically and in accordance with the law. It features several examples of good practice including:

- The London Borough of Hackney—Hackney has a well-established Domestic Violence (Housing) Advice Service. It provides general advice on legal, welfare, housing and benefits issues and offers support to women in need. Referrals are taken direct from women themselves and a wide variety of other sources including GPs and health centres.

- Leeds City Council and Manchester City Council—these are examples of authorities that do not require corroboration that violence or threats of violence have taken place.

Finally, the *Code of Guidance*[2] for homeless people places great emphasis on the importance of joint working between housing and health. The code is currently under review but the emphasis on joint working is not expected to be diluted in the revised version.

In conclusion, although some local authorities already have excellent domestic violence policies, many do not. It is essential that more effective partnerships are developed to break down professional barriers and promote more effective interagency work.

Good practice points

1. Get a copy of your local authority's domestic violence policy.

2. Find out what domestic violence and interagency initiatives currently exist in your district and whether or not the health authority is represented.

3. Make sure that the local joint consultative committee and joint care planning teams are aware of the need to develop joint domestic violence policies and good practice protocol for referrals and confidentiality.

4. Write to the chief executive at your local authority and invite a senior housing officer to visit your practice to give a presentation about housing services for people fleeing domestic violence.

5. Establish named contacts at your local housing authority, housing associations and Women's Aid refuges for onward referral.

6. Display up-to-date literature about housing and domestic violence in your waiting rooms.

7. Be aware of the specialist needs of people from black and minority ethnic groups and make sure that information is available in appropriate languages.

References

1 **Grant C.** *Housing Advice Services: a Good Practice Guide.* Coventry: Chartered Institute of Housing, 1996.
2 **Department of Environment/Department of Health.** *Code of Guidance on Parts VI and VII of the Housing Act 1996, Allocation of Local Authority Housing, Homelessness.* London: DOE/DOH, 1996.
3 **Victim Support.** *Domestic Violence: Report of a National Inter-Agency Working Party.* London: Victim Support, 1992.
4 **Home Office/Welsh Office.** *Inter-Agency Co-ordination to Tackle Domestic Violence.* Interagency Circular. London: Home Office/Welsh Office, 1995.
5 **Malos E, Hague G, Dear W.** *Inter-Agency Initiatives as a Response to Domestic Violence.* Social Policy Research Findings No. 101. York: Joseph Rowntree Trust, 1996.

6 London Borough of Greenwich, Directorate of Housing Services. *Domestic Violence Policy Procedure.* London: Borough of Greenwich, 1996.
7 Chartered Institute of Housing. *Housing and Health: a Good Practice Briefing.* Coventry: CIH, 1998.
8 Chartered Institute of Housing. *Housing Management Standards Manual.* Coventry: CIH, 1996.

Chapter 13e

Onward referral to social services

Bridget Penhale

The context

The process of onward referral by the primary health care team (PHCT) to social services departments of women who have experienced domestic violence is not a simple and straightforward one. Much will depend on the circumstances of each individual situation and how knowledge of the violence and the violent situation has come to light. For example, this could be the result of the woman receiving treatment by the PHCT for physical injuries, or the result of disclosure by the woman to a member of the PHCT that abuse is occurring, or the result of notification concerning violence to the woman being sent to the GP following a visit to a local accident and emergency department by the woman for treatment of injuries caused by an incident of domestic violence.

Possibly the GP will be the first person (either outside of the family or even at all) with whom the woman discusses her situation; therefore it is necessary that a sympathetic and unhurried approach is adopted by the doctor and other members of the PHCT. The woman will need time to disclose, will need to be believed and feel supported throughout her disclosure and afterwards. The GP will need to assess particular aspects of the situation concerning the level of danger to the woman and to any children involved and also whether the woman has made any decision concerning her future or has sufficient information and knowledge of the possible options to enable her to do so. In conjunction with other members of the PHCT, the need for any onward referral (to social services or elsewhere) of the woman will need to be carefully considered. A protocol developed by the PHCT in connection with responding to domestic violence, covering such areas, is likely to be of use within individual situations of abuse presented to the team.

Issues of consent

The consent of the woman concerned to referral to social services is a critical component within situations where onward referral is felt to be likely to be necessary. Paramount consideration must be given to the views of the individual concerned. If consent is not given and the woman is capable of taking that decision (i.e. where there is no evidence of significant cognitive impairment) then no referral should be made by the team. In this type of situation, however, information could and arguably should, be given by a member of the PHCT to the woman explaining how she can access assistance from social services and other local agencies in future should she change her mind.

This discussion with the woman could also usefully serve an educational function in detailing local services and also, perhaps, outlining some of the issues surrounding domestic violence—a gentle exploration of the facts:

- that many women are subject to domestic violence;
- that violence can take many different forms and is not purely physical in nature;
- that she is not to blame for the violence;
- that violence usually becomes more severe and more frequent over time;
- that although it is difficult, women can and do leave violent situations;
- that assistance is available to her should she seek it in future.

Safety planning

It may also be possible to discuss with the woman some of the possible options open to her and to help her to identify a network of safe places and safe people to whom she could turn for assistance when necessary; to assist her to develop her own safety plan. Empowering the woman to make her own decisions and providing support to her in taking them and acting on them are essential elements here.

There is no statutory obligation on health care professionals to refer a woman who has experienced domestic violence to social services, or indeed to the police. The only exception to this would be a situation in which the violence was known or strongly suspected to extend to children within the setting and the children were at risk of further abuse. In this type of situation an investigation concerning the children would need to be conducted by the social services department and a referral should be made even if the woman does not agree to the referral. Ideally the woman will consent to the referral being made. Good practice suggests that the woman should be aware of the referral being made, even in situations when she has not given her consent to the contact with social services.

Traditionally, social workers have not been certain of their role in situations of domestic violence and whether they should become involved or not.[1] This has been mirrored by a lack of clarity about the extent to which social services departments should be involved, perhaps following the general perception of social services as not being of general relevance to women who have experienced abuse and abusive situations. However, a contrary view from research conducted in the early 1980s suggests that although there are limitations in the response of social workers, when women have been involved with social workers they have found it helpful and were satisfied with the response they received. For example, Binney and colleagues[2] found that over half of the sample looked at were broadly satisified, whilst a later study[3] found that the reported satisfaction was higher if the social worker was perceived as having assisted in practical matters such as securing a place in a refuge.

Reluctance about social services

It is necessary, however, for members of the PHCT to be aware and mindful of the fact that a woman may be hesitant and reluctant for social services to become involved in her situation because of a fear that social services will immediately remove the children, even in situations when the violence is not being directed at them. This is clearly a sensitive and difficult area. There is some evidence that social services departments have in the past not responded appropriately to the needs of women who have experienced domestic violence.[1,4] Women have either been referred on elsewhere by social services departments, or those departments have indeed acted overzealously.

It would seem that there has been a tendency for social services departments to see themselves almost exclusively as sources of information and advice for women, unless there were issues concerning the protection of the children. The position adopted centred on a perceived lack of statutory responsibility for women and children experiencing domestic violence unless the children were at risk. However, there are also clear suggestions that departments have not been aware of the effects of domestic violence, especially in the longer term, on both women and children, and have therefore provided insufficient assistance.[5] In this respect, social services are in something of a 'no win' situation: either they act too hastily and remove children unnecessarily, or they are seen as ineffectual, not acting to protect women and their children when this is necessary. This perception, of course, is also apparent within the field of child protection, and it was ever thus. Indeed, members of the public, as well as members of the caring professions, are aware of this 'double bind' situation for social workers.[6]

What is helpful?

Women appear to find the following aspects helpful from their contacts with social services: good, clear, accessible information and advice; help with obtaining accommodation; and, later, support in setting up on their own. Also highly valued is what is perceived as the ability of social workers to act in the role of advocate on behalf of the woman in dealing with other agencies in a liaison and negotiation capacity.[1]

Local authorities are now expected to define their own areas of responsibility, reflected through plans for community care and children's services that are responsive to the needs of the local communities served by social services. This obviously includes the needs of women and their children (if any) who may be vulnerable by virtue of their experiences of domestic violence. It would seem, therefore, that social services departments may need in future to adopt a somewhat more proactive approach towards women who have experienced domestic violence than they have previously.

The currency of this view was expounded from a central level in a recent publication. In 1995, the Social Services Inspectorate of the Department of Health held two seminars concerning the issue of domestic violence and social care, and following this produced a report.[7] This report proposed that social services departments should redress the fact that they were not very involved in this type of work as a matter of some urgency, and should do more to assist women who have experienced violence from a known man. Included within the report were the following suggestions that social services departments should be working towards:

- Developing and implementing policy concerned with working with those who have experienced domestic violence.

- Developing and implementing guidelines for good practice for social workers and other staff to follow.

- Including the issue as part of the basic practice of social workers (as part of referral and assessment processes).

- Publishing and providing information for staff and the general public about domestic violence and responses to it.

- Developing practical services and options for women and children, such as groups, crisis centres or counselling services in hospitals.

- Using legislation, where appropriate, to assist women who have experienced violence (using sections of the Children Act 1989 or the Mental Health Act 1983).

- Monitoring the use of services by women who experience or have experienced domestic violence.

- Establishing and cooperating in multiagency projects to provide information on referral routes, service provision and the respective roles of each agency involved in working with domestic violence.

- Financing non-statutory initiatives, such as work with children or counselling services concerned with domestic violence.

Social services departments have lead responsibility for the provision of community care and as such should assist in meeting the needs of individual women—however those needs occur. Domestic violence may occur in any health or welfare context. It has been suggested that many women who are already in contact with social services (and health services) have experience of abusive situations; perhaps one in five of current cases active to social workers have direct references to domestic violence on the case file (Mullender in [7]). Clients of social services who have other areas of need through disability, age, mental health or substance abuse-related problems may have experience of domestic violence; indeed their difficulties may even have been caused by or resulted from the domestic violence (for example, addiction, mental health problems or physical disability through injury).

Conclusion

The prime needs of a woman experiencing domestic violence can be summarized as follows. Firstly, the woman needs to be believed, listened to and supported by any agency she approaches for assistance. Her experiences must be validated and noted. Secondly, once a decision has been taken by the woman to seek permanent changes, she must be able to do so quickly, and may well require effective protection under the law. Thirdly, she, and any children, should she have them, will need a safe place to go and may need assistance in obtaining this; longer term safe accommodation will also be a priority for her. Fourthly, financial and other practical forms of support will be necessary, but emotional support and on occasion advocacy are also likely to be needed.

When approached by a woman for assistance, social services departments should be responsive and supportive. Clarity is necessary from the outset, however, over such issues as confidentiality, child protection (if necessary) and the limits to the amount of assistance that can be provided, both short and long term. The PHCT should also have a clear understanding about these aspects, developed through effective liaison with social services.

Whilst social services are well placed to provide assistance in meeting some of the needs of women who experience domestic violence, what is also apparent is that no single agency can provide all the appropriate responses and that a number of agencies are likely to be involved. All agencies involved must develop sensitivity and responsivity to meet the needs of women who have experienced or are still experiencing domestic violence.

References

1 Lloyd S. Social work and domestic violence. In: Kingston P, Penhale B, eds. *Family Violence and the Caring Professions*. Basingstoke: Macmillan, 1995: 149–77.

2 Binney V, Harkell G, Nixon J. *Leaving Violent Men: a Study of Refuges and Housing for Battered Women*. Bristol: Women's Aid Federation, 1981.

3 Pahl J, ed. *Private Violence and Public Policy*. London: Routledge & Kegan Paul, 1985.

4 Hague G, Malos E. *Domestic Violence: Action for Change*. Cheltenham: New Clarion Press, 1993.

5 Mullender A, Morley R. *Children Living with Domestic Violence*. London: Whiting & Birch, 1994.

6 Harding T, Beresford P. *The Standards We Expect*. London: National Institute of Social Work, 1996.

7 Department of Health/Social Services Inspectorate. *Domestic Violence and Social Care: a Report of Two Conferences held by the Social Services Inspectorate*. London: HMSO, 1996.

Chapter 13f

Asian and Ethnic minority women's groups

Hannana Siddiqui

South Asian women are up to two or three times more likely to commit suicide than women in the general population. They are also more likely to attempt and contemplate suicide and self-harm.[1,2] Why do Asian women feel they have no other option? We need to ask ourselves why this may be the case, and what needs to be done in order to prevent such tragedies.

Research and our experience at Southall Black Sisters shows that the reasons for suicide and self-harm amongst Asian women is not linked to psychiatric disorders, as it is for women generally. It is associated with pressure on Asian women to conform to strict traditional roles.[3,4,5] They are also often subject to abusive and oppressive practices within the family. These include domestic violence, which can be made up of the following components: physical, sexual and mental abuse; forced marriage; abduction and imprisonment within the home; restrictions placed on lifestyle and freedom of movement, dress and association; denial of education and career choices; and other controlling or belittling behaviour, such as oppressive financial practices and constant criticism undermining their independence and sense of self-worth.

Domestic violence is a serious problem in all communities. It cuts across race, class, caste and age boundaries. Domestic violence is as prevalent in black and minority communities as it is in the majority, white community. Black and minority women, however, have a greater number of obstacles to overcome before they are able to obtain assistance and protection. These obstacles act as extra constraining factors, which exist both within and outside their tightknit communities. For example, South Asian women may experience more intense cultural and religious pressures within their communities, which prevents them from leaving violent situations within the family. Traditions such as 'family honour' are extremely powerful where the honour of the family rests on the expectation that women will adhere to prescribed forms of acceptable female behaviour. Failure to conform to traditional norms and values leads to a stigma attached to the woman. She is ostracized for having shamed her family honour by challenging male violence.

Factors outside the community involve an ignorance or lack of awareness amongst agencies on the needs of black and minority women, or a failure to address their specialist needs, such as providing language facilities. In addition, black and minority women may experience racial harassment and discrimination. Women with an insecure immigration status may not leave violent husbands because they fear deportation. This is often the case where their right to remain in the UK is dependent on marriage. Many women also find that agencies refuse to intervene in minority cultures. They hold the view that problems are resolved within the community by the extended family or community leaders. Outside agencies are fearful of interfering in minority communities or to be seen to be criticizing their cultural practices. In addition, black and minority women share all the same problems as women from the majority community, such as homelessness, poverty and the tendency to deny or trivialize domestic violence rather than treating it as a serious criminal offence.

Health agencies, like other professional agencies, share these problems and perspectives, compounding the difficulties Asian and minority women experience when attempting to escape domestic violence. All agencies must adopt policies and protocols to empower women to escape domestic violence. It is essential that all health agencies establish good practice guidelines for patients experiencing domestic violence. The needs of Asian and other black and minority women must be addressed and integrated into other policies and procedures, such as those dealing with confidentiality, patient welfare and domestic violence more generally.

The following are some suggested guidelines with a particular focus for general practitioners.

- *Recognize the signs.* Domestic violence may not be the presenting problem. A woman may seek help because of 'accidents' causing physical injury, or other illnesses which may be caused by an underlying social problem such as frequent headaches and other aches and pains. They may also complain of stress-related issues such as sleeplessness, poor appetite or an eating disorder, depression or self-harm. Other signs may include missed appointments or that the woman is always accompanied by someone else, who speaks for her or monitors what she says. The woman may appear as if she is not taking care of herself, is frightened or withdrawn and quiet. Avoid stereotyping: do not assume that all Asian women are normally passive and submissive, or that all African-Caribbean women will speak up and express their anger and fear.

- *Private interview and asking question.* Whenever possible, attempt to interview the woman alone, in the absence of those accompanying her. Ask for her expressed permission if she wants someone else in the room. Make this request when she is alone. If this is not possible, try to talk to her when she is alone, for example when carrying out a medical examination. Encourage the woman to speak about her problems. Sometimes a woman may disclose domestic violence immediately, whilst others may require more time. They need to be asked several times over a long period before they feel ready, confident and trust enough to discuss these problems.

Many Asian or minority women speak out after years of remaining silent and in many cases, simply being asked about the abuse by a sympathetic person may help her to reveal a hidden history of abuse. Once the woman has disclosed, ask specific questions about the nature of the abuse, its history, recent incidents and her fears about the future. It is important to believe the woman and not be judgemental of her. Questions should also be asked about the effect of domestic violence on children or other dependants, such as the elderly and vulnerable adults, both as witnesses to or as victims of domestic violence.

- *Interpretation.* Consider the need for an interpreter where there are language difficulties. Whenever possible engage the help of an independent professional interpreter, preferably female. Do not use a child, relative or friend of the woman. Generally avoid using other staff in the surgery. Ensure the interpreter abides by a professional code of conduct. Some interpreters may give inappropriate advice or make negative judgements about Asian/minority women speaking out about domestic violence. If this becomes apparent, do not use the interpreter and complain about their conduct to their professional disciplinary body.

- *Information and advice.* If a woman reports abusive behaviour, advise her to obtain help. Although health professionals may not be best placed to give specialist advice, they should at least inform the woman about approaching an appropriate agency for protection—such as the police, social services, a solicitor or a woman's organization. Stress the need to act urgently in order to prevent further abuse and even more serious abuse from occurring to her, her children or others who may be at risk. Offer to make contact with these agencies for her, or if she remains unsure, give her the contact numbers of these services. Make sure that written information is only handed over if the woman is confident that it would not be discovered by the abuser(s). Otherwise the woman should be asked to memorize basic information. Information in leaflets and posters, translated into various common local languages, should also be displayed in the waiting area, toilets or medical examination rooms.

- *Appropriate agencies.* An appropriate agency includes Asian or other black/minority women's organization, such as a refuge and resource centre, offering specialist services for women experiencing domestic violence. However, these agencies must provide a service where the protection and safety of the woman is of paramount importance. Only those women's groups which adhere to these policies should be used. Services which offer mediation or organize along religious or communal lines may compromise equality of provision and the safety of the woman. The best services provided are those available from women's groups who have a track record and an expertise in dealing with domestic violence, offering a safe space for women to lead independent lives free from violence and abuse. In areas where such services are not provided by Asian or other black/minority women's organizations, contact a Women's Aid group that caters for women from all racial backgrounds.

It is also crucial for other agencies, such as social services and the police, to offer services that aim to protect women from further violence and abuse. In our experience, these agencies often fail black and minority women experiencing domestic violence, despite recent improvements in the policing of domestic violence in some areas. Health professionals who refer women to these and other agencies must ensure these services fulfil their duties and responsibilities by protecting women and children. Agencies must hold each other accountable by making official complaints when services fail to adhere to their own policies and legal obligations.

- *Mediation.* All agencies, including health services, must not attempt to mediate between the woman and her partner or family as this often creates extra pressure on the woman to reconcile back into a violent relationship. Extensive informal networks involving community leaders and members of the extended family already engage in mediation, placing women under consider pressure to return home. Mediation rarely leads to the cessation of violence and places women at risk of further abuse as any agreements made are not enforceable by agencies. Mediation therefore compromises the principle of maximizing safety and protection. The role of law enforcement, social welfare and health agencies is to provide women with alternative services and protection from further abuse. Abuse following reconciliation through mediation by an agency amounts to negligence and a failure in their duty to protect.

- *Referral.* When so requested, contact the appropriate referral agency. Any appointments made or information gained should only be communicated to the woman by a mechanism already approved with her beforehand. For example, only inform her on the telephone if she has made it clear that her calls are not monitored. Sometimes women are imprisoned in the home and kept isolated, only allowed out for visits to the GP or other health services. Such a visit could be the only opportunity for a woman to discuss her problems with an agency, who should be asked to attend the same visit to the surgery in order to meet the woman. Where this is not possible, arrange for a telephone interview with the agency. If this cannot be done in an existing appointment, make one specially for the purpose. Care must be taken to ensure that anyone accompanying the woman is not alerted to the nature of the appointment, unless the woman explicitly states it is safe to do so in their absence.

- *Recording incidents.* Medical records must reflect details of physical and mental injuries caused by the abuse. The reported cause of the injury should be noted. Women should be encouraged to state the true cause, i.e. domestic violence rather than an 'accident'. These records may be essential in providing supporting evidence in a court case or for other purposes, such as immigration applications. Where there is a possibility that medical records may be revealed to the woman's family, such as at appointments also attended by relatives, a separate record of history of domestic violence should be kept.

- *Confidentiality.* Women must be assured of confidentiality, and informed of instances where information may have to be shared with other professionals; for example, when a child is at risk. Many minority women are wary of talking about domestic violence with their family GP, particularly if they are from the same community, because of fears concerning breach of confidentiality. In our experience, many Asian family GPs are judgemental of women and breach confidentiality to their partners and family members, placing women at risk of further abuse. There are also increasing number of networks within Asian communities that are becoming more organized in tracking women down and forcing them to return home to abusive situations. These networks often use corruption or poor confidentiality procedures within agencies to find women. Good confidentiality procedures and safeguards are therefore essential in ensuring protection.

- *Training.* All staff, including reception staff, should be trained on procedures and protocols adopted to deal with domestic violence. The training should include an understanding of the needs of black and minority women.

- *Monitoring and follow-up.* It is important to monitor a case where a woman needs time to make a decision or has decided to continue to live in or return to an abusive situation. A woman may also continue to attend their local GP where the abuser has left the matrimonial or family home, or she may join a practice having left home. It is worth noting that many abusers continue to harass women following separation and through contact arrangements for children. Indeed, research and our experience has shown one of the most dangerous times for women is when they are about to, or have separated from, their partners. Another dangerous time is during pregnancy. For young Asian women, their teenage years and the early stages of marriage are also periods when women may be most at risk of abuse and suicide. However, although there are periods when women are at greater risk, it is important to keep a constant watch on the situation with regular questioning and monitoring. Women who remain in or under pressure to return to violent situations must be regularly encouraged to protect themselves and their children. Such protection procedures require collaboration with other health and welfare agencies involved, such as health visitors, hospitals, schools, social services and women's groups. Women should be encouraged to give their consent for information to be shared between these agencies and to report domestic violence to them themselves.

References

1 **Raleigh VS.** Suicide patterns and trends in people of Indian sub-continent and Caribbean origins in England and Wales. *Ethnicity and Health* 1996; **1** (1): 55–63.

2 **Bhugra D, Desai M, Baldwin DS.** Attempted suicide in west London, I. Rates across ethnic communities. *Psychological Medicine* 1999; **29** (5): 1125–30.

3 Bhugra D, Baldwin DS, Desai M, Jacob KS. Attempted suicide in west London, II. Inter-group comparisons. *Psychological Medicine* 1999; **29** (5): 1131–9.

4 Merrill J, Owens J, Wynne S, Whittington R. Asian suicides. *British Journal of Psychiatry* 1990; **156**: 748–9.

5 Merrill J, Owens J. Ethnic differences in self-poisoning: a comparisons of Asian and white groups. *British Journal of Psychiatry* 1986; **148**: 708–12.

Chapter 13g

Solicitors and law centres

Tamsin Morris

Doctors whose patients suffer domestic violence have a two important relationships with the law. *First*, doctors can very usefully record what they see and are told by their patients about the consequences of domestic violence, and doctors can then be ready to provide that information when requested. *Second*, doctors may discover that their patients are suffering the effects of domestic violence, and can then suggest to them that they are able to stop this in their lives, and can suggest where to go for advice on how to do this.

These are two really important opportunities for helping to relieve suffering, which may come the way of a doctor. We will look at them in turn, because although the second may lead to the first, they are separate functions for the GP.

Confirmation of medical history

Doctors are asked by solicitors for medical reports. There are two golden and simple rules.

1. *Be quick.* Particularly in domestic violence cases, the hearing may be very soon indeed. Get a short reply ready as soon as you can. Your patient can always be asked to collect the report from the surgery. Even if the hearing is not obviously very imminent (like the next day) it will help the advocate considerably if there is a proper chance to read and reflect on your report, however short it may seem to you. Points need to be looked at and weighed, and, if needs be, backed up by some other sort of evidence.

2. *State all you have seen or heard.* Understandably doctors are sometimes worried about making definite statements because they fear they are being asked to make some sort of judgement and are reluctant to do that. However, this is a misconception as it is the court that judges from all the facts that are put before it. If facts are left out, these facts cannot play their part in the picture that the court considers.

Doctors have sometimes said, 'Well, she said the bruises were caused by her husband but obviously I don't know that'. Of course, this is true but you should say she told you that. Women can sometimes be not believed in court because it is understood that 'they never told anybody'. Similarly doctors sometimes are reluctant to report their recorded notes because they say, 'Well, she was very depressed and she said her husband drank a lot, but I don't know his side of the story'. Again, just record what you saw and observed and heard. It is for the husband to put his side of the story before the court and add to 'the whole story' for the judge. The husband will have his lawyers putting forward his side of the story—which may include what he told his doctor!

Doctors are not judges, and they do not make a judicial finding. Of course they make clinical and medical judgements all the time, so it may be hard for them to disentangle their judgement-making capacity when asked for records for a court case or legal application. Just be glad this is one judgement you do not have to make.

However, as doctors know from their own judgement-making work, having as much information as possible is vital, and it is therefore important to provide all the facts you can.

Going to court

Doctors may understandably be anxious that, if they write a court report, they will be asked to attend court. Only those very rare people who love litigation choose to go to court. Everyone else avoids it like the plague. Doctors usually do not want to go to court either.

More often than not, if a doctor writes a report, they will not then have to attend court. The writers of reports are only asked to go to court if the content of their report is challenged in some way. Factual extracts from patient's records are rarely disputed. Therefore, only if a clinical interpretation has been requested is a doctor likely to be asked to attend and explain their reasons for their interpretation or clinical judgement.

Three things may encourage a doctor to go to court:

1. Any adult member of the community has a duty to give knowledge to the court that adult possesses and that the court needs.

2. Doctors are lucky enough to be paid for their knowledge when required by the court. Ordinary eye witnesses are not.

3. If a doctor does have to go to court, the court will usually arrange, as far as possible, to accommodate the doctor (speak to someone who has lost a week at work waiting

to give evidence in a contested family matter and doctors will learn that this is the rare privilege of the experts). The doctor should inform the solicitor who asked for the original report and attendance, about fees and about their availability for court. That solicitor is their point of liaison with the courts.

In court all a doctor has to do is truthfully answer the questions asked. That includes saying if you do not know the answer, or cannot know the answer. You have nothing to hide and only the truth to tell. That is a strong position to be in. A helpful maxim is 'put nothing extra in, but leave nothing out'. What *you do not tell* the judge (or magistrate) *they cannot know*.

Helping a patient sufferer of domestic violence

Patient has two meanings here. First, the doctor is concerned with their 'patient'. Second, the sufferer of domestic violence is almost always very 'patient' indeed in their wait for relief and freedom from their destructive torment. It is that time of waiting, suffering and vainly hoping, that does so much damage to a person, and that a doctor can be very instrumental in identifying.

Doctors may see bruises, black eyes, hair pulled out, concussion, lacerations from broken glass, wrenched joints, twisted limbs, fractures, broken noses and missing teeth. Doctors should record them all, ask how they were caused and if told they were caused by a domestic partner the doctor can tell the patient the choices they have (see below).

The doctor will also see the patient whose hair falls out through stress, the over or undereater, the very depressed, the agoraphobic, the sad headache sufferer, the sufferer from panic attacks, and all those other symptoms of stress that doctors know so well. When a woman presents with one or some of these symptoms, ask how long she has had them and try to prize out an accurate reply.

As lawyers we hear from our clients of the long years of violent abuse that have ground down the spirit, confidence and self-esteem of the woman. Something has happened to make her seek legal advice (a last straw, a supportive relative finally finding out, realizing the damage done to the children, police involvement, etc.) and we ask if she is depressed. Often she will say 'yes, terribly'—she cannot go out, she sits and cries, she cannot do anything, she dare not 'confess' and she has panic attacks/headaches/ 'bad nerves', or has a problem with substance abuse herself. We now suggest she goes to the doctor. Her doctor may be able to prescribe something to help the depression that has now taken hold of her. She will need all the help she can get to make the life changes necessary. We ask if she has been to the doctor before and she may say 'no'—because she had not felt she was worth doing anything about, and she felt helpless, and she had stopped thinking about herself because she was told she was bad and worthless and selfish and it was too painful to think about herself, so she did nothing.

So, when she finally comes to the surgery with these symptoms of anxiety or nervous tension or depression, ask how long she has felt this way, had these symptoms, and suffered these effects. That doctor can then record how long she says she has had these symptoms. It can be reported in a factual report to the court, that she told the doctor that in fact she had her 'stress pains' for several years (or however long). It all adds to the whole picture.

However, something else may have sent her to the doctor, a different sort of final straw, and the doctor may see the sad woman, and *no lawyer is on the scene.*

What causes this misery, where has this depression come from, what is the presenting source of all this stress manifesting itself in different ways? Poverty may sometimes seem an immediate answer. Indeed, it may bring extra stress in the form of bullying, blaming and tormenting, as well as its own grinding anxieties. However, there are poor women in families who are hard up and struggling with a very tight budget, but who are not depressed. If your patient tells you, or lets you know that her partner is a drinker, be alert to the likelihood of domestic violence in that family. If she has drink or drug-related problems when did they start and what were the likely reasons? How does her partner react? Be alert to the prevalence of domestic violence in all its forms.

There are three ways that the doctor can pass on helpful information, to enable a patient to begin to take charge of her life and make choices.

1. *She tells you she is hit or threatened with being hit or is insulted and degraded in other ways, perhaps verbally or sexually.* You can tell her that every adult can be protected from abuse in all its forms and that abusers can be punished. Tell her she can get legal advice, housing advice, welfare rights advice and emotional support. Tell her there are professionals who will work on her side to stop the bullying. Tell her that she can take control by getting information and deciding what she wants to do.

2. *Her symptoms suggest domestic violence but she does not identify herself as a sufferer.* Note down what she says (it may be needed later). Suggest that she may feel better if she talks to someone who can counsel her or give her advice about some of her problems. Let her know about relevant agencies. In her own time she may find that invaluable.

3. *Let your patients absorb information passively.* A mother may be in your waiting room with her child for immunization or the child's headaches or tummyaches and she may see a notice on your wall that (within the privacy of her own mind) she can take on board as describing her, and being relevant to her.

    Have some information that identifies domestic violence as *always unacceptable,* and as including bullying, threatening, taunting and belittling as well as beating. Have an example that she can recognize, and then have the sources of information, e.g. Women's Aid, counseling services, legal advice services, welfare rights agencies, housing advice agencies, police family support units, rape crisis centres, Asian women's support groups, AfroCaribbean women's support groups, and incest survivors groups. Have phone numbers large, clear and easy to read, so that she can see them and remember them, without anyone knowing, or seeing her look at them or write them down.

Make sure that all your staff are alert to the dangers and extent of domestic violence in all its forms, and know where advice can be found, so that if a patient turns to them they can immediately give information in a supportive and accessible way to that patient. Doctors and their staff are used to confidentiality. This is very important because often a sufferer needs to confide in safety first, and then later may need to hide or move, or make contacts back within the area, without the abuser knowing.

What are the courses of action a sufferer can follow?

1. *Call the police at the time of an assault or likely assault.* Assault is a crime, whether it is within a domestic context or not. The police can remove a violent man, or take a woman to safety from a threatening man. The police may refer the matter to the Crown Prosecution Service for the man to be charged with assault. The abuser can be bailed to keep away from the victim until his case is resolved before the court.

2. *The sufferer can go into a refuge.* A refuge is a safe, secret shelter for families and women fleeing domestic violence.

3. *The sufferer may be eligible to be rehoused.* If a mother finds it really impossible to go home because of the danger of domestic violence she can be given temporary accommodation by her local council homeless persons department. Try your local shelter or housing advice centre as well as the council.

4. *Consult a solicitor.* The sufferer can take legal action to stop the bullying and to protect herself and her home and family. She should consult a solicitor who is known to be competent and empathetic in the field of domestic violence. Various legal remedies are available and she should be fully advised so that she can choose the appropriate action for her situation. Her situation will vary according to the following factors:

   - Does she want to terminate her whole relationship or simply the violence or destructive behaviour?

   - Does she want to move to a new safe home, or be safe in her present one?

   - Are her children at risk?

   - Is her partner to be stopped by a salutary, simply worded solicitor's letter?

   - Is he so violent or so obsessed that she must hide and hide well?

   Accordingly she may seek a warning letter, an injunction (an order by the court to *stop doing something*—e.g. hitting her, being there, harassing her), an order to remove a man from the house permanently (transferring ownership or tenancy), an order that he cannot snatch away the children (a very controlling threat by many men), or she may need to flee away and change her name.

So long as she can be clear about her problem, she can find an answer. If she feels better, she can think more clearly, and take her own decisions for her life. Some of these decisions might lead to actions, which may involve confirmation from her doctor of what she has suffered. Taking a decision and following a chosen course of action will make her feel better.

After the change

Making life changes to escape domestic violence usually involves a lot of upheaval, nervous energy, learning and liaising with all sorts of different agencies (courts, voluntary organizations, housing associations, solicitors, benefits officers, teachers, social workers, etc.). It is very difficult and stressful and a woman longs for the peace of when it is all over.

However, frequently when the court case is long closed, the new house has curtains, contact between the father and children is sorted out, her benefit is paid, then she becomes very depressed and does not know why. It is very common, tell her so, and let her know about support groups.

Going back to the abuser

Many people who are in contact with domestic violence sufferers are exasperated because, having had the advice, moved, gone to court and been in the refuge, they then go back to their violent partner.

Why do they do this?

Everyone has an individual story and we are talking about personal relationships, so we must beware of generalizations. But a domestic violence sufferer has lost much confidence, self-esteem and sense of self-worth during all those occasions of being rubbish, abused, blamed and belittled and these dreadful feelings are not cured overnight. Having the courage to construct your own life means you must believe that you are worth it and capable of it. A domestic violence sufferer has had it drilled into them that they are neither.

No-one chose a bully or a brute. That abuser was once a cherished lover, valued husband or perfect partner, sharing dreams of a lovely future together. Losing dreams is an achingly hard loss. Very often the abusers are extremely charming (it has been suggested that the more charming a man is, the more dangerous he is). How wonderful if after all the fear, loneliness, hurt and humiliation, it turns out the lovely future can still beckon, if only you forgive and understand, and change a little? No wonder the sufferer gives it another go (particularly as families, churches, etc. are often urging them to 'try again').

What can you do?

Be consistently there again when the dream repeatedly shatters. Note the symptoms. Give the information. Show neither surprise nor say 'I told you so'. Give any help that is asked for, and that you can properly and professionally give. Be glad it is not you in that position.

How to use the law to stop domestic violence

Here we talk about your patient using the civil law to protect herself. *Civil law* means using the courts where one individual takes action against another (husband vs. wife, father vs. mother, customer vs. supplier, pedestrian vs. council, patient vs. doctor). Civil law is dealt with in a county court (with a judge) or family proceedings court (with magistrates).

This is in contrast to the *criminal law* where the police take action, on behalf of the Queen, to investigate crime. A crime is where an individual has broken the rules of society (broken the law). The criminal law is concerned with punishment, and is dealt with in a magistrates court or crown court. The sentence is the punishment.

The civil law is about one person compensating another for doing wrong to them, and about the victim being able to stop the wrong doer carrying on doing wrong. A patient may sue a doctor for negligence and get a payment of compensation for their resultant injuries. An injunction is to stop a husband assaulting his wife.

Your patient should go to a solicitor and ask for help in stopping domestic violence. She should be ready to tell the solicitor a lot about what has been done to her and what she has suffered and what she is afraid of. It is a good idea if someone goes with her to help take it all in. If she is on income support or family credit she should be eligible for legal aid, otherwise she is likely to have to pay something. This should be sorted out at the start so that she knows where she stands.

The solicitor may suggest sending a warning letter to the perpetrator of the violence. For some men, this is enough to stop the domestic violence.

Legal Aid can help a woman by paying for the solicitor to do the work she needs doing. Before a woman can get Legal Aid, she has to show that she has used the police and they are not effective enough, and that a letter has already been sent warning her abuser (except in extreme and unusual circumstances).

If a woman can pay for her legal work she can go to court straight away and the court have wide powers to help and protect her. Her solicitor must tell her how much it is likely to cost, and how she can arrange to pay.

If she cannot pay, and Legal Aid is not available, but she wants a court order (an injunction), she could make her own application to court, using a clear self-help pack which is produced by Rights of Women (tel. 020 7251 6577, e-mail: info@row.org.uk).

An injunction is a court order that orders a stop to violence or harassment or threats or intimidation (called a *non-molestation order*), or an order that controls who lives in a house (called an *occupation order*). If the injunction is broken, the perpetrator of the violence is punished for contempt of court, because they broke a specific court order, and contempt of court is a serious offence.

The procedure for getting an injunction is now quite straightforward. The person who is making the application to the court and who is the victim of the violence, who is now seeking an injunction, is called 'the applicant'. The perpetrator of the violence, against whom the order is sought and whose behaviour is to be controlled by the injunction, is called 'the respondent'. A preprinted court form has to be filled in saying who wants the order (the applicant), against whom the order is to be made (the respondent), and what the order is to say. The form comes with explanatory notes from the court. Either her solicitor, or the self-help pack will help a woman fill in the form, or she can do it by looking at the notes herself.

The order can say that a man is to move out of the house (occupation order), or he is not to come within 50 metres of the house, or he is not to make any threats over the phone (non-molestation order). The injunction can say what is needed for each woman in each situation. The injunction may be made against a son, brother, boyfriend or ex-boyfriend, grandfather, daughter, sister, girlfriend, etc. The injunction can be made against someone 'in the family' abusing someone else.

The injunction can say that the behaviour that is violent and threatening must stop, and it may also say that the perpetrator must go and live somewhere else. A woman can get a non-molestation order *and* an occupation order. Quite often a woman might want only a non-molestation order, but it would be unusual for her to get an occupation order without a non-molestation order as well. Quite a lot of women may need an order to stop violence or harassment from a man who does not live with her, because he is an ex-husband, a former partner or a threatening brother-in-law (non-molestation order). But if a woman needs an injunction to get a man out of the house they share (occupation order), then she will almost certainly need an order to stop him threatening to assault or harass her as well.

To ask for an injunction, the woman has to go to court herself (with her solicitor, friend or supporter). The perpetrator has the chance to be there too, although the applicant can go and get the order first, to protect her before she is in court with the respondent himself. Because this is the civil law, the applicant only has to persuade the court that on the balance of probabilities the events have happened as she described, and she therefore needs the injunction. This is much easier to do than in criminal law, where the court must confirm guilt 'beyond all reasonable doubt'.

If the respondent does not choose to go to the court, then once the order is made he should be given a copy of the order.

The police should be told about the order if there is a *power of arrest* attached to the injunction. If the respondent breaks the order he can be arrested by the police, taken back to the court and punished. He can be sent to prison for disobeying a court order, or he might be fined or perhaps strongly warned.

If an injunction says that a man (the respondent) must not come within 50 metres of a house and that clause has the power of arrest attached, and he comes within 20 metres of the house, he is then in breach, no matter how peaceful he seems, and he can be arrested and taken to court for contempt of court. This is important because his very presence can be threatening and intimidating.

This is stronger protection than the criminal law remedy where, pending trial or sentence, a man can be bailed to keep away from the victim. An injunction can last much longer than a bail condition, and it is up to the police whether to prosecute for breach of bail or not. The woman herself controls the injunction and how it is used. An injunction has legal teeth that can be made to bite and can stop cruelty and oppression in the home.

The injunction laws were improved and made much stronger and easier to use from October 1997 onwards. Unfortunately this coincided with much tighter control of Legal Aid, so as the remedies and help got better for the sufferers of domestic violence, so the ability to use them was made more difficult.

However, a woman can take heart, getting an injunction is possible and affordable in most cases, so long as she gets the right help and support. The courts powers are wide and strong and the procedure is quite straightforward.

Chapter 14

The future

Iona Heath

Changing attitudes

The pioneering work of Women's Aid over the past 25 years has gradually but profoundly shifted attitudes to domestic violence within society. The 1989 Report from the Home Office Research and Planning Unit[1] led directly to the Home Office circular which was issued to police in 1990.[2] This made clear the responsibility of the police to treat violence perpetrated against women in their own homes as seriously as violence occurring in a public place. Incidents were to be properly recorded and investigated, appropriate arrests made, and abused women offered protection, information and support. The police response to the circular has included the widespread development of domestic violence units within police stations, staffed by officers with special training and growing expertise.

Now perceived as the victims of crime, many abused women were referred by the police to Victim Support, and as a direct result of their increasing awareness of the problems faced by women, Victim Support convened a National Inter-Agency Working Party which reported in 1992.[3] This was followed by the House of Commons Home Affairs Select Committee on Domestic Violence which met from 1992 to 1993, and eventually by the Home Office Report on Inter-Agency Co-ordination.[4]

Interagency working

Interagency forums have now developed in many areas, bringing together professionals and workers from a wide range of different agencies in the attempt to provide a coordinated and sensitive response to the needs of abused women and their children. However, it has proved difficult to involve primary health care professionals, and particularly general practitioners, in the work of these forums, and many have remained marginalized from, and unaware of, the changing service provision.

As a result, many general practitioners remain unaware of the horrifying prevalence of domestic violence, and continue to struggle to find an adequate response to women presenting the resultant injuries or complications. However, it is essential to acknowledge the very real difficulties that general practitioners face in collaborating with interagency working. As self-employed independent contractors with an ongoing, continuous 24-hour responsibility for the health care of a registered list of patients, general practitioners face conditions of service which are very different from those of most of the other agencies involved. If general practitioners wish to take time away from the practice to attend meetings, they have to provide locum cover for the care of their patients. This means that they incur a personal financial cost in attending meetings. Further, most meeting times that are convenient for other agencies tend to coincide with general practice surgery times, making it doubly difficult for general practitioners to attend.

It is clear that different methods are needed to properly involve general practitioners and primary health care teams in coordinated work with other agencies. The Leeds Inter-Agency Project has piloted the attachment of advice workers to individual general practices.[5] The project appears to have been successful in establishing good working relationships with the primary health care teams, and in reducing surgery attendances and psychiatric referrals of abused women. In other areas, health visitors have been able to establish effective links with the interagency forum, but falling health visitor numbers and the pressure of rising caseloads of vulnerable children and families are making this alternative less and less viable.

Practice education and training

If the practice team is to be optimally effective in supporting and offering help to women attempting to survive domestic violence, every member will need an awareness of the extent and damaging health consequences of domestic violence. Practices need to learn actively and explicitly from their experiences of trying to care for women who present with histories of violence, and, in so doing, base education in the real challenges of the team's daily work, bridging the gaps between different members' areas of expertise to the benefit of individual patients who are known to all. Every practice is a learning organization. Everyone whose working life brings them into contact with patients learns something new about life, health, illness and disease every day. Yet in present circumstances, this learning occurs by default and against the odds. The world is not divided between the good people who reflect on their practice, and the bad people who do not. Everybody reflects on what they do, but often in a very disorganized and unfocused way. When things are bad, we may learn more about survival skills than about how to do better for our patients. Practices must be enabled to make time for reflection and education: only in this way, can services to the most vulnerable be improved. The postgraduate education of primary health care professionals needs to be completely transformed so that regular educational sessions, which are properly resourced, can take place in each practice.[6] A full half day every 2 months would seem to be a good starting position. To achieve this, each primary health care team will need protected time for all its members. This can be achieved only by bringing into the practice additional workforce to undertake the clinical service provision that would normally be undertaken by the primary health care team members engaging in educational activity.

Everyone working in primary care needs to be aware of the prevalence, dangers and consequences of domestic violence. An abused woman may reveal her situation, for the first time, to a receptionist, a practice nurse, a practice counsellor, a district nurse, a midwife, a health visitor or a general practitioner. Each needs to know how to respond safely and effectively. Significant event auditing,[7] considering the explicit presentation of domestic violence as a significant event, may offer a useful starting point for an appraisal of the practice's current care of abused women, and how this care might be enhanced.

Educational resources

Information to support practice-based education can be obtained from a range of sources. These include, most usefully, Women's Aid and the huge information resource available from the government website: http://www.open.gov.uk/. Use the website's search facility, entering 'domestic violence'. Women's Aid, local domestic violence units and other relevant agencies can be invited to contribute to practice-based education. Cooperation within educational settings, and exploration of the different areas of expertise of each agency and professional group, can do much to promote good working relationships and effective interagency collaboration.

Undergraduate and postgraduate curricula

The increasing presence of undergraduate medical students within general practice settings should lead to their exposure to practice-based education and an exploration of the issues arising from the presentation of domestic violence in general practice. Vocational training for general practice registrars should offer similar opportunities, augmented by such techniques as random case analysis in tutorials and on the half-day release course. However, there remains an urgent need for the health implications of domestic violence to be explicitly included in educational curricula at both undergraduate and postgraduate levels. Questions relating to the care of abused women presenting in health care settings should be included in both undergraduate and postgraduate examinations.

Research

Although past research has already done much to inform and improve the response to women attempting to survive domestic violence, much remains unknown.[8] We still do not know the prevalence of domestic violence in women presenting in routine general practice in the UK, and whether this varies according to geographical area and/or the socioeconomic profile of the practice area. Many questions remain about the natural history of the physical and psychological ill-health which follows exposure to violence, and what could be done to mitigate the damage. We need to understand more clearly the factors that prevent women extricating themselves from violent relationships and how they might most effectively be supported and helped. When men are violent towards women within the context of an intimate relationship, it is essential that the violence is recognized and censured as a crime. However, while recognizing the dangers of the medicalization of crime, it is important to know whether violent men can be successfully rehabilitated, and if so how this might be most effectively done.

Society

The existence of domestic violence reveals crime and brutality at the heart of our society, and makes a huge contribution to the totality of violence in our lives. The health consequences, both direct and indirect, are devastating.

> It is a problem of the health of our whole society: domestic violence affects the future, through its effect on children and the home. Women and children have the right to live unthreatened by violent personal assault. Unless we can construct a society in which they can do so the problems of violence in our society will reproduce themselves for the foreseeable future.
>
> It is woman's unequal position in society, too often still dependent on men, socially and economically, which makes them vulnerable to domestic violence. Cherished social values and stereotypes of the roles of men and women are very influential. Too often men are portrayed as the only strong and assertive sex; women as dependent and meek, or solely sexual beings. The economic dependence of women on men continues to be a fundamental feature of British society. Attempts by women to leave violent men are influenced and constrained by this basic inequality. It is essential that an understanding of this inequality and its effects informs responses to domestic violence.[9]

General practitioners have a responsibility, not only to respond sensitively and appropriately to the needs of individual abused women presenting to them, but also to be part of the campaign to address the wider causes of domestic violence. Information made available to patients, who will include both survivors and perpetrators of violence, in the form of both posters and leaflets, can support the message of zero tolerance,[10] make clear the position of the practice in relation to domestic violence, and provide information about other sources of help and support.

Violence builds on, and perpetuates, inequality. Only a fundamental shift in the relationships between men and women, and the distribution of power and resources between them, can offer the hope of a less violent and healthier future.

References

1 Smith LJF. *Domestic Violence: an Overview of the Literature.* Home Office Reasearch Study No. 107. London: HMSO, 1989.

2 Home Office. *Guidance to Chief Officers of Police in Dealing with Domestic Violence.* Circular 60/1990. London: HMSO, 1990.

3 **Victim Support.** *Domestic Violence: Report of a National Inter-Agency Working Party.* London: Victim Support, 1992.

4 **Home Office, Welsh Office.** *Domestic Violence: Don't Stand For It: Inter-Agency Co-ordination to Tackle Domestic Violence.* London: Home Office, 1995.

5 **Tara Chand A.** *Pilot Work in General Practitioner Practices.* Leeds: Leeds Inter-Agency Project (Women and Violence), 1996.

6 **Gillam S, Eversley J, Snell J, Wallace P.** ed. *Building Bridges: the Future of GP Education – developing partnerships with the service.* London: King's Fund, (in press).

7 **Pringle M, Bradley C, Carmichael C, Wallis H, Moore A.** *Significant Event Auditing.* Occassional Paper No. 70. London: Royal College of General Practitioners, 1995.

8 **Richardson J, Feder G.** Domestic violence: a hidden problem for general practice. *British Journal of General Practice* 1996; **46**: 239–42.

9 **Tuck M.** Introduction. In: Victim Support. *Domestic Violence: Report of a National Inter-Agency Working Party.* London: Victim Support, 1992: 2–3.

10 **Zero Tolerance.** *Zero Tolerance Leaflet.* Glasgow: Zero Tolerance Campaign, 1995 (20 India Street, Glasgow G2).

Part 4

Violence against older people

Chapter 15

The context

Paul Kingston and Chris Phillipson

Introduction

The extent and nature of abuse against older people has become a major topic of concern over the past decade.[1,2] This development reflects issues relating to the care and treatment of vulnerable adults; and, as well, anxieties about the pressures facing formal as well as informal carers. To provide a context to the debate, this chapter has four main objectives: first, to present an overview of the background to research in the field of elder abuse and neglect; second, to examine some problems with definitions; third, to summarize findings on the nature of its incidence and prevalence, and fourth to explore areas for future research.

Background to the recognition of abuse

In Britain, the first discussion about elder abuse occurred in the mid-1970s, with the publication of articles by Baker[3] and Burston.[4] Subsequently, Eastman's monograph[5] reviewed existing research and highlighted a number of disturbing case studies of abused elders. This preliminary work, however, failed to establish elder abuse as a major topic of concern. This almost certainly reflected, first, the dominant focus on child abuse within the work of health and social services[6,7] (see also Part 2 of this volume); and second, the low status of work with older people, an acute problem within professions such as nursing, health visiting and social work.[8]

This situation changed in the late 1980s, with a number of factors combining to push elder abuse further up the agenda. On the one hand, organizations representing older people became more assertive, improving their ability to influence policy and research discussions. On the other hand, policies such as community care raised concern both about the greater pressures facing informal carers, and problems accompanying the use of market forces in the field of social care.[1]

Reinforcing both the above factors was a greater recognition of violence as endemic in society (and the family in particular). In this context, older people joined children and women as a group recognized as being subject to abuse and neglect—in domestic as well as non-domestic settings. The phenomena of elder abuse thus became accepted in the early 1990s,[9,10] even if precise definitions proved difficult to develop.

Defining elder abuse and neglect

Amongst researchers and practitioners there is still extensive discussion about the precise nature of abuse and neglect, with a range of definitions circulating in the literature. Following the work of Wolf and Pillemer,[11] the main elements of elder abuse are generally agreed to comprise:

1. *Physical abuse*: the infliction of physical harm or injury. It includes physical coercion, sexual molestation and physical restraint.

2. *Psychological abuse*: the affliction of mental anguish.

3. *Material abuse*: the illegal or improper exploitation and/or use of funds or resources.

4. *Active neglect*: the refusal or failure to undertake a caregiving obligation (including a conscious and intentional attempt to inflict physical or emotional distress on the elder).

5. *Passive neglect*: the refusal or failure to fulfil a caretaking obligation (excluding a conscious and intentional attempt to inflict physical or emotional distress on the elder).

Glendenning[12] concludes from his review that a number of uncertainties still remain in defining abuse. These he identifies as: first, the relationship between domestic and institutional abuse; second, the issue of whether elder abuse can be clearly differentiated from the abuse of other adults; and third, the relationship between neglect and other forms of abuse. Further questions could be added to this list. In particular, there is the issue of whether we should restrict the concept to a limited range of actions (focusing, say, on physical and psychological abuse), or whether a broader focus (taking in more general social problems facing older people) is justified.

Kingston and Penhale[2] make the case for broadening the definition of abuse with the following:

> Abuse of elders is human-originated acts of commission or omission and human-created or tolerated conditions that inhibit or preclude unfolding and development of the inherent potential of elders (from [2], based on [13]).

This definition thus encompasses structural and developmental areas that have hitherto been excluded from the arena of elder abuse, focusing on all manifestations of abuse—individual and institutional as well as societal. In the context of the social and economic pressures facing older people, this broader definition is likely to prove of increasing interest in terms of capturing some of the issues and concerns raised by the phenomenon of elder abuse.

The nature and incidence of elder abuse: research from case–control studies

There is now an extensive research literature purporting to explain the causes and risk factors associated with elder abuse. The risk factors reported below are drawn from the most scientific method found in the literature, namely, the use of case–control studies. The five factors that consistently appear in the literature are: intra-individual dynamics; inter-generational transmission of violence; dependency; stress, and social isolation. The research basis for each of these risk factors will now be reviewed.

Intraindividual dynamics

Clear evidence of either mental health difficulties or alcohol use and abuse amongst abusers is found in the work of Bristowe and Collins,[14] Pillemer,[15] Homer and Gilleard[16] and Anetzberger *et al.*[17] However, as Anetzberger suggests, more questions than answers emerge from the research. In relation to alcohol use these include:

1. Does alcohol render individuals prone to abuse by its ability to remove inhibitions and increase impulse response, including aggression?

2. Does prolonged alcoholism foster a dependency between adult children and their elder parents, which distresses and disturbs both, leading to the occurrence of abuse?

3. Do individuals with tendencies towards alcoholism turn to increased alcohol consumption in an attempt to cope when frustrated with elder care?

Intergenerational transmission of violence

The research evidence for this much-quoted risk factor is extremely tentative and evidence of the intergenerational transmission of violence does not appear in any of the case–control studies quoted. However, what does appear in the research is a history of longstanding relationship difficulties that continue into later life, sometimes with 'inverted abuse', that is, situations where a male perpetrator of domestic violence becomes impaired, with the female partner seeking revenge for past misdemeanours. In Grafstrom *et al.*'s research[18] one wife remarked: 'That her husband had been an evil husband, now she was paying him back'. Whilst another wife complained about being abused herself, and a third talked about: 'Sexual demanding behaviour of the husband throughout their lives'.

It is suggested therefore that:

> It may be pertinent at this time to suggest that although intergenerational transmission of violence cannot be stated as a risk factor, graduated domestic violence perhaps can.[1]

Dependency and stress

This risk factor is clearly affected and reinforced by the myths and stereotypes that surround much of the literature on ageing, and is also closely linked to the view that caring is always a stressful occupation. The evidence from case–control studies suggests that if dependency exists in cases of abuse, it is predominately dependency of the abuser on the victim for accommodation and finance.[15] Furthermore, the notion that victims of abuse have greater levels of impairment compared with elderly people who are not victims is again not borne out in the literature. Pillemer's study[15] clearly found that in activities of daily living (ADLS) the abused group had higher functional levels than their non-abused counterparts.

Although the notion of carer stress leading to abuse seems logical, there is little empirical evidence to support the hypothesis. However, it is perhaps necessary to differentiate between 'intrinsic stressors' and 'extrinsic stressors', and the relative effect on the caring situation and the social role. The only case–control study with reference to stress was the work of Grafstrom.[18] In this study, however, the carers themselves reported higher levels of ill-health and psychotropic drug use than the control group.

Social isolation

The evidence for social isolation as a risk factor is rather contradictory. Two of the research studies suggest that social isolation is found as a risk factor for elder abuse.[15,18] In contrast, Phillips[19] and Homer and Gilleard[16] did not find evidence to support isolation as a risk factor. These findings are confounded by the different populations utilized in each study. Grafstrom[18] used a general population study, whilst the other three studies used populations known to health and welfare providers. One way of making sense of this confusion may be to differentiate between family isolation, community isolation and professional isolation in future research studies.

The prevalence of elder abuse and neglect

A limited number of prevalence studies have been carried out in Britain, North America, Finland and Australia. The Boston study of Pillemer and Finkelhor[20] involved interviews with 2000 older people and focused on three types of maltreatment—physical abuse, verbal aggression and neglect. The study found that slightly more than 3 per cent of the population aged 65 plus had been mistreated: 20 cases per 1000 were physically mistreated; 11 per 1000 were psychologically abused; and four per 1000 were neglected. The authors estimate that if a national survey produced similar results, these numbers would represent almost a million people in the USA.

The survey in Britain by Ogg and Bennett[21] reported on results of structured interviews with almost 600 people aged 65 and over, as well as 1366 adult members of households in regular contact with a person of pensionable age. One in 20 reported some kind of abuse, but only one in 50 reported physical abuse. Although 10 per cent of adults admitted to verbal abuse, only 1 per cent acknowledged physical abuse.

A national survey on elder abuse in Canada was carried out by Podnieks.[22] Data were collected through a random sample telephone survey of 2008 elderly persons living in private dwellings. The survey uncovered 80 persons who had been maltreated according to one or more of the study criteria. For the study sample, this translated into a rate of 40 maltreated elderly per 1000 population. Material abuse emerged as the most widespread form of maltreatment in the survey, with a prevalence rate of between 19 and 33 victims per 1000. Chronic verbal aggression was the next most prevalent, affecting 8–18 persons per 1000. The rate for physical violence was 3–9 cases per 1000.

The studies cited are at least indicative of the existence of abuse. On the other hand, the figures—as most of the authors of such studies admit—do need to be treated with some caution. Questions need to be asked about the methods of even the more rigorous research. The American and Canadian work relied either wholly or in part on telephone surveys; some types of abuse may be under-reported using this type of approach. Additionally, certain groups are likely to be under-represented in survey data—the very frail, the disadvantaged or people from ethnic minority groups. Such groups may show a different pattern of abuse and neglect. None the less, all three studies confirm the reality of abuse in the lives of significant numbers of older people.

Unanswered research questions

Whilst the abuse of elderly people is acknowledged to exist, our understanding of the complexities of the phenomenon are clearly underdeveloped. The following list suggests areas where our understanding needs expanding:

- factors that distinguish abused from non-abused, by perpetrator and victim;
- the extent of abuse in minority ethnic elderly groups;
- the types of abuse in minority ethnic elderly groups;
- the prevalence of financial abuse amongst various groups, focusing on socioeconomic status and vulnerability;
- the extent to which domestic violence is a form of elder abuse in later life;
- a risk factor study to test the US risk factors in UK studies;
- the effectiveness of intervention strategies by type of abuse.

Clearly this is not an exhaustive list and many other questions could be noted. However, the list is important because we are aware of the demographic changes in minority ethnic groups, whilst having little knowledge of the caring processes in later life. Financial abuse is often stated to be the most prevalent form of abuse, yet it is perhaps the most difficult to prove. It is also necessary to analyse the extent to which domestic violence is presented as a form of elder abuse: in the US over 60 per cent of elder abuse cases were spouse abuse.[15] With regard to risk factors, most UK policies and procedures include US data that may not travel culturally, therefore urgent replication of the US studies is needed in the UK. Finally, we need to know what works and what does not work as intervention strategies, especially in relation to different types of abuse.

References

1 **Biggs S, Phillipson C, Kingston P.** *Elder Abuse in Perspective.* Buckingham: Open University Press, 1995.

2 **Kingston P, Penhale B.** *Family Violence and the Caring Professions.* Basingstoke: Macmillan, 1995.

3 **Baker A.** Granny bashing. *Modern Geriatrics* 1975; **5** (8): 20–4.

4 **Burston G.** Do you elderly parents lie in fear of being battered? *Modern Geriatrics* 1977; **7**: 20–4, 54–5.

5 **Eastman M.** *Old Age Abuse.* Mitcham: Age Concern, 1984.

6 **Hallett C, Stevenson O.** *Child Abuse: Aspects of Interprofessional Cooperation.* London: George Allen/Unpin, 1980.

7 **Carver V.** *Child Abuse.* Buckingham: Open University Press, 1978.

8 **Biggs S, Phillipson C.** Elder abuse and neglect: developing training programmes. In: Eastman M, ed. *Old Age Abuse: a New Perspective.* London: Age Concern/Chapman & Hall, 1994: 215–28.

9 **Bennett G, Kingston P.** *Elder Abuse: Concepts, Theories and Interventions.* London: Chapman & Hall, 1993.

10 **Decalmer P, Glendenning F.** *The Mistreatment of Elderly People.* London: Sage, 1993.

11 **Wolf R, Pillemer K.** *Helping Elderly Victims.* New York: Columbia University Press, 1989.

12 **Glendenning F.** What is elder abuse and neglect?. In: Decalmer P, Glendenning F, eds. *The Mistreatment of Elderly People.* London: Sage, 1993: 1–34.

13 **Gil D.** The United States versus child abuse. In: L. Petton, ed. The Social Context of Child Abuse and Neglect. New York: Human Services Press, 1981.

14 **Bristowe E, Collins J.** Family mediated abuse of non-institutionalised frail; elderly men living in British Columbia. *Journal of Elder Abuse and Neglect* 1989; **1** (1): 45–64.

15 **Pillemer K.** Risk factors in elder abuse. In: Pillemer K, Wolf R, eds. *Elder Abuse: Conflict in the Family.* Dover, MA: Auburn House, 1986: 239–60.

16 **Homer, A, Gilleard C.** Abuse of elderly people by their carers. *British Medical Journal* 1990; **301**: 1359–62.

17 **Anetzberger G, Korbin JE, Austin C.** Alcoholism and elder abuse. *Journal of Interpersonal Violence* 1994; **9** (2): 184–93.

18 **Grafstrom M, Nordberg A, Wimblad B.** Abuse is in the eye of the beholder: reports by family members about abuse of demented persons in home care: a total population based study. *Scandinavian Journal of Social Medicine* 1992; **21** (4): 247–55.

19 **Phillips L.** Abuse and neglect of the frail elderly at home. *Journal of Advanced Nursing* 1983; **8**: 379–92.

20 **Pillemer K, Finkelhor D.** The prevalence of elder abuse: a random sample survey. *Gerontologist* 1988; **28** (1): 51–7.

21 **Ogg J, Bennett G.** Elder abuse in Britain. *British Medical Journal* 1992; **305**: 998–9.

22 **Podnieks E.** National survey on abuse of the elderly in Canada. *Journal of Elder Abuse and Neglect,* 1992; **4**: 5–58.

Chapter 16

The nature of elder abuse

Claudine McCreadie

Elder abuse is a single or repeated act or lack of appropriate action occurring within any relationship where there is an expectation of trust which causes harm or distress to an older person.[1]

Introduction

In 1987, under the chairmanship of a local geriatrician, members of the Birmingham branch of BASE—the British Association for Service to the Elderly (a forum to further better care for older people)—decided that the issue of abuse to older people was a topic which they wanted to pursue at one of their bimonthly meetings. That first meeting became a catalyst for a series of wide-ranging discussions based on members' experience, the record of which was later published.[2] One of the major purposes of the document was 'to bring to people's attention the widespread occurrence and great variety of abuse within a relatively small geographical area and known to a small number of professional people'.

Although a small and selective sample, involving cases known to members of the group, the nature of elder abuse is well illustrated by the 32 case examples given in this publication, since they bear out most of the conclusions that research has reached to date about the abuse of older people.[3,4] They show the diversity of abuse, its seriousness and its complexity. There are examples of psychological abuse, physical abuse and financial abuse, examples of abuse in institutional settings, and examples of abuse by relatives, friends and paid careworkers. Some illustrate the longstanding nature of the abuse, what Homer and Gilleard[5] call the 'elderly graduates of domestic violence', where long-term violence in a relationship may be exacerbated by the ageing process and/or by illness or disability in either or both parties. Some illustrate that the victim of the abuse is the carer—of a partner or adult child with problems relating to illness or disability. Some show the significance of alcohol as a warning 'red light' in households. Some demonstrate the vulnerability of an older person to financial abuse. Dementia features prominently, as it does in many case examples (see, for example, [6]). Many of the examples show that the older person is already in touch with social services. The examples also draw attention to aspects of abuse in communal settings that distinguish it from abuse in people's own homes—lack of privacy when toileting, nakedness in front of strangers, infantilizing or threatening speech by nurses and the compulsory wearing of hospital clothes.

Risk in the Community

A comprehensive review of research on elder abuse suggests that any notion of risk needs to be related both to the different types of abuse, and to the different settings in which it may occur.[3] Some of these areas remain almost completely unresearched, so little can be said about them. It is important to distinguish different types of abuse, in conjunction with different patterns of living arrangement for older people. The nature of the risk of abuse is almost certainly different according to whether people live on their own or are co-resident with others. The most thoroughly researched area of elder abuse relates to physical and verbal abuse in people's own homes. Somewhat obviously this suggests that risk is higher for people living together. It has to be remembered that the majority of men of all ages in the UK live with a partner, but vastly larger numbers of women, particularly over the age of 80, live on their own.[3] The somewhat limited research suggests that the risk of financial abuse increases for people living on their own,[3] a living arrangement in which mental impairment may render them more vulnerable. There is some evidence that financial abuse is more likely to be perpetrated by more distant relations. The financial affairs of older people with dementia appear invariably not to be correctly ordered in a way that will minimize the risk of financial abuse.[7,8] Doctors may well be approached to advise on this and need to know to whom to refer people for appropriate guidance.[9]

Sexual abuse has been very little researched, but such work as there is suggests that the victims are overwhelmingly female, and dependent on others for their care. Dementia may be an important risk factor. Finally, although research suggests that neglect is the least prevalent of the different types of abuse, it is the type, apart from sexual abuse, that most nearly fits what has been the popular picture of abuse. Neglected older people are invariably in poor health, dependent on a carer, and may be mentally frail.

One of the most important relationships to consider is whether the risk of abuse is related to impairment or disability in the older person. Research suggests that dependency in the abused person, measured in terms of their need for help with activities of daily living, is not a significant risk factor in itself, but dependent older people will be at risk in the sense that there is a greater potential for harming those who are physically or mentally most impaired.[10] Table 16.1 comes from one of the few pieces of solid research that have been done in the UK on the abuse of older people.[5] Homer interviewed 51 carers looking after very dependent older people, all of whom were receiving respite care in a geriatric ward. Half the patients had had a stroke, almost half had dementia, and further problems such as Parkinson's disease, blindness, amputations and severe musculoskeletal disorders were also suffered by many of the patients. Standard research definitions of abuse were used (Table 16.1).

Table 16.1 Reported abuse from a group of 51 carers and 48 patients, London, 1989. (Homer and Gilleard 1990)

Type of abuse	Abuse by carer, reported by:		Abuse by patient, reported by:	
	Carer	Patient	Carer	Patient
Physical	7	1	9	3
Verbal	21	9	17	10
Neglect	6	9	n/a	n/a

Source: Homer and Gilleard, 1990. Table II.
Definitions used by Homer and Gilleard 1990
Physical abuse: 'being pushed, grabbed slapped, hit with a weapon etc'.
Verbal abuse: 'chronic verbal aggression, repeated insults, being sworn at, threats at least 10 times in the preceding year'.
Neglect: 'deprivation of some assistance that the elderly person needed for some important activites of daily living such as getting meals and drinks, washing, and going to the toilet'.

Carers who admitted to abuse were compared with those who did not. The research brought out strikingly, despite the small and particular size of the sample, the widely replicated finding that physical and verbal abuse has less to do with the condition of the person who is abused and more to do with their *family and living situation*. That is to say, the factors giving rise to the abuse stem from household circumstances and relationships and personalities, rather than from conditions common to ageing such as immobility, incontinence and dementia. The research also brought out another increasingly recognized fact, namely that carers can be at risk from the behaviour of the dependent person. Studies of patients with dementia, in particular, have shown significantly higher levels of violence, both towards the carer and from the carer.[11] A postal survey of carers of dementia sufferers in the London Borough of Ealing, while limited by a low response rate of 34 per cent, used the same definitions as Homer and Gilleard.[12] Approximately half the respondents (35 out of 67) admitted to verbal abuse, an eighth (eight out of 67) to physical abuse and the same number to neglect. Like Homer and Gilleard, the authors found that there were different associations with the different types of abuse:

> Verbal abuse and neglect but not physical abuse were associated with a poorer premorbid relationship with the patient. Carers who admitted to verbal abuse noted frequent arguments with the patient as a feature of their interactions with the patient before the onset of dementia.[12]

The importance of premorbid relationships was brought out strongly in a recent study in Northern Ireland,[13] again focusing on the carers of patients with dementia and using the same definitions as the Cooney and Mortimer study. This study found a significant difference in the severity and frequency of problem behaviour by the abused group. Cooney and Mortimer[12] found that although carers who admitted to physical abuse

Table 16.2 Results from an Australian case series documented at an area-based geriatric and rehabilitation hospital between July 1989 to June 1990 (Kurrle *et al.* 1991).

Definition of physical abuse: observed physical injury inflicted by another on an older person
Definition of neglect: conduct by the carer that results in deprivation of care necessary to maintain physical and mental health.
Number of documented cases: 12 soft tissue injury (including 2 with fractures, 1 with laceration); 2 malnutrition, 1 decubitus ulcer.
Characteristics of abused people: 6 men; 9 women; age range: 66—91.
Impairments in abused people: dementia, 6 cases; stroke with aphasia and hemiparesis, 1; osteoarthritis, 2; rheumatoid arthritis, 1; paranoid delusions and mild cognitive loss, 1; ischaemic heart disease, 1; no impairments, 3.
Characteristics of abusers: 8 men (7 husbands), 7 women (2 wives). Age range: 36 (son) to 84 (husband). Neglect cases: 1 daughter (mild developmental disability). 1 wife (schizophrenia), 1 son (drug and alcohol dependency). Physical abuse cases: 7 husbands (4 dementia, 2 sociopathic personality disorders, 1 paraphrenia); 2 friends (1 sociopathic personality disorder; 1 'carer stress'—caring role moderate for 1 year); 1 daughter-in-law ('carer stress'—caring role moderate for 9 months), 1 wife ('uncertain', carer role slight for 5 years), 1 grand-daughter ('carer stress', caring role extensive for 2 years).

---

were more likely to note physical abuse by the patient, 'overall levels of behavioural disturbance using an "objective" rating scale did not differ between abused and non-abused patients'. Like Homer and Gilleard, they found no relationship between the level of formal or informal support and the existence of abuse.

Early studies focused on the stress imposed on the carer by the burden of caring and therefore explained abuse by reference to the dependency of the abused person. However, there is little evidence that the stress of caring for a dependent elder is on its own a cause of abuse. Large numbers of carers are 'under stress' but do not abuse their relative. The crucial issue is to try and discriminate between abusing and non-abusing situations. Research on physical and verbal abuse consistently finds that characteristics associated with the abuser—particularly their physical and mental health and notably, in many studies, their consumption of alcohol—are those that discriminate. An Australian case series provides an excellent illustration.[14] Fifteen cases of elder abuse presenting during a year at an area-based geriatric and rehabilitation hospital were examined. In only three cases was 'carer stress' identified as the major characteristic and in only one case—that of a 42-year-old granddaughter caring for her 90-year-old grandmother (with obesity and osteoarthritis)—was the caring role said to be 'extensive'. Further details are shown in Table 16.2.

Risk in institutions

There is little evidence about abuse in institutional settings.[3] Although the definitions used in the domestic setting apply to the communal one, methods of caring assume significance, particularly as the prevalence of physical and mental disability is generally so high amongst older people in communal settings. Research in 57 residential and nursing homes in the USA found that 10 per cent of 577 staff admitted to at least one act of physical abuse in the preceding year: excessive restraint was the most frequently recorded form. Thirty-six per cent of respondents had observed at least one act of physical abuse by others in the preceding year; restraint accounted for around two-thirds of reports.[15] Respondents reported a very much higher rate of verbal abuse than of physical abuse. Significant factors in explaining both kinds of abuse were staff burn-out, patient aggression and staff–patient conflict. Numerous enquiries in Britain into grave deficiencies in various areas of institutional care for all age groups have shown that abuse flourishes within a culture which allows it to be acceptable. Clough,[16] after an analysis of these enquiries, suggested that there are a number of warning signs. It has been suggested in the United States that greater attention should be paid to the risk of sexual abuse in residential and nursing home settings.[3] Within institutional settings, very little is known about financial abuse. Again there is an important issue over whether the appropriate arrangements for handling older people's financial affairs are in place and whether there is someone responsible for seeing that these protect the elderly from financial exploitation.[7]

Intervention

It is now clear that there are a diversity of often complex situations under the general heading of abuse.[17] For the general practitioner, the majority of cases, whether in domestic or instititutional settings, are likely to arise as part of some other presenting problem. There is widespread agreement that prevention depends on an awareness that abuse is a possibility and that identification requires a high index of suspicion.[18] Abuse is frequently denied. Physical symptoms may be common to frail older people suffering from chronic disease and can be unreliable indicators.[19,20] Psychological symptoms similarly arise from a wide range of causes and so in themselves are no indicator of abuse. All the evidence points to the need to view the patient in the context of his/her lifestyle and family or institutional environment.[18] Research by McCreadie et al.[21] used logistic regression techniques to predict a 'diagnosis' of abuse by GPs in two locations. GPs were seven times more likely to have identified a case of physical or verbal abuse, or neglect, if they had also identified patients in five or more risk situations for abuse. The most commonly identified risk situations involved alcohol consumption, dementia and problems of a household member, including problems of a carer in their own right. Variables relating to the GP—gender, experience, home visiting rates, size of practice, or number of older patients had no significant effect. The research was replicated in Sweden with remarkably similar results.[22]

Conclusion

General practitioners face both opportunities and dilemmas. The opportunities arise from the GP's knowledge of particular households, their history, the quality of their relationships and the physical and mental state of their members, although doubt has been cast on how thorough this knowledge is.[23] The dilemmas—shared often in relation to domestic violence—arise from pressures on the doctor's time (not only time with the patient, but time to make contact with colleagues elsewhere); the conflicting loyalties that may arise in relation to different members of the same household; the sometimes acute shortage of resources of some vital community services that may address the needs of the abuser; and in the sheer perceived intractability of some of the situations— particularly if there is an only too understandable reluctance by older people to move themselves, or to see a partner or adult child moved.[24,25] However, there is some evidence from domestic violence research that people would welcome factual questions about abuse, and the evidence from elder abuse research is that carers invariably are relieved to have the opportunity to talk about their situation and how they respond to it.[26]

References

1 **Action on Elder Abuse.** *Everybody's Business: Taking Action on Elder Abuse.* London: Action on Elder Abuse, 1995.

2 **British Association for Service to the Elderly.** *Old Age Abuse: Lifting the Lid.* Birmingham: British Association for Service to the Elderly/West Midlands Institute of Geriatric Medicine, 1991.

3 **McCreadie C.** *Elder Abuse: Update on Research.* London: Age Concern Institute of Gerontology, King's College London, 1996.

4 **McCreadie C, Tinker A.** Elder abuse. In: Tallis RC, Fillitt H, Brocklehurst J, eds. *Brocklehurst's Textbook of Geriatric Medicine and Gerontology,* 6th edn. Edinburgh: Churchill Livingstone, 2002.

5 **Homer A, Gilleard CJ.** Abuse of elderly people by their carers. *BMJ* 1990; **301**: 1359–62.

6 **Decalmer P, Glendenning F.** *The Mistreatment of Older People,* 2nd edn. London: Sage, 1997.

7 **Langan J, Means R.** Financial management and elderly people with dementia in the UK: as much a question of confusion as abuse? *Ageing and Society* 1996; **16**: 287–314.

8 **Tueth MJ.** Exposing financial exploitation of impaired elderly persons. *American Journal Geriatric Psychiatry* 2000; **8** (2): 104–11.

9 **Al-Adwani A, Nabi W.** Financial management in patients with dementia: their adult children's knowledge and views. *International Journal of Geriatric Psychiatry* 1998; **13**: 462–5.

10 **Lachs M, Pillemer KA.** Abuse and neglect of elderly persons. *New England Journal of Medicine* 1995; **332**: 437–43.

11 **Cooney C, Howard R.** Review: abuse of patients with dementia by carers—out of sight but not out of mind. *International Journal of Geriatric Psychiatry* 1995; **10**: 735–41.

12 **Cooney C, Mortimer A.** Elder abuse and dementia—a pilot study. *International Journal of Social Psychiatry* 1995; **41**: 276–83.

13 **Compton SA, Flanigan P, Gregg W.** Elder abuse in people with dementia in Northern Ireland: prevalence and predictors in cases referred to a psychiatry of old age service. *International Journal of Geriatric Psychiatry* 1997; **12**: 632–5.

14 **Kurrle SE, Sadler PM, Cameron ID.** Elder abuse—an Australian case series. *Medical Journal of Australia* 1991; **155**: 150–3.

15 **Pillemer KA, Moore D.** Abuse of patient in nursing homes: findings from a survey of staff. *Gerontologist* 1989; **29**: 314–20.

16 **Clough R.** *Scandals in Residential Care: Report to the Independent Review of Residenital Care, Chaired by Lady Wagner.* London: National Institute of Social Work, 1988.

17 **Kerr J, Dening T, Lawton C.** Elder abuse and the community psychiatric team. *Psychiatric Bulletin*, 1994; **18**: 730–2.

18 **Fisk J.** Abuse of the elderly. In: Jacoby R, Oppenheimer C, eds. *Psychiatry in the Elderly*, 2nd edn. Oxford: Oxford University Press, 1997.

19 **Bennett G, Kingston P.** *Elder Abuse: Concepts Theories and Interventions.* London: Chapman & Hall, 1993.

20 **O'Brien JG.** Screening: a primary care clinician's perspective. In: Baumhover LA, Beall SC, eds. *Abuse, Neglect and Exploitation of Older Persons: Strategies for Assessment and Intervention.* London: Jessica Kingsley, 1996: 00.

21 **McCreadie C, Bennett G, Gilthorpe MS, Houghton G, Tinker A.** Elder abuse: do GPs know or care? *Journal of the Royal Society of Medicine* 2000; **93** (2): 67–72.

22 **Saveman B-I, Sandvide A.** Swedish general practitioners awareness of elderly patients at risk of or actually suffering from elder abuse. *Scandinavian Journal of Caring Sciences* 2001; **15** (3): 244–9.

23 **Gulbrandsen P, Hjortdahl P, Fugelli P.** General practitioners' knowledge of their patients' psychosocial problems: multipractice questionnaire survey. *BMJ* 1997; **314**: 1014–18.

24 **Noone JF, Decalmer P, Glendenning F.** The general practitioner and elder abuse. In: Decalmer P, Glendenning F, eds. *The Mistreatment of Elderly People.* London: Sage, 1997: 136–47.

25 **Richardson J, Feder G.** Domestic violence: a hidden problem for general practice. *British Journal of General Practice* 1996; **46**: 239–42.

26 **Homer A.** *Elder Abuse.* Royal College of General Practitioners Members Reference Book. London: Royal College of General Practitioners, 1996.

Chapter 17

The presentation and diagnosis of elder abuse

Gerry Bennett

Introduction

Most relationships older people have in a domestic (and institutional setting) are positive, some are not. Violence against older people has been a consistent thread through world literature but public discussions of these private events is a recent phenomenon. From initial 'response' letters and articles to child abuse,[1,2] elder abuse has more recently been addressed within a family violence framework reference. The only United Kingdom random sample, community-based epidemiological study of elder abuse to date took place in 1992.[3] This study allowed for cautious projections concerning abuse and the British population indicating that up to one million older people could be at risk of verbal /psychological abuse and up to half a million at risk of either physical or financial abuse. The Action on Elder Abuse telephone helpline analysed the first 3919 calls[4] and found that of the 1564 calls seeking information and support about incidents they considered abusive, the majority of callers were women, 30 per cent identified themselves as victims of elder abuse, 40 per cent of callers were relatives and 20 per cent paid careworkers. Over two-thirds of cases of abuse occurred in people's own homes while a further 22 per cent occurred in either residential or nursing homes. Psychological abuse predominated (39 per cent), with 23 per cent of cases being physical abuse and 23 per cent financial abuse. Ten per cent of calls concerned neglect and 2 per cent sexual abuse. Nearly as many women as men perpetrated abuse with 46 per cent being a relative (child, spouse or in-law), while paid workers committed 29 per cent of abuse cases. This study does not allow extrapolation of figures to the national picture (because callers remain anonymous and their motivation for calling the service is unknown). The number of calls to the helpline is now many thousands more and the statistics remain very similar[5] making it the largest sample of potential cases of elder abuse in the UK.

This evidence puts the presentation and diagnosis of abuse of older people firmly in a primary care setting. General practitioners' awareness of the topic has been studied[6] and · this work indicates that elder abuse is a clinical dilemma for primary care workers and that GPs recognize the clinical scenarios that have evolved from research evidence and that frame many abuse situations. The clinical situation remains complex and challenging but the importance of this issue in terms of morbidity and mortality should not be underestimated. In a powerful study,[7] the data from an annual health survey of 2812 elders in one US city was examined and merged with reports of elder abuse and neglect made to the local adult abuse agency over a 9-year period. When the mortality rates of the non-abused and abused were compared, by the thirteenth year following the start of the study, 40 per cent of the non-reported (non-abused, non-neglected) group were still alive and only 9 per cent of the physically abused or neglected elders. After controlling for all possible factors that might affect mortality (e.g. age, gender, income, financial status, cognitive status, diagnosis, social supports, etc.) and finding no significant relationships, the researchers speculate that mistreatment causes extreme interpersonal stress that may confer an additional death risk.

Neglect is a poor relation term to abuse in the United Kingdom, yet comes under the broad umbrella of mistreatment. Pressure ulcers (death of skin and underlying tissues from the effect of pressure, friction and shear) are a quality indicator and the development of pressure ulcers implies neglect. The magnitude of this condition is, again, illuminating to health care workers, with approximately 10 per cent of hospital inpatients developing pressure ulcers.[8] The neglect /abuse link is illustrated by research carried out in Germany.[9] In a prospective postmortem study of 10 222 corpses, 11.2 per cent had a pressure ulcer (the majority deep and over the sacrum). The author states: 'The prevalence of pressure sores in a defined population can be seen as a parameter for the quality of nursing and medical care. In bringing these fatalities to light, the field of legal medicine contributes to a general quality control of standards.'[9]

Recognition and assessment

A 4 year old presenting with a fractured arm will, without exception, have non-accidental injury as part of the differential diagnosis—i.e. clinical staff are educated and primed to 'think the unthinkable' and within a structured context include a challenging diagnosis amongst the more classic disease models. How many 84 year olds presenting with a fractured hip will be assessed in the same holistic framework? Abused older people remain outside mainstream medical thinking and unless a condition is recognized it will not be diagnosed (at least not early on).

Primary care physicians will be at the forefront of the presentation or allegations of elder abuse. It is always a challenging situation and GPs are not meant to be (or trained) as forensic pathologists or lawyers. They should, however, feel part of a team and the 'system' being developed post No Secrets[10] should include and support the GP within that management framework. The network involved for each case (real or suspected) should include social services adult protection lead officers, the GP and, where appropriate, hospital consultant specialists, legal advice and police advice. The framework widens where necessary and may include housing, voluntary sector, etc. The older person is at the centre of this network of caring professionals with, hopefully, mechanisms in place for their support (e.g. advocacy schemes) and support for carers /relatives.

All social services must have established formal procedures within their adult protection policies for dealing with suspected /accepted cases of elder abuse post *No Secrets*. They will be the lead agency, though the pathway should involve many disciplines. GPs may refer cases following a clinical assessment or be approached by the lead social services officer to bring a medical perspective if the referral originated elsewhere. Some key points may help keep clinicians grounded in reality and within their depth of expertise:

- It is useful to avoid the term 'abuse'; 'inadequate care' is an acceptable alternative and following investigations may or may not be found to be caused by abuse.
- Understand one's role in the process being undertaken.

If a GP suspects 'abuse' it is important to get basic details and, where possible, discuss the situation with the social services lead officers, i.e. share and benchmark the information. Use the process one is skilled in, i.e. history-taking and examination:

- Interview involved parties separately, asking 'open' questions.
- Document carefully—the importance of record keeping cannot be stressed too highly.
- 'Disclosure'—the term used when a client or perpetrator reveals details of abuse— is common when people feel they can speak about such events, i.e. the holistic communication approach.
- Assess the patient's mental state to give the interview context. (Confusion does not discount reports but it does make the whole situation more challenging.)
- Client autonomy means that many older people stay in abusive situations despite professional advice. In cases where the mental capacity to make decisions that involve significant personal risk appears impaired, further advice and assessment from a psychiatrist is usually required.
- It is the history that usually helps complete the jigsaw. Physical examination may reveal unambiguous marks (burns in the shape of an iron, buckle marks, etc.). These are unusual, although bruises and skin lesions occur for many physiological reasons. It is still important to document them all.
- It may be important to seek a photographic record of marks /injuries. Obtain written consent; in cases of mental incapacity act in the patient's best interests and obtain photographs if you feel it is important and appropriate to do so. Police advice can be helpful here.
- Interviews can be repeated later, when it may require a more experienced investigator.

- Avoid confrontation, e. g. 'I suspect Mrs X has been abused'. Use more open phrases such as 'I am uncertain as to the cause of the marks /bruises and will use the locally established procedures to help me try and reach a diagnosis'.
- Obviously a 'disclosure' may alter the dialogue process.

The focus of attention has been dominated by an analysis of the perceived characteristics of the abused older person (demented, incontinent, faller) and looking for the 'carer stress' trigger. There has been an increasing emphasis away from this simplistic and indeed erroneous approach.[11,12] Some sociomedical features of older people and their carers, which may increase the risk of abuse, have been summarized by Lachs and Pillemer.[12] They are potential risk factors and research evidence for their inclusion has been evaluated. Each includes a view on the mechanism involved:

- Poor health and functional impairment of the victim—disability reduces an elderly person's ability either to defend him or herself or seek help.
- Cognitive impairment—dementia may cause aggression towards a carer and /or be associated with difficult and disruptive behaviour, precipitating abuse. Higher rates of abuse have been found among dementia patients who 'hit out'.
- Abuser deviance—abusers are likely to depend on the victim financially, for housing and in other areas. Abuse often results from the carer's (often adult children) attempts to obtain material resources from the older person.
- Living arrangements—abuse is much less common where elderly people live alone. A shared living environment provides more opportunities for tension and conflict, which generally precede abusive acts.
- External stress—stressful life events (illness, bereavement, unemployment /retirement) and chronic financial hardship decrease a family's ability to cope and increase the likelihood of abuse.
- Social isolation—elderly people with few social contacts are more likely to suffer abuse. Isolation also reduces the likelihood that abuse will be detected and stopped. Social support can act as a buffer against stress.
- History of violence—a prior history of violence in a relationship, especially with spouses, can be a predictor of abuse in later life.

Lachs and Pillemer also summarized the clinical knowledge base available, based on original work by Jones.[13] The presentation may suggest elder abuse and /or neglect:

- Delays between injury or illness and seeking medical attention; examples include lacerations healing by secondary intention, X-rays revealing healing by misaligned fractures.
- Compensated chronic disease presenting *in extremis* where the carer has been monitoring the patient.

- Differing histories from patient and abuser; examples include different mechanisms of injury offered and different chronology (timings) of injuries.

- Implausible or vague explanations provided by either party, e.g. fractures that are not explained by the mechanisms of injury.

- Frequent accident and emergency department visits for chronic disease exacerbation, despite care plan and available resources, e.g. chronic obtrusive airways disease or chronic heart failure due to lack of medicines or their administration.

- Functionally impaired patients who present without the main carer available; an example is a patient with advanced dementia who presents to the A and E department alone.

- Laboratory findings that are inconsistent with the history, or prove subtherapeutic drug levels (e.g. digoxin), despite carer-reported compliance. Toxicology may reveal that psychotropic agents are not being administered.

General clinicians, especially geriatricians, are more likely to encounter the less dramatic forms of abuse, e.g. psychological/emotional, and their task is made even more difficult by such things as the amount of chronic disease (multiple pathology) present in this age group and the altered presentation of disease. United Kingdom geriatricians have championed these facts for over three decades. The message includes the fact that disease may present classically in older age (and hence be recognized by all clinicians) but, crucially, in the older and more frail it may not. This altered presentation of disease was termed the 'geriatric giants' by Isaacs[14] to indicate its importance to elderly people. Any disease process can present in this way:

- confusion;

- incontinence;

- immobility;

- falls.

Unfortunately, few see beyond the presentation state to the ill older person behind, who can usually be restored to better if not full health. It is inevitable that as the education process around elder abuse reaches a wider audience another information gap will become apparent, and the presentation of ill health may mimic some aspects of abuse and hence lead to false positive diagnoses. This process will only be minimalized by all health care workers becoming aware of both sets of issues. Formal protocols are by their nature holistic and multidisciplinary, and are pioneered by those working with older people. More than one assessment may be necessary and the complexity of the cases necessitates mental as well as physical evaluation. Assessment includes the view and needs of the carer's activities of daily living (ADL).

In the USA, some clinicians are using formal protocols to improve the detection rate. These act as an *aide mémoire*, so that unexplained injuries or implausible explanations are not overlooked, and undernutrition or dehydration are questioned when a main carer is present. A formal elder abuse protocol has yet to be pioneered in the United Kingdom. Government initiatives such as *No Secrets*[10] pave the way for integrated pathways developed between social services (as the lead agency), health, police, voluntary sectors, etc. US protocols have been used for over a decade and have developed into targeting and assessment instruments:[15]

- *History from the elderly person.* The patient should be interviewed alone. There should be direct but open enquiries about physical violence, restraints or neglect, and precise details about the nature, frequency and severity of these events. Include a functional assessment (independence with ADL). Note who is the main carer if ADL impairment is present.

- *History from the alleged abuser.* The alleged abuser should also be interviewed alone. This can be a highly demanding situation and is usually best carried out by someone skilled in these interviewing techniques. Confrontation should be avoided in the information-gathering stage. Interview other sources if possible. Enquire about recent psychological factors (bereavement, illness, unemployment and financial hardship). Check the carer's understanding of the patient's physical or mental health (care needs, prognosis) and ask for the carer's explanations for the injuries or physical findings.

- *Behavioural observation.* Look for withdrawal, infantalizing of the patient by the carer, or the carer who insists on giving the history.

- *General appearance.* Note the patient's state of hygiene, general cleanliness and appropriateness of clothing.

- *Skin/mucous membranes.* Note skin turgor and other signs of dehydration (NB skin turgor can be a misleading sign in some elderly people). Check multiple skin lesions in various stage of evolution. Note the presence of bruises and pressure sores and how such lesions have been managed (NB many elderly people bruise easily—senile purpura secondary to photoageing or medication; and pressure sores, in addition to implying neglect, can also indicate underlying ill-health).

- *Head and neck.* Look for traumatic alopecia (distinguishable from male pattern baldness on the basis of distribution), scalp haematomas, lacerations and abrasions.

- *Trunk.* Examine for welts and weals; the shape may suggest the implement used (e.g. belt or iron).

- *Genitourinary.* Examine for rectal bleeding, vaginal bleeding, infestations, and evidence of trauma or pressure ulcers. Recent suspected rape requires expert examination by clinicians used to dealing with such cases and obtaining the appropriate specimens.

- *Extremities.* Wrist or ankle lesions suggest the use of restraints or immersion burns (glove/stocking distribution).

- *Musculoskeletal.* Examine for occult fractures and pain. Observe the gait.

- *Neurological/psychiatric.* This needs a formal and thorough neurological examination to ascertain the focal site of any lesion. Anxiety and depressive symptoms should be assessed. Where symptoms suggest formal testing, depression rating scales should be used or referral to a psychiatrist made.

- *Mental state.* Formal testing should be carried out using the Mini-Mental State questionnaire. Cognitive impairment suggests either delirium (acute confusional state) or dementia (chronic confusional state) is present. This then needs further assessment to rule out treatable causes, but also indicates a question over decision-making capacity. Psychiatric symptoms may be present, including delusions and hallucinations.

- *Imaging.* The tests ordered will derive from the clinical evaluation.

- *Laboratory tests.* Again, the tests ordered will be indicated from the history and examination and may include drug levels, albumin, blood urea and electrolytes, haemoglobin and, occasionally, toxicology.

- *Social and financial resources.* Document the social networks (formal and informal) available to assist the patient. Record all available financial resources. This information may be crucial if interventions are considered later that include alternative living arrangements and/or the provision of home services.

Most clinicians are not expected to be experts in a number of areas. They are expected to keep regularly updated, and be aware of developing and emerging issues in medicine as a whole and the related social impact. Clinical governance includes the above with an expectation of appropriate history-taking and examination skills that lead to a differential diagnosis. This should be followed by an understanding of the procedures to be followed and the clinician's role within them. Violence against older people in all its forms has emerged and is now in the medical practitioner's expected domain of generalist expertise. Process and a knowledge base are available to help clinicians manage these complex and challenging cases—older people themselves would expect this challenge to be taken up. Education will be a key factor, especially as the data from research helps formulate diagnosis and assessment abilities as well as interview strategies. In the words of Benjamin Franklin, 'Tell me and I forget, teach me and I remember, involve me and I learn'.

References

1 Baker AA. Granny battering. *Modern Geriatrics* 1975; **8**: 20–4.
2 Burston G. Do your elderly relatives live in fear of being battered? *Modern Geriatrics* 1977; 7 (5): 54–5.

3 Ogg J, Bennett GCJ. Elder abuse in Britain, *BMJ* 1992; **305**: 998–9.

4 Bennett GCJ, Jenkins G, Asif Z. Listening is not enough: an analysis of calls to the Elder Abuse Response. *Journal of Adult Protection* 2000; **2** (1): 6–20.

5 Bennett GCJ, (unpublished data, 2001).

6 McCreadie C, Bennett G, Gathorpe MS, Houghton G, Tinker A. Elder abuse: do general practitioners know or care? *Journal of the Royal Society of Medicine* 2000; **93**: 67–71.

7 Lachs M, Williams CS, O'Brien S, Pillemer KA, Charlson ME. The mortality of elder mistreatment. *JAMA* 1998; **280** (5): 428–32.

8 O'Dea K. The prevalence of pressure damage in acute care hospital patients in the UK. *Journal of Wound Care* 1999; **8**(4): 192–94.

9 Tsokos M, Heinemann A, Püschel K Pressure sores: epidemiology, medico-legal complications and forensic argument concerning causality. *International Journal of Legal Medicine* 2000; **113** (5): 283–7.

10 Department of Health. *No Secrets: the Protection of Vulnerable Adults—Guidance on the Development and Implementation of Multi-agency Policies and Procedures.* London: HMSO, 2000.

11 Bennett GCJ. Shifting emphasis from abused to abuser. *Geriatric Medicine* 1999; May 20: 45–7.

12 Lachs M, Pillemer K. Abuse and neglect of elderly persons. *New England Medical Journal* 1995; **332** (7) 437–43.

13 Jones JS. Geriatric abuse and neglect. In: Bosker G, Schwarz GR, Jones JS, Sequeira M, eds. *Geriatric Emergency Medicine.* St Louis, MO: Mosby, 1990: 00.

14 Isaacs B, Livingstone M, Neville Y. *Survival of the Unfittest: a Study of Geriatric Patients in Glasgow.* London; Routledge & Kegan Paul, 1972.

15 Mount Senai Victim Service Agency. Elder *Mistreatment Guidelines for Health Care Professionals.* Elder Abuse Project, 1988.

Chapter 18

Onward referral

Chapter 18a

Introduction

Iona Heath

General practitioners express uncertainty about their role in the management of elder abuse[1] and have six areas of concern:

- patient autonomy;
- confidentiality;
- conflict of interest between family members when both are patients;
- powerlessness;
- inadequacy of resources;
- questions about the proper role of GPs in these situations.

Whereas the responsibilities of the general practitioner in relation to both child abuse and domestic violence are relatively clearly defined, the correct response to elder abuse remains elusive (Fig. 18.1). In child abuse, the practitioner must prioritize the interests and protection of the child; in domestic violence, the prime responsibility is to respect and promote the autonomy of the abused women and support her in making her own decisions. In elder abuse, a delicate balance must be struck depending on the mental competence of the abused older person. When the older person is fully competent, no matter how physically frail, the appropriate response to elder abuse parallels that to domestic violence. Indeed, some elder abuse represents the progression of longstanding domestic violence over time so that both the perpetrator and the abused person have become old. In such cases, the abused older person's wishes must be elicited and respected, although much can be achieved by offering extra help within the home, so that the stresses of daily living are minimized and the transactions of care more closely

INADEQUATE
GENERAL PRACTITIONER
RESPONSE

HELPING FACTORS	HINDERING FACTORS
Desire to offer a high standard of service to all patients whatever their health need	Inadequate investment by society in the care of the frail elderly
Long-term relationship of general practitioner and patient	Time constraints within general practitioner service
Long-term relationship of general practitioner and carer who is also often a patient	Hidden presentation that offers the general practitioner the opportunity of collusion
Accessibility, acceptability and lack of stigma of the general practice consultation	Fear of revealing a problem that difficult and time-consuming to tackle
Increasing 'partnership of experts' within general practice allowing empowerment of patient and carer	Sense of helplessness about being able to improve the situation combined with a fear of making things worse
Expertise and support of the primary health care team	Relationship between the general practitioner and the extended family
Placement of social workers within primary health care teams	Difficulty of asking the question
Gradually increasing professional and public recognition of elder abuse in a range of settings	Complications of confusion and dementia
	Inadequate record-keeping
Increasing understanding of the range of presentations of elder abuse	Limited availability of services able to offer appropriate help
Information offered by Action on Elder Abuse, Age Concern and other agencies	Lack of availability of information at the moment of the consultation

EFFECTIVE AND ENABLING
GENERAL PRACTITIONER
RESPONSE

Fig. 18.1 Forcefield analysis of general practitioner role in elder abuse.

supervised. In situations where the older person is rendered incompetent through confusion or dementia, the priority shifts towards the protection of the abused person. However, again, situations can be complicated by relationships in which each party is both a victim and a perpetrator of abuse.

The close relationship between a frail older person and their carer may easily compromise the older person's rights to confidentiality and health care professionals will

Table 18.1 The similarities and differences between domestic violence and elder abuse.[2]

Domestic violence	Elder abuse
Physical and sexual violence, emotional abuse	Also includes financial abuse and neglect
Violence as criminal behaviour	Emphasis on protection
Violence by men towards women	Violence by men and women towards men and women
Violence by partners and ex-partners	Violence by adult children, partners, siblings, friends, neighbours
Clear victim; clear perpetrator	Ambiguities over victim

need to be pay very explicit attention to these rights. When the older person is suffering from confusion or dementia, the situation becomes even more complicated as the imperative to protect begins to override the duty of confidentiality.

McCreadie[2] has usefully tabulated the overlaps and differences in understanding between domestic violence and elder abuse (Table 18.1)

General practitioners may also feel that the usefulness of their intervention is undermined by a lack of clear local policies for the management of elder abuse and inadequate opportunities for effective interagency liaison. However, social services departments are actively developing their role in relation to elder abuse and are now expected to have a local multi-agency code of practice in place. Practitioners may wish to ask for a named contact with responsibility for elder abuse and the protection of vulnerable adults. Every primary health care professional who has contact with older people has a responsibility to identify local resources and named contacts across agencies who are able to contribute to the management of elder abuse. Action on Elder Abuse (tel. 020 8765 7000) has produced a useful information leaflet for doctors which outlines the range of possible interventions.[3]

The following subsections of this chapter have been written by community nurses, a social worker and a lawyer. Each has been asked to describe their role in the management of elder abuse, what they would like or expect from general practitioners and what general practitioners can reasonably expect from them.

References

1 McCreadie C, Bennett GCJ, Tinker A. *General practitioners' knowledge and experience of the abuse/ill treatment of older people in the community. Report to King's Fund.* London: Age Concern Institute of Gerontology, King's College London, June 1997.

2 McCreadie C. *Elder Abuse: Update on Research.* London: Age Concern Institute of Gerontology, King's College London, 1996. p.19.

3 Action on Elder Abuse. *The Abuse of Older People—Information for Doctors.* London: Action on Elder Abuse, 1998 (in press).

Chapter 18b

The role of the community nurse

Lynne Phair and Wendy Goodman

Introduction

The community nurse is ideally suited to be a prime mover in the prevention, detection and management of elder abuse, due mainly to the unique relationship she has with her patient. The nurse is usually welcomed into the home, has the opportunity to see the interactions between other family/carer members where appropriate, will carry out an in-depth verbal assessment and, where necessary, is allowed to carry out intimate treatments. To augment this, the nurse will have close contact with the patient's general practitioner and should have a good working relationship with community nursing colleagues and staff of the social services department.

All first-level registered nurses have undertaken at least 3 years preregistration training and education. Further study at university is needed to gain the qualification of district nurse, health visitor or community psychiatric nurse, which gives registered nurses the skills to assess the nursing needs of patients/carers in the community and to plan, implement and evaluate this care.

All nurses are personally accountable for their practice and are bound by a Code of Professional Conduct.[1] Two particular points from the code are perhaps worthy of further discussion in relation to elder abuse; a registered nurse midwife or health visitor must:

- protect and support the health of individual patients and clients, and protect and support the health of the wider community;
- protect confidential information. Only disclose information outside the team with the patient's consent. If the patient withholds consent or if consent cannot be obtained for whatever reason, disclosures may only be made where they can be justified in the public interest.

The first point should ensure that all nurses are heedful of any 'risk' situations, whether clinical or social. In reality, however, they do need to be aware of what constitutes a risk situation. Elder abuse is a relatively new concept to most people and systems need to be in place to raise this awareness.

The second point ensures that, as with other health professionals, nurses are required to keep a confidence. However, elder abuse is now being recognized as 'a matter of wider public interest', and thus confidentiality may be breached, although judgements such as these can be hard to make. These difficulties must be acknowledged and respected by team members and colleagues. The nurse is also expected to have regard for any physical, psychological and social effects on the patient/carer of any breach in confidentiality.

The community nurses most often found within a primary health care team (PHCT) and having an elderly care remit are district nurses, health visitors and community psychiatric nurses.

The role of the district nurse

The district nurse's role can be summarized as the provision of skilled nursing care for any person living in the community[2] to enable them either to recover from disease or injury or to cope with its effects.[3] A key part of the district nurse's function is to offer support, advice and training to formal and informal carers in respect of the day-to-day management needs of the patient and carers. This might include continence management, handling techniques, hygiene requirements, pressure management and information about the support networks available. The district nurse will manage a skill-mixed team which may include first- and second-level registered nurses who have been trained to certificate, diploma or degree level and nursing auxiliaries or health care assistants. Although certain team members may carry a delegated caseload, it is the district nurse who remains responsible for the overall management of the caseload and the nursing care given to the patient.

The role of the health visitor

The following four principles of health visiting encapsulate the role of the health visitor:

- the search for health needs;
- the stimulation of awareness of health needs;
- the influence on policies affecting health;
- the facilitation of health-enhancing activities.[4]

Health visitors have a universal brief that allows them to visit families without an obvious problem and actively seek out those who need preventative or remedial help[5] thus giving a comprehensive, non-stigmatizing service. At the same time it is probably fair to say that many members of the public are unsure as to their role, particularly towards the older person and many are unaware that they are nurses. Their caseload, whilst weighted towards the under fives should reflect the generic nature of their work and include the elderly. Although there are significant differences between child abuse and elder abuse,[6] work done by health visitors with child protection issues could lay the foundations for work with the older patient. These skills and knowledge must not be overlooked.

The role of the community psychiatric nurse

The community psychiatric nurse (CPN) is a registered mental health nurse, and may also be known in some areas as a community mental health nurse. Their special contribution is to work with people who have psychiatric illness or psychological distress and problems. Their assessment and management skills will enable them to assess the psychological and physical health of the person, including the impact of drugs, the environment and society. The CPN will also be able to manage and advise on simple physical problems and be able to refer to district nurses as appropriate.

Team working in the primary health care team

All community nurses endeavour to liaise and work closely with other disciplines and agencies, which will bring to the fore their communication and interpersonal skills. If the effects of abuse of older people are to be dealt with effectively the PHCT must first accept everyone's contribution to health care and look towards developing a defined system of communication and practice. Ovretveit[7] argues that there is no clear definition for a PHCT. He argues that the team is characterized as having a fairly high differentiation— a variety of disciplines—and low integration, with few if any formal common policies binding the grouping. He also defined a multidisciplinary team as:

> a group of practitioners with different professional training, employed by more than one agency, who meet regularly to co-ordinate their work providing services to one or more clients in a defined area.[7]

The future for the management of older people who are abused will be assisted greatly by members of the PHCT developing an understanding of the unique contribution of all professionals and of the knowledge that can be gained from each member of that team. This can be achieved through a number of different approaches:

- Education of the PHCT about the parameters and function of all disciplines in the team in order to dispel misconceptions surrounding certain roles.

- Education at a multidisciplinary level, which would include the opportunity for all professionals to explore their own feelings in respect of abuse. They will need to develop a trust and understanding of themselves and all members in their team.

- Meeting schedules should acknowledge that GPs are extremely busy. It must be appreciated that they cannot easily alter surgery times or arrange for a stand-in.

- An awareness of the role played by different members of the mutlidisciplinary team when undertaking an assessment for suspected abuse.

Community nursing contracts are currently based on contracts that may not reflect the increasing dependency of their clients. This can put the service under the extra pressure of seeing less patients who require more care whilst not achieving targets. The GP should be aware of the strains arising from ever-increasing workloads and apparently diminishing resources.

What can a GP expect from the community nursing service?

The GP can expect a sound knowledge of the subject and an awareness of local policies and procedures. Initial training should begin at staff induction and continue throughout the career span. This training can also include other team members and be both formal and informal.

It has been found that fear of labelling patients/carers as abusers and differences in interpretation as to what constitutes elder abuse has posed problems for some community nurses.[8] Knowing the risk factors associated with abuse of the elderly should promote vigilance.

Attempts have been made to develop checklists of risk factors, for both for patients and carers. Perhaps risk assessment tools should be developed specifically for the nursing assessment. The annual 'over 75' check offered by GPs to all patients of 75 years old and above, also provides an opportunity to assess risk. Some in-roads have been made in this direction.[9] Multiagency 'guidelines for action', have been developed to help alert workers with the elderly in the community.[10]

Through the holistic nursing assessment, which would look at physical, social, psychological and spiritual needs, the district nurse, health visitor or CPN should be alerted to family coping mechanisms and stressors. This would enable help and support to pre-empt or ease any problems. However, not all patients will be totally candid with a health professional at the first visit and it may take several visits before a suitable relationship is built up.

What the team can achieve together

It is important that all team members appreciate that it is not only the patient that can suffer abuse—carers can be abused by patients. The early intervention of the nursing team can help to prevent either the carer or patient being abused due to lack of support or resources. The relationship the nurse forms with the carer will support their ability to disclose any abuse that they are suffering. Whichever member of the multidisciplinary team first makes contact with the carer should ensure they are offered the opportunity of an assessment in their own right.[11]

Patients and carers often feel that they cannot waste the doctor's time and will take problems to the nurse to be legitimized. Nurses and GPs could capitalize on this to enable facilities for drop-in clinics, perhaps run by a health visitor in her role as promoter of health and preventer of ill-health.

The team also need to be aware that not all carers are relatives and that not all carers, relative or not, may want to care for their 'loved' ones when they are becoming dependent. Relationships may always have been strained or become strained with the increasing dependency. Systems need to be in place to allow carers to opt out without feeling that they have failed. The GP, who may have known the family for many years, should pass on such relevant social information along with the health requirements to other involved professionals, thus assisting with the development of a positive outcome. Multidisciplinary meetings, in the early days, provide a platform to ensure that all team members are aware of local policies and protocols for dealing with suspected elder abuse; the length of time allocated to them needs to be clearly defined. It is essential that all are aware of each others' roles and responsibilities.

The importance of an up-to-date, comprehensive area profile must be stressed; it should include details of the help and support available locally and, even more importantly, the person responsible for updating it should be identified. Someone will also need to take responsibility for the meetings, even if informal, to ensure that notes are taken and any action plans followed through. Another important aspect of team work, highlighted by Gilmore *et al.*,[12] is not only the sharing of knowledge, skills and resources but taking joint responsibility for outcomes. The Chief Nursing Officer of the time added another requirement, as important now as then: 'a mutually agreed system for communication and referral both within the team and between the team and other agencies'.[13]

The most important part a GP can play in helping cooperative, effective working is to respect a nurse's concerns and to take them seriously. It is extremely difficult for any nurse to feel she is informing on a patient or carer who she is trying to support, especially as it may include breaking a confidence. Every support must be given to the nurse and the incident should be reflected upon, preferably by the team, to ensure that the correct procedures are followed and any omissions highlighted and acted upon. Every member of a community nursing team has a unique role in the prevention, investigation, management and support of patients and/or carers at risk of potential or actual abuse.

References

1 **Nursing and Midwifery Council**. Code of Professional Conduct. London: NMC, 2002.

2 **Baly M, Robottom B, Clark J.** *District Nursing*, 2nd edn. London: Heinemann, 1987.

3 **Orem D.** *Nursing Concepts of Practice*, 3rd edn. London: Collier Macmillan, 1983.

4 **Council for the Education and Training of Health Visitors.** *An Investigation into the Principles of Health Visiting.* London: CETHV, 1977.

5 **McClymont M, Thoman S, Denham M.** *Health Visiting and Elderly People: a Health Promotion Challenge,* 2nd edn. Edinburgh: Churchill Livingstone, 1991.

6 **Tomlinson D.** *No Longer Afraid: the Safeguard of Older People in Domestic Settings.* Social Services Inspectorate. London: HMSO, 1993.

7 **Ovretveit J.** *Co-ordinating Community Care.* Buckingham: Open University Press, 1993.

8 **Clarke M, Ogg J.** Identifying the elderly at risk. *Journal of Community Nursing* 1994; June: 4–9.

9 **Davies M.** Recognising abuse: an assessment tool for nurses. In: Decalemer P, Glendenning F, eds. *The Mistreatment of Elderly People.* London: Sage, 1993: 102–5.

10 **Age Concern.** Abuse of elderly people—guidelines for action. In: Decalemer P, Glendenning F, eds. *The Mistreatment of Elderly People.* London: Sage, 1993: 169–73.

11 **Department of Health.** *Carers (Recognition and Services) Act 1995: Policy Guidance and Practice Guide.* London: HMSO, 1996.

12 **Gilmore M, Bruce N, Hunt M.** *The Work of the Nursing Team in General Practice.* London: Council for the Education and Training of Health Visitors, 1974.

13 **Department of Health and Social Security.** *Nursing in Primary Health Care.* CNO(77)8. London: HMSO, 1977.

Chapter 18c

The role of social workers and GPs

Jacki Pritchard

Introduction

In the United Kingdom it has taken a long time to recognize that elder abuse is an important social policy issue; the general public still do not have a general awareness that it exists even though doctors and other professionals have been talking about it since the 1970s.[1–3] Since the early 1990s, the term 'vulnerable adult' has been used more widely and with the advent of the Department of Health's guidance *No Secrets*[4] the issue of elder abuse is now addressed under the term 'adult abuse'. Yet even in the early days of working with elder abuse, there was a general consensus of opinion that we should be working in a multidisciplinary way.

Multidisciplinary working may sound like a cliché to many people and sometimes it does not always work in a satisfactory way, but it can work and this is what we should be striving to achieve. In this section I shall be considering how general practitioners and social workers can work together in dealing with cases of elder abuse, whether suspected or proven.

Many professionals think that when working with elder abuse we should not be going down the same road as with child abuse, that is, not following the same procedural route. However, a great deal can be learnt from what has happened in that field and it is possible to learn by mistakes made. Elder abuse is a different concept in that we are dealing with adults, many of whom are capable of making informed choices about their future. Nevertheless, there are similarities between child abuse and adult abuse; professionals need to have an understanding about abuse across the age ranges. It often takes a long time for a victim to disclose about abuse; older people may have been brought up in a setting where they were taught to keep things to themselves. Even when disclosures are given, many victims choose to stay in the abusive situation.

Sometimes all the professionals can do is listen and support the victim in their situation. Frustration occurs because elder abuse has no statutory framework, therefore professionals have limited powers to intervene.[5] In cases where the victim is confused or cannot make an informed choice, then the work becomes even more complex. The GP may have different roles to play, both in the short term (identifying abuse, referring on) and the long term (monitoring the situation, providing help for the victim and/or abuser).

This section will focus on how social workers and GPs can work together effectively. It is necessary to remember that abuse can happen both in the community and in institutions (day centres, residential/nursing homes, hospitals). GPs are likely to pick up abuse in any of these settings. I want to consider how GPs and social workers can work together:

- when abuse is suspected and situations need monitoring;

- in investigations;

- in the long term.

I intend to include case examples where there has been positive intervention by GPs in elder abuse cases, in order to illustrate the fact that GPs and social workers can work together successfully.

Training

There has been a lack of awareness generally about elder abuse and it is crucial that all professionals who work with older people receive appropriate training. *No Secrets* emphasizes the importance of 'a training strategy for all levels of staff . . . no staff group should be excluded'.[4] GPs need training so that they can develop their expertise in this field and become more confident in recognizing and working with abuse. Ideally GPs should be invited to multidisciplinary training sessions organized by agencies who will be members of the local adult protection committee. By doing this they can increase and share knowledge, but also build up links with the professionals they might liaise with in future cases.

Training sessions need to cover a wide range of issues. It is not enough just to be able to recognize signs of abuse; GPs need to have an understanding of why and how elder abuse may happen. GPs have to come to realize that elder abuse can take many forms and they have a role to play in identifying many different types of abuse, not just physical abuse. Some specific examples are:

- signs of neglect (physical and emotional);
- indicators of malnutrition/dehydration;
- medication abuse (e.g. overmedication and links with financial abuse);
- sexual abuse;
- discriminatory abuse.

Training and raising awareness does not just have to happen in formal training sessions. It is useful for GPs to meet up with social workers to discuss how they can work together on the whole issue of elder abuse. If there is a general practice-attached social worker, s/he should pass on information about how the social services department is addressing the issue. Otherwise, both GPs and social workers need to be proactive in getting together (e.g. inviting each other to practice meetings or team meetings) to discuss what they need to do to work together in a better way. The two professions need to have a clear understanding of their different roles.

Procedures and process

For many years social workers who came across cases of elder abuse did not know what to do. If they were working generically then they tended to transfer their skills from child protection work. For a long time there was no guidance and this is why so many cases were badly managed or not followed up at all. There has been progress in the l990s, which has resulted in the publication of *No Secrets* and the requirement that 'directors of social services will be expected to ensure that the local multi-agency codes of practice are developed and implemented by 31st October 2001'.[6] Every GP should have a copy of the local multiagency policy and procedure; it is important for them to become familiar with local policy and practices.

GPs can be in a position to identify any form of elder abuse, whether it is physical, emotional, financial, neglect, sexual or discriminatory. However, whichever category of abuse it may be, it is often extremely difficult to prove and, in many cases, situations have to be monitored for some time. If a GP has concerns, s/he should make a referral to the local social services area office. Talking and communicating with each other is the way forward for GPs and social workers. In elder abuse cases, there is often a 'suspicion' or 'gut reaction' that something is not right; this needs to be verbalized and discussed.

If a patient already has an allocated social worker, s/he should be contacted to make a referral. If the patient is unknown to social services, a duty worker will deal with the initial gathering of information. Most guidelines state that the referral should be dealt with within a specified time limit, usually within 24 hours. Sometimes, a strategy meeting will take place in order to decide how to proceed.

When making a referral, a GP needs to give as much information as possible, and it is useful to state what basic information is needed:

- name, address and date of birth of alleged victim;
- name, address and date of birth of alleged abuser (if known);
- who is involved with the victim (professionals, volunteers, family, financial advisors);
- what are the concerns and what type(s) of abuse suspected;
- details of incidents (dates, times, location).

Many policies suggest that two people should visit the alleged victim; usually a qualified social worker and another person (one of whom should know the victim). This other person may very well be the GP. Again, this is why GPs need training (for example on interviewing technique—having a lead person, not asking leading questions, taking notes, recording interviews, etc.) and it is crucial for GPs and social workers to build up their links so that they get used to working/interviewing together.

After a proper assessment has taken place (which may involve several visits) a case conference should take place. The purpose of the case conference is to:

- share information in a multidisciplinary forum;
- assess the degree of risk;
- make decisions and recommendations (if an authority has an 'at risk' or 'vulnerable adult' register, a decision is needed regarding registration) that will form the basis of a protection plan.

If the GP has not been involved in the investigation visits, s/he will be invited to attend the case conference, which often takes place within certain time limits (for example 10–15 working days). If a GP is not able to attend the case conference, s/he will usually be asked to send a written report that can be presented to the case conference.

The case conference should be multidisciplinary and the victim is also invited to attend. Some victims may not wish to attend and if this is the case they should be asked if they want an advocate to attend in their place. Sometimes an abuser may attend; this will depend on the wishes of the victim. If an abuser demands to be heard and this is going to cause the victim distress, the chairperson may allow him or her to attend for only part of the conference.

For the case conference the GP will need to present specific and general information about both the victim and the abuser (if known):

- physical condition;
- medical problems;
- social history (important life events, losses);

- family contacts;
- family history if relevant, e.g. important relationships, whether good or bad; it is important to discuss the positives and negatives as this may shed light on the victim's attitude towards the abuser;
- involvement of other professionals/workers/volunteers;
- knowledge of abuse that has occurred;
- evidence of abuse, i.e. signs and indicators.

If a patient is at risk, the case conference may well devise a protection plan which states the objectives, roles, responsibilities and tasks of the people involved. The GP could have a crucial role in monitoring abuse cases and therefore would be included in any plan. The protection plan should be reviewed regularly (for a proforma and examples of protection plans, see [7,8]).

GPs and social workers working together

Although a framework of good practice has been outlined above, it must be stressed that not all referrals become formal elder abuse investigations. It needs to be emphasized to all GPs that it is useful and important for GPs and social workers to talk informally as well as formally. If either one of them has concerns, then they should be shared and possible future action discussed without the fear that formal procedures will be instigated immediately.

It has been said already that GPs may be involved in identifying any type of abuse and they should be part of the monitoring process if it is appropriate. GPs may hold vital information about a victim or abuser, because they may have known the person for some time. This is crucial because often the root cause of abuse is linked to something that happened many years ago rather than the present situation.

Case

Marie was the main carer for her 80-year-old father, who was demented and had suffered several strokes. For a long time, the home care staff suspected that Marie physically abused her father. Eventually a formal elder abuse investigation took place. The GP had known the family for 30 years. He told the case conference (with Marie's permission) that Marie hated her father because he had sexually abused Marie when she was a child.

A dilemma for GPs can be regarding the boundaries of confidentiality. Social workers often complain that when they contact GPs for information, the GP may refuse to discuss the patient because s/he feels that the information is confidential. This is how elder abuse differs from child abuse. There is no statutory framework in place and, therefore, professionals are not bound to share information in the same way as they are under the Children Act 1989. A GP may choose to break confidentiality and divulge some information if and when s/he feels the victim may be in a life-threatening situation. Social workers and GPs need to be aware of any multiagency sharing information protocol that may exist locally, and also of the power under the 'sharing information principle' stated in Section 115 of the Crime and Disorder Act 1998.

GPs are important in working with abuse cases because people usually trust GPs and often confide in them. It may take years for the victim to disclose the abuse they have been experiencing and they usually confide in someone they trust.

Case

Georgina had been physically abused by her husband (all through her marriage) and by her son (since he was a teenager), but she loved them both dearly and did not want to leave the abusive situation. Day care workers frequently rang the GP about Georgina's injuries. Georgina would only talk about the abuse to the GP, who continued to treat her injuries at the day centre, listened to her, offered to arrange a counsellor (but Georgina refused) and respected her wishes that she did not want anyone to intervene.

GPs are in a good position to monitor situations because they, or the district nurses attached to the practice, may be visiting regularly. For example, it may be possible to pick up when a carer is under stress or the carer might in fact admit that they are not coping or disclose they have lashed out in a fit of temper. There are other examples where it has been the GP who has identified abuse.

Case

Mr G was caring for his wife, who was physically disabled and a very demanding woman. Mr G always said he was coping. Over a 6-month period, Mrs G seemed to become quieter and the district nurse who visited to dress her leg ulcers told the GP that Mrs G seemed to be sleeping a lot, which she had not done previously. The GP made several visits and checked Mrs G's medication. Mr G then admitted to the GP that he was overmedicating his wife to keep her quiet. The GP referred onto social services, who, after an assessment, were able to provide more support for Mr G.

Case

Two of Dr D's patients lived in a residential home. The two patients started ringing the surgery frequently for the doctor to visit. Both patients were losing weight and seemed malnourished. They had also become very nervous and withdrawn. On his visits to the home the doctor noticed the physical condition of the other residents. He talked to a local social worker about his concerns. The registration and inspection unit was then contacted and an investigation took place. It came to light that the doctor's patients and other residents were not being fed properly and generally neglected. The staff had also threatened them.

As well as maybe having a role in identifying abuse, the GP can clarify matters for the social worker. For example, an older person may have frequent injuries, which are seen by the home care assistant and day centre staff, who voice their concerns to the social worker. If the older person agrees to see the GP, s/he may be able to say more about the injuries (e.g. confirm an injury is a cigarette burn or bite mark; date the bruising) and whether the injuries are non-accidental.

GPs and hospital doctors/consultants need to develop their expertise in identifying non-accidental injury in older people in the same way GPs and paediatricians have to do in child protection work. Often the right questions are not asked and professionals are too accepting of stories given about what has happened to an older person. Again this is due to the lack of awareness about the prevalence of elder abuse.

If GPs and social workers talk to each other, certain matters can be clarified or questioned further if necessary. Some typical examples are:

- Suspicion of medication abuse: the GP should review medication regularly and can clarify the correct dosage.

- Suspicion that older person is not fed properly: the GP can arrange monitoring of weight loss and confirm whether there is a specific medical problem.

- Suspicion of physical abuse: the GP can keep records of injuries seen, possibly using body charts.

Good indicators of abuse can be changes in behaviour, and this is another constructive way in which a GP can help in identifying abuse. If a GP has known a patient for a long time s/he will know what the person was like previously. Also, the GP can diagnose certain conditions which may rule out or confirm elder abuse for example:

- Sometimes victims become confused—this can be a way of withdrawing from the real abusive world or, in cases of sexual abuse, the onset of confusion can be very sudden and dramatic. The GP can be involved in obtaining a proper diagnosis and answer questions such as: is this dementia or the onset of Alzheimer's disease, or has the patient recently had a chest infection or urinary tract infection, or could it possibly be a case of elder abuse?

- If a patient has frequent infections, urinary/genital irritation or bleeding, an examination will help to ascertain whether this is thrush, piles or sexual abuse.

In many cases where abuse is suspected, the findings of an investigation may not be conclusive, especially if the victim is protecting the abuser or the victim is confused or has severe learning disabilities. But it is still important that the GP and social worker talk to each other and voice their concerns. If there are continuing concerns that a patient is a victim of abuse the GP can help in the diagnosis, but s/he may also be the person to bring in other professionals to help monitor the situation (district nurse, community psychiatric nurse, dietician, psychiatrist, psychologist).

In the long term, the GP may continue to monitor the situation, because it can take months or even years to prove that abuse is occuring. Or in cases where it is known that abuse has occurred and the victim requires help, the GP can be the person to bring in the appropriate resources to help either the victim or the abuser (specialist counsellor, therapist).

Conclusion

We still have a long way to go in working with elder abuse. All professionals are worried about the implications for their workloads. To work with abuse effectively we need more time, personnel and resources. GPs are no different. However, if we are going to address the issue then GPs and social workers must work with each other and help each other. Neither parties should be frightened to voice their concerns or suspicions. If an older person may be at risk, this has to be investigated. If the alleged victim denies that abuse is going on, but there is still suspicion, then the situation must be monitored. The bottom line is that GPs and social workers have to keep communicating whenever they think that an older person may be a victim of elder abuse, otherwise the issue will remain hidden.

References

1 **Baker AA.** Granny battering. *Modern Geriatrics* 1975; **5** (8): 20–4.
2 **Burston GR.** Granny battering. *BMJ* 1975; **3**: 592–3.
3 **Burston GR.** Do your elderly patients live in fear of being battered? *Modern Geriatrics* 1977; **7** (5): 54–5.
4 **Department of Health.** *No Secrets: Guidance on Developing and Implementing Multi-Agency Policies and Procedures to Protect Vulnerable Adults from Abuse.* London: HMSO, 2000.
5 **Lord Chancellor's Department.** *Making Decisions: the Government's Proposals for Making Decisions on Behalf of Mentally Incapacitated Adults.* London: Stationery Office, 1999.
6 **Department of Health.** *No Secrets: Guidance on Developing Multi-Agency Policies and Procedures to Protect Vulnerable Adults from Abuse.* Health Service/Local Authority Circular HSC 2000/007. London: NHS Executive, 2000.
7 **Pritchard, J.** *Working with Elder Abuse.* London: Jessica Kingsley, 1996.
8 **Pritchard J,** ed. *Elder Abuse Work: Best Practice in Britain and Canada.* London: Jessica Kingsley, 1999.

Chapter 18d

The role of the solicitor

Ann McDonald

Introduction

There is no discrete body of law relating to older people in England and Wales; old age, outside the field of pensions and social security, has no legal status. Such law as there is has therefore to be gleaned from other sources: the criminal law, the law of domestic violence and mental health law.[1] This causes particular problems in the area of elder abuse where the paucity of legal provision means inevitably that there are gaps in the law, leaving people unprotected and dilemmas unresolved.

Difficulties in defining the boundaries of elder abuse can no longer be ignored when referral for legal advice is being considered. The law has to operate within exact parameters. Not all situations that may be considered abusive fit neatly into existing legal categories; this is particularly so in cases of neglect, where a duty to provide care may simply not exist. Legal remedies may be draconian in their operation, and require considerable perseverance to pursue; no matter how difficult the situation is, the victim of abuse may decide to exercise their prerogative not to pursue legal remedies.

Who is the client?

It is important for the general practitioner to establish good working relationships with local solicitors and law centres, but it is also important to understand the limitations imposed by the nature of the solicitor's professional relationship with his or her client. The Law Society's *Guide to the Professional Conduct of Solicitors*[2] makes it clear (para. 12.05) that where instructions are received not from a client but from a third party purporting to represent that client (including a family member), a solicitor should obtain written instructions from the client that he or she wishes the solicitor to act. In such circumstances a solicitor must advise the client without regard to the interests of the source from which he or she was introduced. A solicitor must not accept instructions which he suspects have been given under duress or undue influence, and paragraph 12.04 of the guide is explicit that: 'particular care may need to be taken where a client is elderly or otherwise vulnerable to pressure from others'. Paragraph 16.02, which requires that a solicitor should keep his client's business and affairs confidential, prevents disclosure to others except with the express consent of the client, or unless authorized by law.

Although such an authorization extends to certain cases of suspected child abuse, there is no authority to disclose when the client is an adult victim of abuse.

In what circumstances may referral be appropriate?

Referral for legal advice or assistance may arise in a range of circumstances, not necessarily only at a point of crisis. Preventative action is also important, for example to ensure that adequate support services are in place, or to enable the individual properly to put his financial affairs in order. Community care law is a new field of interest to solicitors following the implementation of the National Health Service and Community Care Act 1990. Though this Act did not impose any new substantive obligations upon local authorities to provide services, it did introduce, for the first time, a legally enforceable duty individually to assess people who may appear to be in need of any such 'community care services' (Section 47). Community care services are defined in Section 46(3) of the Act as including residential care, domiciliary care and other support services and aftercare services under Section 117 of the Mental Health Act 1983.

A wide spectrum of need is therefore covered. These are all services that would not only support individuals in the community, but that would also assist carers under stress. In this context, the Carers and Disabled Children Act 2000 entitles any carer who provides a substantial amount of care on a regular basis to an assessment in their own right, upon request. Services are also available under the Chronically Sick and Disabled Persons Act 1970 for those who are physically or mentally disabled.

Growing demand for services has led local authority social services departments increasingly to target resources on those who are in the greatest need and at greatest risk. Though it is clear from the guidance based on the Community Care Act that the targeting of resources is legitimate,[3] the cutting of services across the board without reassessment is not. Referral on for legal advice may thus be of assistance where a service that has supported a potentially unstable situation is threatened with withdrawal. An example might be a threatened reduction in a package of domiciliary care put in place after discharge from hospital. It is not uncommon for local authorities to restrict long-term domiciliary care to a maximum of perhaps 14 hours per week. However, if the need for an intensive package of care remains (perhaps because recovery of the patient has been slower than anticipated) any objective reassessment of the situation would have to indicate that no change was made. Legal assistance may be helpful in reminding local authorities of their statutory duties. The legal adviser would be best placed to consider the relative merits of the different remedies available in such a situation; whether that is use of the local authority's own complaints procedure; referral on to the local government Ombudsman; or an action for breach of statutory duty or judicial review, if a letter before action did not produce a satisfactory response. The role of the GP might then be to encourage people not simply to accept local authority decisions, but to seek advice elsewhere for challenging those decisions, either on the merits or for a failure to follow proper procedures.

Preventative action in the field of financial abuse may include encouraging the patient to enter into either an ordinary or enduring power of attorney, enabling control over his financial affairs to be delegated to a trustworthy friend or relative or professional adviser. An enduring power of attorney will continue to be valid when the donor becomes mentally incapacitated, whereas an ordinary power of attorney will not. For patients who are already mentally incapacitated there is no alternative other than to apply to the Court of Protection for the appointment of a receiver to take complete control of the patient's affairs. Patients even with modest assets should be encouraged to make a will if they express any anxiety about the use of their assets after death; legal aid is available in appropriate cases.

Dealing with neglect

Cases of neglect, including self-neglect or failure to act to prevent a life-threatening deterioration in a person in need of care, pose particular legal difficulties. There may be cases in which compulsory intervention has to be considered. Here the law draws a clear distinction between those who are suffering from a mental disorder, and those who are not. The Mental Health Act 1983 applies to the former; the latter are dealt with under the provisions of Section 47 of the National Assistance Act 1948.

The Mental Health Act makes provision for admission for assessment (Section 2), admission for treatment (Section 3) and admission for assessment in an emergency (Section 4). Section 115 authorizes an approved social worker to enter and inspect any premises, which are not a hospital, and in which a mentally disordered person is living, if he has reasonable cause to believe that the patient is not under proper care. Section 135 provides for the issuing of a warrant by a magistrate authorizing a police constable to enter premises where such a person has been, or is being, ill-treated, neglected or kept otherwise than under proper control (Section 135(1)(a)) or who, being unable to care for himself, is living alone in any such place (Section 135(1)(b)). A warrant will be necessary if forced entry is required, or removal of the person to a place of safety is anticipated. The general practitioner refused entry to premises should consider these provisions.

In a situation where admission to hospital is inappropriate, but a degree of monitoring in the community is thought to be desirable, guardianship is available as an option to be considered. The guardian may require (Section 8(2) of the Mental Health Act 1983) the patient to attend at times and places specified for the purposes of medical treatment, and may require access to the patient to be given to any doctor, approved social worker, or any person similarly specified. Increasingly, guardianship is being seen as an appropriate limited powers order that, at its best, will contain an element of advocacy for the patient in securing access to community care services (Mental Health Act 1983 Code of Practice, para. 13.1).

Where the patient is not mentally disordered, but the situation has deteriorated to the extent that compulsory removal from the premises is being considered, Section 47 of the National Assistance Act 1948 is the provision to be invoked. Section 47 is an obviously ageist piece of legislation with its roots in the slum clearance provisions of the immediate postwar period. It exists 'for the purpose of securing the necessary care and attention' for persons who:

- are suffering from grave chronic disease or, being aged, infirm or physically incapacitated, are living in insanitary conditions; and

- are unable to devote to themselves, and are not receiving from other persons, proper care and attention.

The procedure is initiated by the community physician who certifies in writing his concerns to the local authority. It is common for a case conference then to be held, prior to an application to the local magistrates court. It is thus a judicial and not an administrative process. Seven days notice must be given to the patient. However, there is a more commonly used emergency procedure under Section 1 of the National Assistance Act 1951, which provides for removal without notice. Because it is a judicial process, proper legal assistance for the patient is essential though, surprisingly, legal aid is not available for the court proceedings. The application of the legislation has been much criticized;[4] as only a small minority of those removed under Section 47 ever return to their own homes, careful attention needs to be paid to the quality of life that can be offered elsewhere.

Neglect by persons assumed to be responsible for the physical care of an elderly person, poses particular conceptual difficulties. Moral responsibilities and legal responsibilities do not always go hand in hand. Outside the duty imposed upon the local authority to assess persons appearing to be in need of community care services, it may be that there is no-one who is under a duty to intervene to provide a person, not otherwise able to cope for themselves, with the necessities of life such as adequate nutrition and sufficient warmth. It is in the non-existence of familial duties towards elderly people that the distinction from child protection issues in cases of abuse becomes most apparent. It is otherwise, however, if the duty is voluntarily assumed; for example, by taking a dependent person into one's own home for care. Then a duty of care is assumed to arise; and there will be civil, and in some cases, criminal liability for breach of that duty. In the case of professional carers, such as proprietors of residential homes, general guidelines, such as those in *A New Home Life*,[5] may be used as evidence of minimum standards.

Physical abuse

Physical abuse may constitute both a criminal offence (in which case a referral to the police may be seen as the appropriate course of action), or it may on the same facts be used as the basis of a civil action for assault, for which damages are sought. A civil action would be pursued by a solicitor, who may seek evidence from the general practitioner as to the extent of the injury inflicted and of any subsequent loss of function or disability. This evidence would be used to quantify damages, or to justify an application for an injunction to prevent further incidents of violence occurring.

The use of domestic violence remedies, such as non-molestation and occupation orders, should not be discounted because the parties are elderly. One difficulty is that domestic violence legislation has only been available where there has been a 'matrimonial home' shared by spouses or cohabitees; it has not provided remedies for those who are assaulted or harassed by other members of the family, e.g. adult sons or daughters whether living in the same household or not. The Law Commission[6] therefore recommended that the protection of the legislation should be extended to cover violence by a wider class of 'associated persons', including relatives of different degrees and past or present members of the same household, and there are provisions in the Family Law Act 1996 to that effect. Legal advice will be essential in all these cases; but equally necessary is encouragement and support of people who find it difficult to conceptualize themselves in later life as potential beneficiaries of this legislation.

Instituting proceedings

Normally witnesses will be expected to attend and to give oral evidence on oath. This may cause difficulties where the witness is infirm or incapacitated. Until the coming into force of the Youth Justice and Criminal Evidence Act 1999, there was no provision analogous to that in the Children Act 1989, for the use of video links in court.

Documentary evidence may, however, be admissible if the witness is unable to attend court in person because of physical or mental infirmity certified by a medical practitioner. A further relevant question for the court, however, will be the reliability of the evidence given the degree of infirmity of the witness.

People who are mentally incapacitated can bring litigation only through a third party (their 'litigation friend') or defend an action only through a guardian *ad litem*. Considerable procedural complexities therefore exist when court action is contemplated.

Financial abuse

Financial abuse is probably the area in which cooperation between doctors and lawyers can be most fruitful in preventing as well as in dealing with exploitative situations. Cooperation will most likely revolve around the issue of mental incapacity. Incapacity in decision-making is fundamentally a legal concept, the evidence for which is provided by medical assessment.[7] Confusingly, the legal test of capacity will vary according to the type of legal transaction into which the patient wishes to enter; different tests of capacity are applied, for example, to the ability to enter into a contract for the sale of goods; for the making of a will; and for the granting of an enduring power of attorney.

It is therefore the responsibility of the lawyer to advise the doctor of the correct legal test to be applied in each of these different circumstances.

Being proactive, and encouraging patients to protect their financial affairs by the making of a will, or an enduring power of attorney, demands a degree of legal knowledge on the part of the general practitioner. Clarity about when the stage of self-determination is passed is also important, particularly when others may exert pressure to retain control over the financial affairs of the patient, who is already incapacitated. It is useful to have some knowledge of when intervention is possible to set aside a bad bargain entered into by a confused elderly person, or if a gift is made and later regretted.

The Law Commission and the British Medical Association have jointly published guidance to facilitate liaison in a range of situations.[8] This guidance contains practical suggestions for solicitors instructing doctors (para. 2.3) and practical suggestions for doctors receiving instructions from solicitors (para. 2.4). Both reiterate the importance of asking for further information if in doubt and of keeping the request and the sub-sequent report specific to the particular transaction in hand. If the doctor feels that he has insufficient knowledge or practical experience to make a proper assessment of incapacity he should say so, although paragraph 2.4 does assume that 'a general prac-titioner who sees his or her patient on a fairly regular basis is likely to be in a better position to say what the patient is capable or incapable of doing than a specialist who has seen the patient once or twice'. If the matter is likely to be contentious, and the opinion open to challenge, this should be clearly stated in the request made to the GP by the patient's solicitor. Particular care should be taken when acting as a witness to a signature on a legal document (e.g. a will); it will be assumed that the doctor is signing as an expert witness as to the person's capacity to enter into the transaction effected by the document. Careful reading of the Law Society/British Medical Association guidance is highly recommended for an insight into the range of legal remedies available, as well as different professional expectations.

The lawyer's role

Referral to a solicitor or law centre gives a patient access to the proper exploration of the legal paradigm of rights/duties/powers/remedies in both public (concerning the state) and private (between individuals) law. Litigation in the courts is not the only outcome that may be achieved (in fact it is a very unlikely outcome, and is usually a last resort); but referral on for legal advice opens up to the patient the potential to use all the other skills of the lawyer—in negotiation, in drawing up documents or in seeking clarification of the law. Older people who may have no previous experience of contact with lawyers will need considerable support through the process. Particularly where questions of mental capacity are an issue, active collaboration between medical practitioners and lawyers is fundamental to a holistic response to the problems of abuse.

References

1 McDonald A, Taylor M. *The Law and Elderly People*. London: Sweet & Maxwell, 1995.

2 Law Society. *Guide to the Professional Conduct of Solicitors*, 8th edn. London: Law Society, 1999.

3 Department of Health. *Community Care in the Next Decade and Beyond: Policy Guidance*. London: HMSO, 1990.

4 Tregaskis B, Mayberry J. The Anniversary of Section 47 of the National Assistance Act 1948. Justice of the Peace, 23 April, 1994.

5 Centre for Policy on Ageing. *A New Home Life*. London: Centre for Policy on Ageing, 1996.

6 Law Commission. *Domestic Violence and Occupation of the Family Home*. London: HMSO, 1993.

7 Law Commission. *Mentally Incapacitated Adults and Decision Making: an Overview*. Consultation Paper No. 119, London: HMSO, 1995.

8 British Medical Association, Law Society. *Assessment of Mental Capacity: Guidance for Doctors and Lawyers*. London: BMA, 1995.

Chapter 19

The future

Ginny Jenkins

The future of elder abuse in this country depends on people:

- accepting that it exists and agreeing what it is;
- recognizing the rights of both victim and perpetrator;
- undertaking appropriate interventions.

Acceptance and recognition

Agreeing that elder abuse exists may seem straightforward. However, acceptance that it is more than granny battering or bashing and that its causes are complex has been slow. In 1993, only months after the publication of the national prevalence study by Ogg and Bennett,[1] Virginia Bottomely, then Secretary of State for Health, said that she did not think that elder abuse was a problem. The prevalence study showed that the size of the problem was half that of child abuse, indicating that up to 5 per cent of older people living in the community might be victims of physical, verbal or financial abuse.

Recognition needs to be by everybody though, as with child abuse, professional awareness is likely to come first. Indeed this is essential if people are to get help. Action on Elder Abuse, a national voluntary organization, was established in 1994 specifically to prevent abuse of older people by raising awareness, education, the promotion of research and the provision of information. One of its primary task is ensuring that elder abuse is understand and that workers and others are aware of the wide range of possible action. One of its first actions was to survey all social services departments, health authorities and trusts to identify their responses. The results were salutary. Policys and procedures on elder abuse, together with staff training and education, were much less frequent in health authorities and trusts than in social services departments.[2] Indeed some trusts responded that their geriatricians said that elder abuse did not exist.

In the future, both workers and statutory and voluntary services will understand the issues relating to elder abuse. As a result, older people will receive a sensitive response giving them the help they want. Public acceptance is already growing. Over the last 3 years there have been a number of television programmes and newspaper features on abuse in residential and nursing home settings. Relatives have become ready to speak out about incidents, perhaps as a direct result of concern over standards and requirements to pay for care. Elder abuse in care settings has the added dimension of abusers being paid workers. Changes to the registration and inspection mechanisms as a result of implementation of the Care Standards Act 2000 will hopefully result in better and more coordinated prevention, identification and action.

Unlike abuse within care settings, which is gaining recognition, abuse in the home often remains concealed. The victim's shame if the perpetrator is a family member, or relatives living at a distance and not realizing what is happening, may be parts of the reason. Physical and psychological changes resulting from abuse are too easily dismissed as the results of ageing. In all circumstances the primary health care team have an important role supporting and encouraging those involved to seek help.

Although there is broad acceptance as to what is elder abuse, closer definition is required and outdated concepts must be abandoned if it is to be prevented. Initially, carer stress was thought to be a major contributory factor, though research has now shown that this is untrue. Unfortunately, the continuing image has had two results. The genuinely stressed carer is often reluctant to seek help in case there are accusations that they are an abuser, while actual incidents are unidentified since they do not fit in with preconceptions.

Early definitions focused on the imbalance of power within relationships or the denial of the rights of citizenship. The tight parameters that now define both child abuse and domestic violence have enabled effective service responses to victims in both of these types of violence. At present, the older person is lost in the debate of what the service is responding to and what the service response should be.

The most recent definition, from Action on Elder Abuse, says that 'elder abuse is a single or repeated act or lack of appropriate action which occurs within any relationship where there is an expectation of trust which causes harm or distress to the older person'.[2] Definitions should be modified as our knowledge grows, but it is essential that there is agreement on the basic features. A strength of the Action on Elder Abuse definition is that it clearly defines the limit for a service response as it specifically excludes those people who are abused by strangers. At the same time by inserting the phrase 'expectation of trust' it allows an observer to believe that there is trust between the parties though those involved know that there is none.

It is accepted that all adults may decide their own lifestyle, provided they have capacity and are not subject to any order under the Mental Health Act. However, when this is viewed in the context of an abused person it is often forgotten. At present there is a tendency to view any victim, both with and without capacity, as vulnerable and so in need of protection. Yet the vast majority of older people have capacity and as such can dictate their own future, especially if given help and empowerment.

The rights of the abuser must also be recognized. Currently very little is known about why family members abuse older people. Causes that have been put forward, such as poor long-term family relationships, mental health or drug or alcohol problems, all suggest that the perpetrator needs assistance. It is a continuing danger that in spite of the Carers Assessment Act 1996 too little attention is paid to the ability of the carer to provide care.

A significant number of abusers are workers. Domiciliary care may mean that isolated vulnerable people are cared for by a worker who calls alone. People working with older people are not subject to the systems of checking and vetting of previous employment records that have been designed to protect a child. Regulation of domiciliary care providers and registration of all employees is a provision of the Care Standards Act 2000, but there is no date for implementation. Such safeguards must be introduced as a matter of urgency to protect all involved.

Intervention

At present far too little is known about what interventions work. Some important moves forward have been made, which have mirrored the growth of responses for child abuse and domestic violence. Elder abuse is the subject of specific conferences and a topic in general ones. In the last 5 years a significant number of books have been published and major research has started. In certain parts of the country, specialist adult or elder protection units are being established. These tend to follow American practice, of mandatory reporting and investigation of any incident.

A major area of debate is the role of the law. It is argued that existing civil and criminal legislation does not allow for the right responses to be made and that the victim cannot be adequately protected in spite of full recourse to both criminal and civil legislation. New laws such as the Family Act 1996, although introduced as a measure against domestic violence, is equally applicable to older people abused by family members as exclusion orders can be sought against them.

One dilemma for workers is caused by those with capacity choosing to decline assistance and remain at risk. Workers can find this hard to work with and it certainly limits the response of statutory agencies and the effectiveness of special elder protection services. The government recently proposed adult protective legislation for any vulnerable adult, especially those who lacked capacity.[3] However, concern has been expressed that the proposals are based on outdated concepts of child protection legislation rather than ensuring that abused older people have their access to legislation for adults, such as the Family Act 1996, facilitated and maintained. In 2000 the Department of Health issued *No Secrets*, a multiagency guidance on the protection of vulnerable adults.[4] Implementation of this is patchy and too often local authorities have allocated no specific, or totally inadequate, funding for its effective implementation.

Five main types of elder abuse are recognised: physical, psychological, financial, sexual and abuse by neglect. Interventions in all areas need to be developed, but perhaps there is especial urgency for cases of financial and sexual abuse.

Financial abuse of older people is widespread. Home ownership and private pensions mean that many have significant assets, while even those dependent entirely on state benefits can be intimidated or cheated out of them. While all are at risk, the protection of those who have lost capacity are of especial concern. Banks and building societies are allowing accounts to be operated by people who are no longer competent, while enduring powers of attorney and receivership for state benefits are being granted to people who do not use the money for the benefit of the older person. The Green Paper, *Who Decides*[3] proposed major changes to the Court of Protection, and the Benefit's Agency are currently reviewing the guidance on receivership, which should help reduce social security fraud in this area. However, there seems to be complete lack of political will to give people with mental incapacity a proper legal framework, both for decision-making and protection. Currently all involved, including doctors, with this client group need to be very careful to ensure that they are not unwittingly allowing abuse to take place.

Sexual abuse is often unrecognized and is sometimes denied. Both men and women who live either at home or in care settings are victims. At present they are often disbelieved, given little sympathy and rarely offered access to specialist services. Indeed specialist services for the older victim of rape hardly exist and need to be developed. Where the victim has dementia it is too often assumed that they have not been traumatized by what has happened to them and so no help is offered. The cases are often not reported to the police and prosecutions are rare.

There have been many suggestions put forward to explain the low rate for prosecutions. The victim may be reluctant to lay charges against a family member. It is said that there is an unwillingness by the Crown Prosecution Service to act. It is argued that there may be insufficient evidence, or older people are unreliable witnesses or that the strain of a court appearance is too great for them. This has been said even in cases of sexual abuse where conclusive DNA evidence is available. Successful prosecution acts as a major deterrent and the system must become more sympathetic to the victim. Proposals from the Home Office to help vulnerable witnesses should help[5] but currently have been delayed indefinitely.

Much lip service is paid to multidisciplinary working, but intervention with elder abuse really does require a team which represents all those involved and works together. A major lesson from child protection is the crucial involvement of certain key professional groups. For older people, the primary health care team is perhaps the most important. While agencies are working competitively rather than cooperatively, as market forces are resolved, true multidisciplinary working will be difficult to achieve. A strong lead from members of the primary health care team will mean that older people will not lose out.

Every health care worker is key in taking action on abuse and the right help for the victim will only be offered where they are actively involved. Help will focus on increasing skills to recognize abusive situations and making the appropriate onward referrals. The primary health care team is important because of its unique knowledge of the older person and their social network and family. Not only may both victim and perpetrator be prepared to talk about what has happened, but other family members may be more prepared to raise suspicions with the family doctor's team than with another agency. The lead given by these workers will undoubtedly start to prevent abuse and older people will be freed from the additional abuses of denial and inaction by workers.

References

1 Ogg J, Bennett G. Elder abuse in Great Britain. *BMJ* 1992; 24: 998–9.
2 **Action on Elder Abuse.** *Everybody's Business, Taking Action on Elder Abuse.* London: Action on Elder Abuse, 1994.
3 **Lord Chancellors Department.** *Who Decides? Making Decisions on Behalf of Mentally Incapacitated Adults.* London: Stationary Office, 1997.
4 **Department of Health.** *No Secrets: Guidance on Developing and Implementing Multi-agency Policies and Procedures to Protect Vulnerable Adults from Abuse.* London: HMSO, 2000.
5 **Home Office.** *Speaking up for Justice, Report of the Interdepartmental Working Group on the Treatment of Vulnerable and Intimidated Witnesses in the Criminal Justice System.* London: Home Office, 1998.

Index